MANAGING IN HEALTH AND SOCIAL CARE

Vivien Martin and Euan Henderson

Department of Health

management education
scheme by open learning

The Open University
BUSINESS SCHOOL

Institute of
Healthcare
Management

Routledge
Taylor & Francis Group

LONDON AND NEW YORK

First published 2001
by Routledge
11 New Fetter Lane, London EC4P 4EE

Simultaneously published in the USA and Canada
by Routledge
29 West 35th Street, New York, NY 10001

Reprinted 2003

Routledge is an imprint of the Taylor & Francis Group

© 2001 The Open University

Designed and typeset in Futura and Sabon by Keystroke,
Jacaranda Lodge, Wolverhampton
Printed and bound in Great Britain by TJ International Ltd, Padstow, Cornwall

Managing in Health and Social Care is the prescribed text for
students from health and social care registered for the Professional
Certificate in Management (B630) of the Open University Business
School. Details of this and other Open University courses can be
obtained from the Course Reservations Centre, PO Box 724, The
Open University, Milton Keynes, MK7 6ZS, United Kingdom;
tel: +44 (0) 1908 653231; e-mail: ces-gen@open.ac.uk. Alternatively,
you may visit the Open University website: http://www.open.ac.uk,
or the Open University Business School website: http://oubs.open.ac.uk

British Library Cataloguing in Publication Data
A catalogue record for this book is available from the British Library

Library of Congress Cataloging in Publication Data
Martin, Vivien, 1947–
Managing in health and social care / Vivien Martin and Euan Henderson.
p. cm.
Includes bibliographical references and index.
1. Human services–Management. 2. Health services administration.
I. Henderson, Euan S. II. Title.
HV41 .M286 2001
362′.068–dc21   00-054871

ISBN 0–415–25189–3 (HB)
ISBN 0–415–25190–7 (PB)

CONTENTS

ILLUSTRATIONS

FIGURES

TABLES

INTRODUCTION

This book should be of value to all those with management responsibilities for health and social care – whether as departmental managers, team leaders or project managers. It is not only for those who are full-time managers, but also for those who have management roles alongside their professional roles.

Its focus is on practical approaches to management and leadership in the particular context of the need to modernise health and social care services for the twenty-first century. The emphasis is on ensuring that services are responsive to the needs of service users, integrated across traditional professional and organisational boundaries, effective in achieving the outcomes that both individual service users and society as a whole are seeking, and inclusive in identifying and meeting the needs of disadvantaged groups.

This includes understanding what effective management and leadership mean, developing shared values with service users and other stakeholders, and managing performance by setting quality standards, monitoring progress against them and leading the drive to seek service improvements. It includes managing teams, managing projects and managing change. It also includes making the best use of available resources – people, money, facilities and, not least, information.

All the chapters are drawn from learning materials prepared for the Management Education Scheme by Open Learning (MESOL), a project that has involved close collaboration between the National Health Service Executive, the Social Services Inspectorate, the Institute of Healthcare Management and the Open University Business School. Since they first appeared in 1990, the MESOL materials have been frequently redeveloped and updated by a broadly based team of practising managers and management developers (see list of contributors at the end of the book) to meet the changing needs of health and social care services.

Over the past ten years, over 20,000 managers in the United Kingdom have benefited from studying courses based on the MESOL learning materials – some in open-learning sets within their workplaces, others through supported distance learning with the Open University, and yet others in programmes offered by local universities, colleges and training organisations. The MESOL materials have also been extensively used overseas, adapted and translated where necessary – in Hong Kong, Australia, Malaysia, the Cayman Islands, Slovakia, Russia, South Africa and, most recently, Namibia and Egypt.

Although the chapters have been designed to follow a logical sequence, management learning is not a linear process, and each chapter can be studied as a free-standing topic. Effective management learning is also a reflective process, and each chapter includes activities to encourage the reader to pause and consider the implications for his or her work as a manager.

OVERVIEW OF THE CHAPTERS

Chapter 1 – Your job as a manager in health and social care – focuses on what managers do. It offers some examples of how managers in health and social care work, and invites you to compare your work with theirs. You are invited to analyse the main roles you play as a manager and consider the demands these make on you.

Chapter 2 – Improving your effectiveness as a manager – sets you thinking about managerial effectiveness and how managers in health and social care today achieve effective results. You are asked to consider what effectiveness means for you in your job and to set or review your key objectives.

Chapter 3 – Management and leadership – considers what is meant by leadership and the extent to which managers are expected to show leadership. We discuss some ways in which you can develop your management style to improve your effectiveness as a leader.

Chapter 4 – Values and vision – discusses the values that shape your organisation and influence the ways in which services are delivered. Vision should be at the heart of any organisation, and the direction in which it is travelling is described by its mission.

Chapter 5 – Mapping the service environment – sets out to map the service environment by dividing it into the 'internal environment', the 'near environment' and the 'far environment'. It explores the boundaries of the internal environment and the stakeholders that comprise the near environment. We consider how organisations can influence their near environment and how health and social care services respond to needs and demand.

Chapter 6 – Developing effective performance – considers how effective groups and teams work and how their performance can be improved. We consider multidisciplinary and multi-agency working and some of the tensions that can emerge. We discuss how you can plan systematically to meet training and development needs and some ways in which you can manage poor performance.

Chapter 7 – Managing change – examines the stages of the change process. We consider diagnosis, the change process and some approaches that can be helpful in ensuring that you understand the current situation fully enough to implement a change. We invite you to consider using these approaches to manage a change in your area of work and we demonstrate the application of several useful techniques in a case study of a change process.

Chapter 8 – What do your customers and service users want? – focuses on the ultimate customers of health and social care – patients, service users and their carers. It distinguishes between what the end-users of services *need* and what they *want*, as well as what their expectations are. It examines how you can collect feedback from the users of your service, as a basis for making service improvements. It considers your role in handling complaints, and how these can be another useful source of feedback.

Chapter 9 – Managing outcomes for service users – stresses the importance of being clear about the purpose of the services for which you are responsible and their intended outcomes. We discuss the range of different ways in which service users can participate in identifying desired service outcomes and designing services to achieve them. We explore the need for collaborative working to ensure that services are effectively integrated for the benefit of patients and service users. This involves you, as a manager, focusing on the boundaries between your service and other related services, within and outside of your organisation.

Chapter 10 – Quality in services – sets out to help you to identify what quality means to managers in health and social care and to those who use health and social care services – both for services in general and for your area of work in particular.

Chapter 11 – Working with standards – is about quality standards. We discuss what standards are and how they can be developed, and invite you to think about how you can develop standards for your own area of work.

Chapter 12 – Management control – is about controlling quality. Once you have established standards for your area of work, you can monitor progress against each standard and take action if standards are not met. This is the process of *management control*.

Chapter 13 – Managing processes – considers the importance of managing the service delivery processes that are part of your everyday work. Once you are able to map the flow of the processes in your work area, you will be able to identify potential areas for improvement.

Chapter 14 – Planning and managing projects – introduces some of the techniques available to you in planning and managing projects. Using these techniques will help you to ensure that outcomes are achieved within the time-scales and budgets available.

Chapter 15 – Service planning, accountability and risk – reviews the planning frameworks within which health and social care organisations plan their activities and describes the process of business planning. This leads us to consider the concept of accountability in health and social care and how managers are accountable for themselves, for their staff and for their area of work. We examine the responsibility that you have as a manager for assessing and managing risk.

Chapter 16 – Working with a budget – discusses the different ways of setting budgets and the implications for budget holders within health and care services. We give some suggestions for approaches to negotiating a budget and for making a proposal for funding.

Chapter 17 – The flow of work and information – invites you to identify the core tasks that constitute the rationale for your section's or department's existence, as opposed to other tasks that, while they may also be important, support the main purpose of your work rather than delivering it. These core tasks may need to be carried out either sequentially or in parallel, and the requirements for co-ordination and information flow may differ accordingly.

Chapter 18 – Evidence and investigation – examines the nature of evidence and focuses on how investigations can be carried out to collect evidence to support decision making and to demonstrate that standards have been achieved. We introduce some basic research approaches in the context of planning a consultation with patients, service users and their carers.

The book concludes with a list of all of the people from health and social care who have contributed to the course materials from which this book is drawn.

YOUR JOB AS A MANAGER IN HEALTH AND SOCIAL CARE

In this chapter we consider the nature of a manager's work. We begin by inviting you to compare your work with that of other managers in health and social care settings and to consider the extent to which your activities are similar to or different from theirs. This will help you to identify your activities and roles as a manager, and thus to gain a better understanding of the job of a manager in health or social care. Whatever your area of work, it is essential to understand the contribution that you can make as a manager, so that you can contribute more effectively to the delivery of high-quality services for patients, service users and carers.

A MANAGER IN ACTION

There are many different types of manager in health and social care. Not all of them have the title of 'manager', but they include people who manage service provision, who manage delivery teams and who manage the various support systems for service delivery. Although management responsibilities may be very different in different types of work and in different types of organisation, the focus of the work is the same for any manager in health and social care – the delivery of high-quality services to those who need them. The activities which managers undertake to carry out their work have many similarities, although the contexts in which they work may be very different.

Let's begin by looking at a manager in action. We asked some managers in health and social care to describe their work. All their reports illustrate the wide range of activities that managers undertake and the correspondingly wide range of skills and knowledge that they use. Second, they show that a lot of these skills are common to many management jobs, irrespective of the level or functional specialisation involved. Third, they illustrate how the various skills and compe-tences described may complement each other to produce an effective managerial approach.

ACTIVITY 1.1

What, exactly, does a manager do? The following passages are descriptions of the work of four different managers in health and social care:

- Case Study A – a Cancer Clinic Co-ordinator
- Case Study B – a Practice Manager
- Case Study C – Manager of a Resource Centre for Children with Disabilities
- Case Study D – Manager of a Day Centre for Older People.

Glance through all of them and choose one to read carefully – you might like to choose someone who works in a context similar to your own or to focus on the work of a manager in a very different setting.

As you read the description, consider what the manager did and how he or she achieved outcomes. You may like to highlight the activities or to make brief notes.

Case Study A – a Cancer Clinic Co-ordinator

I am Clinic Co-ordinator at North Bridge Hospital, a specialist cancer hospital in the north of England. I manage 22 medical secretaries and 8 clerical staff. My role involves responsibility for inpatient admissions, clinical coding, the case-note library, income from private patients, referrals, overseas visitors and the management of cancer clinics at the surrounding district general hospitals.

In 1995 The Calman–Hine Report *Commissioning Cancer Services* recommended the designation of cancer centres and cancer units. Cancer centres would provide expertise in the management of all cancers, including common cancers, within their immediate geographic locality and less common cancers by referral from cancer units. Centres would also provide specialist diagnostic and therapeutic techniques, including radiotherapy. Cancer units were to be established in many district general hospitals, with clinical teams with sufficient expertise and facilities to manage the common cancers.

The cancer centre for my region was formed through a partnership between the two large acute teaching hospitals, as well as North Bridge Hospital, the Children's Hospital and the Community Health Services Trust. This cancer centre is associated with cancer units in five district general hospitals in the area.

A foundation stone of the Calman–Hine Report was the provision of at least five non-surgical sessions per week in cancer units. The regional office of the NHS Executive wanted to provide dedicated clinics for breast cancer, colorectal/intestinal tract cancer, lung cancer, gynaecology, head and neck oncology, and general oncology. These clinics needed to include joint and parallel clinic sessions involving consultant oncologists from North Bridge Hospital working alongside specialists at each cancer unit. The overall objectives were to increase the number of patients having a consultation with an oncologist with an appropriate sub-specialty interest and for those patients who needed it to be able to receive therapy nearer to home.

My objective was to manage the conversion of the general cancer clinics into the clinic sessions for the sub-specialties. This might seem fairly straightforward, but the fragmented system in the National Health Service did not encourage co-ordinated, cross-organisational changes. A lead clinician was appointed from among the consultants at North Bridge Hospital to implement the changes for each of the five district general hospitals we visit, and each of the five hospitals nominated a lead clinician to take responsibility for organising and co-ordinating its cancer services.

The time-scale was incredibly short. Contracts for the new financial year were being finalised and I was given the go-ahead just 16 working days before the first district general hospital was scheduled to start running the new clinics. The changes within the four other district general hospitals were to take place over the following twelve months.

I began by meeting with the North Bridge consultants to confirm the types of cancer conditions they would see at the district general hospitals. I then searched through the case notes of patients being cared for at these five hospitals to determine which consultants would take over their care under the new arrangements. This would allow patients to see a North Bridge consultant with an appropriate sub-specialty, for example an oncologist with a special interest in melanoma. I then met each of the North Bridge consultants again:

- to get their agreement to take over the care of patients in the district general hospitals
- to check the length of consultation they would require in the new clinics
- to find out who would carry out radiotherapy on patients if the consultant was not a radiotherapy specialist.

I was conscious that decisions on sub-specialisation are sensitive matters for consultants and that they were experiencing a change that would not necessarily be easy for them. I found myself coaxing, consoling and reassuring the consultants in order to get their agreement to the new arrangements.

I also met those responsible for organising clinics at each of the district general hospitals. It was important to establish a shared understanding with them of what we were trying to do. The type and consultant staffing of each clinic had been planned by the relevant lead clinician from North Bridge.

The purpose of these meetings was to find the best way of achieving the changes and to schedule action.

The objectives were clear, but their practical implementation was complex. For example, in one district general hospital there were to be four half-day clinic sessions during which one or two local consultants and a consultant from North Bridge Hospital would see patients, together with a further six clinics to be run solely by North Bridge consultants. Whereas most district general hospitals had previously had one visiting North Bridge consultant, there would now be four. Some consultants' work plans had to change so that they could attend the new clinics – not an easy matter to negotiate when two or three consultants from different hospitals had to attend clinic sessions at the same time. One new clinic session involved a consultant surgeon from a district general hospital in another city changing the day of his visit for a clinic. The managers at this hospital were reticent about approaching him, so I contacted him and gained his agreement to the change.

I was able to delegate the task of finding sufficient examination and consulting rooms to the local hospital staff. I developed booking rules for clinics and obtained the agreement of the local managers to these arrangements. Booking patients into jointly run clinics was complicated by the fact that both North Bridge Hospital and the district general hospital concerned needed to be able to book patients in, and this was resolved by each organisation having a one-hour slot in the session for their patients. Information technology systems varied between the district general hospitals and I included their IT managers in the discussions at each hospital. I established guidelines to determine whether the patients were recorded on the district general hospital's patient administration system or the North Bridge system. I wrote up notes of the agreements reached at each meeting and faxed them to the appropriate people. As the programme of changes rolled out, I was dealing with several district general hospitals at the same time and I took responsibility for checking progress on the actions being taken locally.

Prior to the clinics becoming operational, I delegated their detailed operation to my team of North Bridge medical secretaries, who had been involved as the planning progressed. To aid this process, I arranged and led meetings at each district general hospital with the appropriate medical secretaries and the local clinic staff. I started each meeting by outlining the changes and describing the different responsibilities of each organisation and the relevant people within them. The meetings provided opportunities for staff to ask questions and to meet people whom they had previously only spoken to on the telephone. I produced notes afterwards and circulated them to all attendees. I also held individual discussions with my medical secretaries to check their understanding of what was required of them.

Once the clinics were operational, I maintained contact with the managers at the district general hospitals in order to monitor progress. There were some teething problems, and I sometimes visited the district general hospital concerned with the relevant medical secretary to sort the problem out. In one case, we had been booking patients into a clinic at a district general hospital but the patients who came in by ambulance were not arriving on time. I met with the managers at the hospital and the ambulance liaison officer and we agreed to designate a period during the clinic which would be reserved for patients coming by ambulance.

The motivation of all those involved with these changes was helped by the fact that this was a high-profile programme and its successful achievement relied upon a wide range of people co-operating to put the detailed arrangements in place. My own staff's motivation and confidence rose as they became more involved and took responsibility for the clinics. I had taken the lead without having formal authority over most of the people involved, including people in different organisations. It was a satisfying experience to have influenced the provision of care which involves collaboration across organisational boundaries.

We suggested that you tried to identify the activities that this manager carried out and we think that these include the following list. The Cancer Clinic Co-ordinator:

- arranged and led meetings
- collected data
- negotiated with hospital consultants
- made plans
- delegated tasks to others
- developed rules and established guidelines
- wrote up and circulated notes of meetings
- monitored the progress of her project
- kept her staff informed
- motivated others
- influenced people.

Case Study B – a Practice Manager

The Beach Medical Practice is situated in a seaside resort on the south coast which attracts over 2,000 temporary residents each year. Its nine partners are responsible for 12,300 registered patients. There is a thriving local community hospital and the practice has a contract with the local Community Trust to provide 24-hour cover in its casualty department, as well as cover for inpatients and day-case patients. One of the GPs visits the hospital every morning and also has an advisory role, and the other partners assume responsibility for the hospital when they are on call.

The practice works from a health centre purchased from the Health Authority in 1991. The partners own the practice and I am the Practice Manager. All the partners are involved in the management of the practice: we have a committee for each area of management – finance, staff, purchasing, premises, training and computers – with two GPs on each committee alongside other professionals. I am a member of all the committees, to provide an overall perspective and to ensure continuity.

We have now become part of a primary care group preparing to become a trust. However, we are fairly isolated geographically and tend not to have close contact with the other practices for day-to-day matters. Our health visitors, district nurses and community psychiatric nurses were employed by the local Community Trust (the same one that manages the community hospital). Because of our geography, none of these worked in other practices.

Our vision was to manage an extended primary health-care team based in our practice and working only for our practice so that we could improve our services for the benefit of our patients. For example, the trust's health visitors concentrated on the under-5s whereas the practice has a large number of older patients. Also, practice nurses and district nurses were undertaking the same tasks (such as treatment of ulcers), leading to duplication of resources. There was lack of continuity of care, with too many different individuals and organisations caring for patients. Lack of resources meant we were unable to provide patients and carers with, for example, night-sitting services. Patients who would have preferred to remain at home therefore had to be admitted to hospital. We wanted to support a wider range of patients in their own homes, including patients requiring terminal care and those discharged early from hospital. We could also have a major role in preventing admissions to hospital. All this would mean extending the team and bringing in additional professionals. To transform the vision into reality, I formed a small working group consisting of the two most enthusiastic GPs and myself. We called this the Community Services Committee and it met weekly. Its task was to develop proposals for approval by all the partners.

The Community Services Committee drew up a plan which involved several stages. We agreed to write a business plan to submit to the Primary Care Group and to invite them to a meeting with all the partners and me to discuss our proposal. Each of the stages of our plan had set time-scales and we identified who would take the lead in implementing each one. However, we had to review each stage constantly and reset the time-scales because the process often took longer than we had anticipated. A key problem was to decide at what stage to involve the full practice team. Too early with too many suppositions and too few answers would create uncertainty. Too late and we could lose credibility and create suspicion.

Writing a business plan took a considerable amount of time and management effort over a number of weeks. Our first negotiations with the Primary Care Group were very positive. They were keen to try this approach, although many issues remained to be addressed and resolved. The proposals were then put to a meeting of all the partners, agreed and minuted.

Next, we had to concentrate on the potential impact of the proposed changes on all the staff of the practice. What we were proposing would result in some very major changes to the operation of the practice and thus for the staff. We knew that we had to communicate the vision to the whole team and seek to eliminate the obstacles to change. We realised that there had to be varying levels of communication. We firmly believed that the more team members were involved, the better the outcome would be: change is most threatening if it comes as a surprise. The whole team needed to be aware of the proposals, but more detailed discussion and negotiation would need to take place with some than with others – especially the staff from the Community Trust for whom we would be taking management responsibility. The health visitors and district nurses understandably felt very threatened. There was no local role model with which they could identify. Keeping them informed through regular meetings, stressing the positive aspects and offering them a choice were important, as was involving them in the planning of future services and in how the new enlarged team was going to work.

At that time the number of employees of the practice was approximately 30. We were proposing to double that number, and most of the additional staff would have a clinical background. An urgent issue was to decide who would manage the community team. Up to this time all the practice staff were accountable to me, either directly or indirectly through the team leaders, who in turn were responsible to me. We had three team leaders – Practice Manager, Senior Sister and Administrative Manager, each of whom managed a team of receptionists, nurses and administrative staff. We decided to employ a Community Team Co-ordinator who would manage the community team. He or she would have to have a clinical background and would be accountable to me. My role would be strategic, having an overview of the whole organisation and taking responsibility for all financial matters.

We drew up a job description and a person specification for this new senior member of staff, placing some emphasis on seeking some-one who could not only manage the team at an operational level, but who would also be keen to develop new services and to have a role in research and development. We advertised in the national press, shortlisted and interviewed. We appointed a health visitor who had had some management experience. Her first few months with us were a learning experience for her and for me. From the very beginning, our working relationship was strained. We agreed to meet off site to try to resolve this. She admitted that she found it difficult to have a manager without a clinical background. I recognised that I had not given her sufficient support and had not empowered her to do the job she had been employed to do. We were able to agree a list of objectives for both of us. Over a very short period of time, we resolved our differences. Our working relationship is now excellent and built on mutual respect and trust.

As well as taking on the management of staff employed by the Community Trust, we wanted to recruit additional nurses to enable more patients to be cared for in their own homes and to provide 24-hour cover. In addition, the team needed a generic community psychiatric nurse, a community physiotherapist, an occupational therapist and a welfare worker. In order that the trust would feel confident with our choice of new recruits – and because we had no previous experience of selecting new team members from these professions – we invited the trust's heads of department for the appropriate professions to be present at the interviews. The other two panel members were the Community Team Co-ordinator and me.

Because we would be providing community services, we needed to enter into a contract with the Primary Care Group. This contract covered financial allocations and detailed how the contract would be monitored, with what frequency and by whom. It also contained service specifications for each of the professions employed in the primary health care team. An initial meeting was held with representatives from the Primary Care Group and the practice to agree the basic principles of the contract. The Community Team Co-ordinator and I then produced a draft which was amended by the two GPs on our Community Services Committee and submitted to the Primary Care Group. This process went through several iterations until both parties were satisfied. The contract was drawn up before any of our new team were in place and setting levels of activity for each profession for subsequent monitoring proved difficult: it had to be based on what had been achieved through the trust. The activity levels had to be realistic and achievable and yet sufficient to ensure that the Primary Care Group was getting value for money.

However, as our first year progressed, I became convinced that we should be monitoring our service in a different way. Activity levels were essential data, but they did not tell us anything about the quality of the service we were providing. In addition to activity measures, we are now developing – with the team members for each profession – a system for monitoring clinical outcomes.

Now that the processes of change have been completed, the main role of the managers of the practice is to monitor and evaluate and to continue to explore ways of improving our service provision. This is a never-ending process. However, it is clear that the local community is pleased with the additional services we are now providing. We survey our patients from time to time and we frequently meet with local community groups.

We noted the following activities carried out by the Practice Manager who:

■ set up a working group
■ identified the need for change
■ consulted with those involved

- made plans
- negotiated with the Primary Care Group
- presented proposals
- communicated with staff
- wrote job descriptions and person specifications
- advertised, shortlisted and interviewed for new staff
- drafted a contract
- identified the information needed to set up a monitoring system.

Case Study C – Manager of a Resource Centre for Children with Disabilities

I manage the Wood House Resource Centre for children with disabilities. We are based in a converted bungalow in a small Midlands town, and we provide a range of services to 40 children and their families. Some of the children have profound and multiple disabilities and/or severe learning difficulties, some have sensory impairments, and some have very disturbed behaviours which are very hard for families to cope with at home.

Our service was moved to the bungalow about seven years ago by the County Council's social services department. We're about 25 miles from the nearest city, where my line manager is based, and where the senior managers are grouped together in County Hall.

We provide:

- short-term residential care
- outreach – offering time-limited support in the child's home to help parents and children to establish sleep, feeding and play patterns
- staffing for a youth club for 14–18-year-olds once a week in a local youth centre
- a fortnightly session with 9–12-year-olds, offering opportunities for social interaction and working together
- a range of day care from three hours to whole days
- support to families – siblings' days, pre-school work, training for parents in lifting and handling.

Each child has personalised care. We visit the family home and find out how they are cared for, their likes and dislikes, and special diets and equipment. Our aim is to make sure that they are treated as individuals when they come to us. I have to ensure that their needs are properly assessed and that each has a care plan. I match the staff and the children, and ensure that we have sufficient staff available, with appropriate skills, for the children who are with us.

We have to be very careful that the living environment we provide is both homely and safe and hygienic for the children and the staff. A large part of my job therefore involves ensuring that these requirements are met – that the kitchen is properly run and that all the equipment (including hoists and wheelchairs) is properly maintained so that, as far as possible, we protect staff from injury. I delegate as much of this work as possible to my senior staff.

Some of the children have great difficulties expressing themselves and their behaviour can be very difficult and sometimes aggressive. All our staff are trained both in the techniques of physical care for children and in ways of handling them to keep aggression to a minimum and to protect themselves and other children from harm. The senior staff carry out a risk assessment each day, looking at the children who are with us and their needs, and checking that we have the skilled staff available to meet them. We normally have one staff member for each child, and occasionally two.

A large part of my job involves liaison with other people, especially parents. Our role is to share the care of the children to reduce the strain on parents and siblings. We see parents every time they bring their children to us and we listen to how things are going at home, as well as making sure we keep them informed of what is happening at Wood House. We keep in regular touch with the children's care managers, with the medical staff who work with the children and with the special schools that they attend. We are part of a county-wide service to children with disabilities, and I meet regularly with the managers of the four other centres in the county to keep up to date with changes and developments and to make sure that we all provide a consistently good service.

Each member of staff has a regular meeting with his or her line manager, at which they discuss the care of the children they are responsible for, deal with any problems arising in practice or care, and plan training and development. We call this 'supervision'. I supervise the four senior members of staff and they each supervise other members of staff.

My deputy prepares the staff rotas, always making sure that there is a senior member of staff on duty. All the senior staff take a turn at 'sleeping in' – providing cover on the spot at night in case of emergencies.

I am responsible for Wood House's budget. I have some freedom in how I use it to maintain staffing levels, although restrictions are sometimes imposed centrally when there are county-wide budget problems. The County Council has been under severe financial pressure for some years, and this has meant that our budget has been progressively reduced, leading to reductions in the services we provide. This year, the financial crisis is severe, with proposals for reductions of services of all kinds across the county. One proposal is to close three of the five resource centres for disabled children unless a suitable arrangement can be made for independent financing of the services we provide. At the moment, we don't know which three would close if no rescue plan is forthcoming.

We have always had a strong parents' group, who have elected representatives to speak on their behalf in relation to matters affecting the centre. This group has been particularly active over the past three years. I support them and the county-wide parents' group by providing clerical help, a meeting place and any other support I can. They have recognised the threat to the service that is posed by budget problems. Two years ago we took a 16 per cent cut in budget, which meant that we had to choose between reducing the number of children we could take at any one time or closing for one day a week. We asked the parents to help in making this decision, and they opted for closing for one day a week. Over the past two years, the parents' group has lobbied local and national politicians, worked with the local press and made a very moving *Newsnight* programme. The county has no wish to close Wood House or reduce our services, but has to make cuts or go into the red. Senior managers are happy to support our activities by bringing the needs of these children and their families to the attention of opinion formers and people who may be able to offer financial support.

Managing the resource centre in these times presents major problems. Stress is taking its toll on parents and staff alike, and we have several staff on long-term sick leave, all with stress-related problems. I have permission to recruit more staff, but we are in an area of low unemployment: qualified staff are hard to find and potential recruits are not attracted to a job without a firm future. It is easier to recruit temporary staff, but they need more support and training and cannot take the same level of responsibility. The summer is always a difficult time because of staff holidays, but this summer has been particularly difficult, and I have sometimes had to withdraw services because of having insufficient staff. I recently had to send all the children home over the weekend because we did not have sufficient staff to meet their needs safely. Each time we have to reduce our services, parents have to reorganise their lives to accommodate the change. This can involve complicated arrangements for the transport and care of their children, adding to the stress of their lives.

Sustaining morale is hard in these times of uncertainty. We do not know whether we are preparing to close or preparing to be taken over by a new organisation. My mood – and that of my staff – swings from optimism to pessimism and back again, with occasional bouts of exhaustion. I try to offer the staff as much choice as possible in how they work so that they do not feel too pressured. However, with staff in short supply, much of my time is spent in keeping the basics going.

The good thing is the sense of common cause between staff and parents. We are all committed to providing an effective service. We will fight hard to keep Wood House open because we know how much it is needed.

We noted the following activities carried out by the Resource Centre Manager who:

■ ensured that needs were assessed and care plans made
■ delegated tasks to others

- ensured that risk assessments were carried out
- listened to and informed parents
- liaised with those providing related services
- supervised staff
- planned staff training and development
- managed a budget
- recruited staff
- maintained staff morale
- promoted the service.

Case study D – Manager of a Day Centre for Older People

I am the Manager of Eastways Day Centre, a resource for older people living in the community. The Community Healthcare Trust and the Social Services Department jointly manage the centre. The building itself is owned and managed by the Borough Council.

We have 200 clients who attend on a part-time basis, either at the centre or at outreach groups. The majority are over 65, although we can provide for younger people, for example, those suffering from dementia. Many of our clients have social needs rather than – or in addition to – medical needs. They are referred to us from many different sources, for example, by health visitors, GPs, the Social Services Department, or as part of a hospital discharge plan. They may also self-refer or be referred by their carers and relatives.

I am employed by the Community Trust and am the only registered nurse among the 22 staff of the centre. I manage a secretary, an occupational therapist, two physiotherapists, a chiropodist, and a speech and language therapist, all of whom are employed by the Community Trust. In addition, I have two assistant managers, four support workers, four catering staff and a cleaner who are employed by the Social Services Department.

Prior to my appointment at Eastways, a planning group consisting of representatives of the three stakeholders (the Community Trust, the Social Services Department and the Borough Council) had identified a need for more collaborative working. They saw the appointment of a nurse as manager of the centre as a means of developing common working practices for the different staff groups. I was given a clear mandate to translate the stakeholders' vision of improved cross-boundary working into an operational reality. Their emphasis was on changing the culture within the centre rather than on changing the service to clients. I was not set specific objectives, as I had been in all of my previous jobs. From the beginning, I was given considerable freedom to effect changes in line with the planning group's vision.

The expectation that I would bridge the health and social services sectors was demonstrated by the fact that I was given managerial responsibility for all employees in the centre, as well as responsibility for managing both health and social services budgets. In this I differed from my predecessor, who had not managed the staff employed by the Social Services Department and had had no budget management responsibilities.

I have two distinct lines of accountability. Although I am employed by the Community Trust and my line manager is the trust's Community Services Manager, I am also accountable to the Social Services Department's Adult Services Manager. I meet with my two managers fortnightly to review developments and any issues that may have arisen for clients or staff. My performance is formally reviewed regularly by the trust's Community Services Manager.

Both of my managers are very supportive and there is a real sense of working to a common purpose. I think we have a shared understanding that what we are trying to achieve depends very much on each of us making an effort to see the benefits of perspectives other than our own.

However, there are differences in the underpinning philosophies and values of the Community Trust and the Social Services Department, and these could give rise to problems if we are not prepared to compromise when necessary. For example, individualised care and care planning are a very prescriptive part of the Community Trust's philosophy, in that all clients should have a personalised care plan and every attendance and activity should be documented. The Social Services Department's philosophy is 'management by exception' – it is only necessary to record problems in a log book. Also, the Community Trust monitors clients' attendance at the centre in terms of their reasons for attending – i.e. by illness. The Social Services Department monitors attendance simply by the number of clients attending, thus avoiding 'labelling' them in this way. If, for instance, someone is attending the centre following a stroke, the disease process is irrelevant to the Social Services Department – he or she is simply an individual attending for day care.

My central task as manager of the centre is to act as a bridge between the health and social care sectors – drawing upon the best of both systems while working towards a commonality of approach whenever it is possible and desirable to do so.

One very practical thing I did during my first few months at the centre was to become an Accredited Nurse for Placement in Nursing Homes. Having that qualification means that I can assess a client attending for day care – for example, one whose condition is deteriorating – much more quickly than would otherwise be the case. Because I am working as part of both the health and social services teams, I have a more complete picture of clients and their needs. I can pass relevant information from one sector to another and can be used as a resource by both.

I identified as an early priority the need to harmonise the terms and conditions of service for the centre's two staff groups. When I arrived, these were very different for the employees of the two organisations. For example, they had different pay scales, different holiday entitlements and different working arrangements for bank holidays. I've negotiated changes so that both groups now work on bank holidays and all work a one-in-eight weekend rota. In the past, the staff employed by the Social Services Department were paid at a higher rate than the staff of the Community Trust, but the latter did not work unsocial hours. Introducing weekend and bank-holiday working has brought the two staff groups up to almost identical levels of pay. This has not been easy to achieve, but it has had the effect of improving working relationships to a very significant extent. I've also developed an equal opportunities policy for the centre, drawing on the different policies of the Community Trust and the Social Services Department.

There are also differences relating to staff support. The Social Services Department has a system of supervision whereby all staff have a one-to-one session with their manager for 1½ hours each month. The Community Trust has adopted the 'individual performance review' system, which is used widely throughout the National Health Service to appraise its staff. I've incorporated both of these support systems. I now have a monthly supervision session with all staff. I've also put the individual performance review system into place, which operates in harmony with the supervision system. This gives all staff explicit objectives to work towards in a way that hadn't happened before. My objectives are formulated in discussions with my line manager and her counterpart in the Social Services Department. My two assistant managers and I then identify their objectives, and team objectives are agreed by discussion with the rest of the staff. These practical steps are having a significant impact on the culture of the centre: we're changing 'the way things are done around here' and we are creating an Eastways identity.

It is important for me to be mindful of the implications for staff of changing systems, expectations and roles. I encourage them to undertake further training and development. Most of my staff, though very experienced, have little in the way of formal qualifications. Some are now completing vocational qualifications in care and two have done the Open University course *Working with Older People*. We set aside days to meet common training needs such as 'moving and handling' and 'food hygiene'. We've also had visits from health professionals to inform staff on the impact of strokes and disability. I try to encourage staff to be aware of initiatives which will improve our service users' quality of life. I want to move away from the notion that day care is little more than institutionalised 'minding'.

I believe it is very important that all staff, regardless of their employing authority, feel confident in taking responsibility for client care. For this to be possible, systems must be in place that are robust enough to support their decision making, without the need to refer either to me or to one of the assistant managers. For example, I've changed the way in which the out-reach groups are run, encouraging staff to take ownership of these groups and to organise them in ways that best meet the needs of their clients. Though I remain ultimately accountable if there is a problem, I have delegated authority to the staff running them, whereas previously the assistant managers had explicit day-to-day responsibility for the outreach groups.

This approach is very much a reflection of my personal management style. I've been fortunate in having been appointed to a post in which there is ample scope for me to take an active part in the delivery of the service as well as being involved in more strategic planning. This is facilitated by the way in which my managers have given me a high degree of autonomy while also giving me support when I need it.

In my experience, the positive aspects of working with two different organisations far outweigh the negative ones, and I have a real sense of achieving something worthwhile through joint working. This is certainly the case for me personally: my job satisfaction is high and I enjoy the diversity of the day-to-day work in the centre. I feel it is important for the manager of a service like ours to be visible by taking part in the centre's activities as well as carrying out my management duties. So on some days I can be found playing dominoes, ironing or driving the minibus, and on others writing the criteria for accreditation of day hospitals. For me, effectiveness depends on being available and being an active member of the team providing a service to our clients. I'm trying to create an environment in which my staff are afforded as much job satisfaction as I enjoy.

I'm currently continuing this process by empowering clients to determine what they want from the service we provide. We've set up a user group in order to obtain feedback from clients; this has not been done in the past. In an effort to improve our service to clients, we now have a system of planned activities; this previously operated on a rather *ad hoc* basis. Another development has been a more flexible approach to allocating places at the centre. Originally, the 20 places were divided equally between health and social services. Clients referred through the Community Trust had access to additional services such as physiotherapy and occupational therapy, but those referred through the Social Services Department were denied such facilities. There is now no fixed division of places and all clients can access our additional services.

Having freedom to initiate changes like these, which improve the experiences of both clients and staff, really motivates me. The fact that my employers recognise the value of closer collaboration – and are prepared to work in a way that enables potential difficulties to be overcome – is enabling me to translate their vision into a practical reality.

We noted the following activities carried out by the Day Centre Manager who:

- met regularly with her managers
- developed her skills
- negotiated changes in the staff's terms and conditions of service
- developed an equal opportunities policy
- set up supervision and appraisal systems
- encouraged her staff to undertake training
- set up systems to support decision making
- delegated tasks to others

- took an active part in the work of the centre
- developed criteria for the accreditation of day hospitals
- set up a user group.

An impressive number of activities were carried out by the manager in each of these studies. A manager's work often appears very busy and muddled because many of the activities are interrupted and progress is made on several issues in parallel rather than in a neat and logical sequence. Reading between the lines, we might deduce many other things that all four of these managers must have done, which are only implicit in the case studies. They must certainly have:

- built and developed their teams
- developed a network of contacts
- consulted and persuaded other decision makers
- made some deals
- listened to people's complaints and worries
- sorted out innumerable problems
- made many decisions
- compromised on occasion
- written papers and letters
- written reports
- studied other people's reports.

ACTIVITY 1.2

Now use a highlighting pen to mark every activity on our summary lists that these managers undertook which you also carry out at some time in your own work as a manager.

It would be surprising if your activities were exactly the same as the ones in these examples. It would be equally surprising if you did not find a significant number of similarities between your activities and those described by these managers (though the similarities are more likely to occur in *how* they did their work than in *what* they did). For example, most managers, whatever the context of their work, do some planning and some monitoring or supervision of the work of others, and all communicate in a variety of different ways. These are some of the skills and activities that are the very essence of management, and you probably find yourself doing them day after day.

One likely difference is that your work as a manager might seem to be more of a jumble of events concerned simply with keeping your department running. The list of activities and skills involved in your daily tasks may seem to be endless. In the remainder of this chapter, we encourage you to search for coherent patterns among the things that you do. This should help you to gain a better understanding of the nature of your job and this, in turn, will open the way towards improving your effectiveness as a manager. To be more effective, you need to understand the purpose of your job and to be able to achieve the outcomes required in a way that is appropriate to the setting in which you work.

THE NATURE OF YOUR JOB

What are the things that you do – and what should you be doing – to make sure that you are an effective manager? Your chances of doing the job effectively will certainly be improved if you have a good understanding of what you should be doing. There are several different ways of looking at your job, and each provides its own particular insights.

Many researchers have attempted to identify the elements of management work. Colin Hales (1993) made a comparison of eight studies of management work which were carried out between 1959 and 1988. Although he found that there were variations, he summarised the similar elements which had been found in all these different studies.

ACTIVITY 1.3

The elements Hales identified are listed below. Consider whether each one is something that you do as part of your work as a manager and tick the ones that you can recognise to some extent in your own work.

1 Acting as a figurehead or leader of a work unit, representing it and acting as a point of contact ❑
2 Monitoring and disseminating information flowing into and out of the work unit ❑
3 Negotiating with staff at different levels, other managers, other work units and outsiders ❑
4 Monitoring the flow of work by handling disturbances, solving problems and dealing with disruptions ❑
5 Allocating resources in the form of money, materials and people ❑
6 Directing and controlling the work of other staff ❑
7 Forming contacts and liaising with others ❑
8 Innovating, by looking for new objectives and methods to improve the work of the unit ❑
9 Planning what is to be done and when ❑

Many of these characteristics indicate that the work that managers do is complex and involves a great deal of interaction with other people. The range of work is often summarised as:

- managing people
- managing activities
- managing resources
- managing information

and doing all these through *managing yourself*.

Not every manager has all of these responsibilities: it depends a great deal on the context in which he or she works. It would also be unusual for all of the activities to be equally important: a manager's work depends on the purpose of the organisation in which he or she works.

There are also differences in how managers are expected to work. In some settings a manager will be expected to look smart and behave in a formal way; in others informal dress is expected and behaviour may be similarly informal. Many other expectations reflect the 'culture' of the organisation. However, some features are typical of any manager's work. They flow from the responsibility held by managers for work processes and for the people who perform the processes. Hales recognised that much of the research into how a manager works demonstrates frenetic activity.

ACTIVITY 1.4

Here is the list Hales made from his research into the activities that are typical of how a manager works. Think about whether any of these descriptions remind you of your own work and tick those which apply to your work.

1 Fragmented – short, interrupted activities ❑
2 Reactive – responding to, rather than initiating, events and requests ❑
3 Concerned with *ad hoc*, day-to-day matters ❑
4 Negotiated – bargaining over the boundaries, content and style of work ❑
5 Eclectic, with rapid commuting between activities ❑
6 Thinking-in-action, with decisions and plans developed while engaged in other activities ❑
7 Interactive, involving a high level of face-to-face communication ❑
8 Concrete, concerned with practicalities rather than abstractions ❑

All these features indicate responsiveness – noticing what is happening around you and responding to people and events. Much of a manager's work involves responding to other people and to situations. However, a manager is expected to do more than just respond to day-to-day issues and manage routine work. Managers are also expected to make progress towards particular objectives. It is all too easy for a manager to be very busy but not necessarily to have achieved what he or she had intended. This may mean that progress is not being made towards achieving key objectives. If you ticked most of the boxes in the previous Activity, you will need to manage your time well to be effective.

Henry Mintzberg has been researching and writing about the nature of management work since the early 1970s. He became dissatisfied with a classification of management roles which consisted of a list of disconnected activities and developed an integrated model. This model emphasises that managers must apply six roles – controlling and communicating, leading and linking, doing and dealing – to all their work. He applied these ideas when observing how a symphony orchestra conductor managed highly skilled professional musicians. He commented: 'Taken together, the various constraints within which the orchestra conductor works describe a very common condition among managers – not being in absolute control of others, nor being completely powerless, but functioning somewhere in between' (Mintzberg, 1998).

If you work in a setting where there is frequent change – and most people do these days – it is unlikely that you will be effective unless you take enough control over your time to make sure that you are able to achieve your key objectives. This is not to suggest that your time is more important than that of the people you manage. However, if you can demonstrate that you manage your time in a way which helps you to be effective, it will help others to respect and value their time as well as yours.

REFERENCES

Hales, C. (1993) *Managing through Organisation*, Routledge.
Mintzberg, H. (1998) 'Covert leadership: Notes on managing professionals', *Harvard Business Review*, November–December.

IMPROVING YOUR EFFECTIVENESS AS A MANAGER

If you have just moved into a managerial position, clarifying your objectives and the means of achieving them will be one of your first concerns. It doesn't make a great deal of sense to contemplate how you will set about doing a job if you are not clear about what it is you are trying to achieve. If you have been a manager for some time, you should not overlook the importance of reviewing your objectives. Objectives can be used to clarify the purpose of your management activities, and they can also help to identify the processes through which you will make progress.

Setting clear objectives and planning how they will be achieved are fundamental to managing effectively. But you will usually need to allow for some flexibility in how objectives are pursued so that you can accommodate other people's views and adjust to changes in circumstances.

A sense of direction and purpose is critical to effectiveness. In this chapter we discuss what is meant by effective management and the factors upon which effectiveness depends. We consider the needs to which you and your organisation respond and the priorities between them. This leads to identifying key objectives to ensure that you address these priorities. We examine the process of setting objectives in three stages: reviewing what you need to do to be effective, determining your priorities in terms of objectives, and planning how you will achieve your objectives.

REVIEWING WHAT YOU NEED TO DO TO BE EFFECTIVE

You may already have some idea of what being an effective manager means, even though we have not yet precisely defined 'effectiveness'. Before proceeding further, we'll attempt to define it now. Managerial effectiveness is a measure of the extent to which the results one sets out to achieve are achieved. However, just achieving what you have set as targets is not enough in itself. It is very important that the targets that you set are ones that will really add value to the area of work for which you are responsible. The quality of your objectives is as important as the fact that you set objectives at all. There are two important stages in achieving your planned results. The first is to set clear objectives so that you know what you are trying to achieve; the second is to review your progress against these objectives so that you know how you are doing and can take action to keep on track if necessary.

But setting and reviewing objectives are not as straightforward as they might appear at first glance. Even in a well regulated manufacturing process, many factors make this procedure difficult to apply. In health and care services, the variables are numerous and situations are often in a state of frequent change. If we are to judge the performance of an individual, a team, a department or a whole organisation, we must know against what criteria the judgement is to be made.

ACTIVITY 2.1

Let's say that effective management is performance measured against intentions. Using this definition, tick the boxes which show how accurately you are currently able to assess managerial effectiveness for:

	Accurately	*Loosely*	*Not at all*
Yourself	❐	❐	❐
Your team	❐	❐	❐
Your service area	❐	❐	❐
Is this satisfactory for effective management?	*Yes* ❐	*No* ❐	*Partially* ❐

It would be unusual if you found that the current approach to evaluation of effectiveness is entirely satisfactory. You might feel that having a loose definition of managerial effectiveness has its advantages. However, if people are to be judged on the extent to which they achieve the outcomes that are expected of them, it is important to have a common understanding of what these outcomes include. Your answer to the final question might suggest that you need to set some clearer objectives for yourself or for your team, if only to ensure that everyone has a similar understanding of what is expected.

It is also interesting to consider whether service users would be entirely happy with your current approach to reviewing effectiveness. Staff may all be working very hard, but are they achieving the high quality of service delivery that everyone would like to be part of?

Effectiveness is not easy to pin down because it has to be considered in relation to the ever-changing needs and expectations of service users.

However, you should now have a clearer picture of what we mean by effective management. You are also probably aware from your own experience that, to be effective, managers need a very wide repertoire of skills and competences to carry out the many different tasks that they are asked to do. However, important as these skills are, effective management does not come automatically from having the right skills. The reality is much more complex than that.

A number of factors influence your effectiveness as a manager, not all of which are under your control. Let's consider five such factors.

In the first place, *you* are a factor. You are unique. You bring a unique blend of knowledge, skills, attitudes, values and experience to your job, and these influence your effectiveness to some extent.

Then there is *your job*. It will have many features in common with other management jobs but, just as you are unique, so your job is likely to be unique both in its detailed features and in the unique demands it makes upon you. The match between your skills and the demands made on them by your job shapes your potential effectiveness.

The resources you have to work with exert a major influence on how effective you can be as a manager. The most important of these resources is people – your staff. You may have come across such definitions as 'a manager is a person who gets work done through other people' or 'managers are people with so much work to do that they must get other people to do it' or 'a manager is the person who works out what needs doing and gets someone else to do it'. Some of these definitions are a bit tongue in cheek, but nevertheless get close to the truth with their emphasis on the importance of other people in the achievement of a manager's work. One measure of your effectiveness as a manager is the extent to which you can motivate your staff and co-ordinate their efforts to achieve optimum performance. However, you do not control people in the way that you can control the other resources – such as finance and information – that are needed to get work done.

Your organisation is another major factor in determining how effective you can be. Both the structure and the culture of the organisation, whether it is large or small, place limits on what you are able to achieve as a manager. The structure, and your position in it, make an impact on the nature of your authority and your responsibilities and impose constraints on what you are able to achieve. Similarly, the culture of the organisation – its norms and standards, its written and unwritten rules, and its style of working – also has a direct bearing on your ability to be effective as a manager.

Finally, your work can be affected by influences from *the world outside your organisation*: by social trends, changes in technology, the state of the economy, and in general by the people and other organisations with whom your organisation must interact. Health and social care services are delivered by many different types of organisation. To improve the integration and quality of services for users, patients and carers will require more co-operative working and the formation of partnerships.

So effective management does not come just from learning a few skills and techniques. Skills and techniques are important and necessary, but effective management is more complex than that. It depends on you, the job you do, the people you work with, the other resources you have at your disposal, the organisation you work in, and the wider world with which your organisation must interact.

ACTIVITY 2.2

This activity will help you to identify some of the factors upon which effectiveness depends.

Think about a piece of work you recently carried out as a manager. This might have been an improvement in your area of work or an occasional, but more routine, activity. Choose something that was fairly complex, something that you had to think about and plan to some extent and something that involved other people. Answer the following questions about the activity.

- To what extent was the outcome influenced by your own level of competence?
- Did you bring particular skills or knowledge to the situation?
- To what extent were your actions influenced by personal or professional values?
- What contribution did your staff, colleagues and line manager make to the outcome, positively or negatively?
- How critical were the abilities and attitudes that others brought to the situation?
- Did you have the influence in your organisation that was required to achieve the task?
- Do you feel that your job allows all your abilities to be brought into play?
- Does it make demands that you feel unable to respond to?

All these questions refer to aspects of work that you can think about before taking action. Preparation for a complex task can be, to some extent, a rehearsal for the real thing. If you start a major task by considering what is involved and what you are trying to achieve, this will clarify the direction and purpose of your work. It is then possible to consider how the desired outcomes will be achieved – what steps are needed to achieve each of the outcomes. This is the planning stage.

A simple recommendation for effective management is:

- Plan
- Do
- Review.

Once these steps are expressed as separate tasks, you have created an agenda for action. You can then think about who should carry out each of the tasks. Your planning at this stage will include consideration of who has the necessary skills and experience or who could be supported to develop the necessary skills with appropriate supervision. In health and social care settings you will also have to consider who has the appropriate professional or clinical background and qualifications for some of the activities, and this may raise the question of your ability to bring people from different backgrounds together to work effectively. You might also need to have sufficient influence in your organisation to secure other necessary resources. All this may seem daunting, but much of your effectiveness as a manager will result from your ability to plan and co-ordinate the work of other people.

When you have reached the stage of carrying out activities, there is still a further stage – review. This is crucial in making sure that your actions are leading in the direction you intended. The simple sequence of plan, do, review is a useful way to remember these stages.

One approach to becoming effective as a manager is to set objectives and to review them to make sure that you are progressing in the right direction and at the right speed to achieve them. However, it is never quite this easy because other people are always involved. There is a stage before planning which involves making sure that you understand the situation well enough to inform your planning. You may think that you know what is needed, but deciding what needs to be done is not simply a matter of indicating your perception of those needs. You must also give careful consideration to other people's views about what needs to be done (which may mean the perceptions of service users, your team, your manager, other managers, people in collaborating organisations).

Your perception of what needs to be done

If you are to be effective as a manager you will be concerned to ensure that you clearly identify what you see as the needs of those you are serving – your target groups. If you are the manager of a Help the Aged day centre, for example, the needs of the users of your service will be crucial, but so will those of your management committee and of the staff of the social services department to whom they are contracted to provide this service. If you are a nurse or therapist, your patients will be an important target group, but so will be the doctors and consultants with whom you are working. If you are a finance officer, your target group may be the staff for whose pay cheques you are responsible, or senior management to whom you are providing budgetary information. If you have line management responsibility for other staff, these staff will be an additional target group. You will find it useful to devise a system for identifying needs, and Activity 2.3 suggests one possible approach.

ACTIVITY 2.3

Consider *one* of the target groups of the service for which you are responsible. Identify and list the different types of needs to which you try to respond.

If your chosen target group is your patients or service users, your list might well include their physical, emotional and social needs. Remember that, as a manager, you also provide a service to your staff, so you could choose your staff as your target group.

You have probably drawn up an impressive list of the needs of this target group that you try to meet in your work. Your knowledge and experience and that of your team allow you to understand and attend to the detail of your day-to-day service provision.

Identification of needs is more difficult if you are a manager new to an area of service provision or if you have responsibility for areas of work with which you are unfamiliar. It is also sometimes difficult for those supporting direct service providers to see how they contribute to the quality of service to the patients and service users. Managers and staff in finance, personnel, audit and all the other support areas have other staff in the organisation as their target groups and do not always find it easy to recognise the importance of providing them with a good service to enable them to deliver services to patients, service users or carers.

In health and social care nowadays, the boundaries around service areas are changing. Many managers have responsibilities for broad service areas or for multiprofessional teams and it is inevitable that they will be more familiar with the service areas in which they gained their own experience. Few managers of complex services will have had wide enough experience to understand fully all of the detailed work carried out by members of their teams. If you are in this position, it is important to spend time with each different area of service provision to understand more about why they deliver their part of the service as they do and how they perceive the needs of the users of their service.

One of the reasons why more multidisciplinary teams have been formed is that, in the past, some services were very good at one part of health or social care but did not link with the next stage needed by the user. For example, people could be treated in hospital and become well enough to go home, but would be sent home without provision being made to ensure that they had adequate support and help to stay well. Your service may be excellent at achieving its immediate results, but less effective in ensuring that the overall purpose of the intervention is achieved.

Other people's perceptions of what needs to be done

The needs you identified for the users of your service are likely to be only part of the work of your organisation. Organisations often deliver a number of services and, unless you are a manager in a very small organisation, there will be other considerations to take account of. Before you begin to identify what you believe ought to be done in response to the needs you have identified, you must take careful note of other points of view. An efficient organisation will normally have gone through a similar process of identifying needs of target groups in developing its policies. It will have identified the needs that it perceives to be important, and will have developed statements about what the organisation ought to do to respond to them. These are likely to be in the form of corporate objectives – often referred to as aims or goals.

It is the responsibility of senior management to communicate their corporate objectives to the people whose responsibility it is to achieve them. In large organisations with several layers of management, each level of management bears the responsibility for communicating the objectives, strategies and implementation plans that apply at their level to those below so that they, in turn, can plan accordingly. This 'cascade' process is illustrated in the ladder diagram (Figure 2.1). Each rung on the ladder represents a separate level of objectives, the number and nature of the levels reflecting the site and structure of the organisation.

At the corporate level, objectives are likely to be identified in very broad terms, but as they are transmitted down through the hierarchy they will be translated by departments and units into increasingly

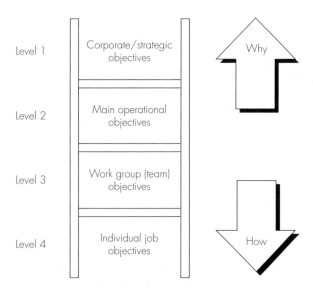

Figure 2.1 The ladder approach to the analysis of objectives

specific terms. You must study any statements of objectives that come down to you, for they may determine to a large extent both what you can do and what you can't. In some organisations, they may simply provide you with broad guidelines within which you have great freedom to think for yourself. In others, the guidance provided might be much more specific.

At the level of your work group or team there may be clear overall objectives for your team to meet, or you may need to develop your own objectives from a broad statement of the purpose of your team's work. The guidelines you are expected to work within may require your objectives to meet some of the following requirements:

- contribute to the overall strategy of the department or organisation
- be within the constraints of the budget
- be at an acceptable level of risk (to be defined)
- make use of, or reinforce, organisational strengths
- meet a major need that has been identified as a local priority
- avoid, reduce or mitigate major threats or hazards
- be consistent with other major strategies
- be capable of implementation.

Not all organisations are as organised or directive as this. Some may not even explicitly identify their corporate objectives. Nevertheless, they will have philosophies which guide their direction and their objectives will be implicit in what they do or try to do. Unless your organisation is completely adrift, it will have some objectives at a strategic level, but these may be implicit rather than explicit.

ACTIVITY 2.4

Think about the objectives of your organisation (or your part of the organisation).

Do you know the objectives of your organisation?	Yes/No
If not, do you believe that they exist?	Yes/No
Are they in writing?	Yes/No
Do you know where to find them?	Yes/No
Do you know who determined them?	Yes/No
Do you know the arrangements for reviewing them?	Yes/No
Did you (or will you) help to formulate (or review) them?	Yes/No

'Windowless cubicle 3217. Drone 466–N–3567 speaking. In order to continue achieving immediate goal, I will need clues to the overall plan.'

If you answered 'no' to several of these questions, you should try to find out more from your line manager or colleagues. Part of your effectiveness as a manager is determined by the extent to which you are seen to be contributing towards achieving the objectives of your wider service or organisation. This will inevitably be difficult to do if you are not sure what they are!

Objectives almost certainly do exist in some form or another within your organisation, even if only as ill-defined and unarticulated ideas inside the heads of the senior management group. Your service may have a strategic plan, such as a community care plan, in which the key objectives will be stated. A smaller or less formal organisation might produce an annual report in which the aims and objectives are outlined. If your organisation is large and provides many different services, you may only need to know about the objectives for your service area (for example, if you work in learning difficulty services, you may not need to know the objectives for the services for older people).

DETERMINING YOUR PRIORITIES IN TERMS OF OBJECTIVES

Once you have a list of important needs categorised in a meaningful manner (for example, according to different types of needs and with regard to different target groups), you can start to convert this list of perceived needs into statements indicating what you might aim to achieve in response to each need.

ACTIVITY 2.5

Convert the list of needs you made in Activity 2.3 into statements of what you intend to do to respond to them. For example, you might have determined that one of your groups of service users needs information about your service. Your aim might be 'to give accurate information about the service'. Use your previous list to write a few more statements of aims.

But identifying your aims is not enough. The aim 'to give accurate information about the service' describes what you want to achieve in relation to a particular need – it sets out your direction – but it does not indicate how you are going to achieve it, when you are going to do it, or how you will know that you have been successful in doing it. So you need to convert the *aims* into *objectives*. Objectives need to be as precise as possible if they are going to help you to become more effective. This means that they should have some particular characteristics. An easy way to remember these characteristics is to think of them as 'SMART'. They must be:

- *Specific* – clear about what is to be achieved
- *Measurable* – state how success will be measured
- *Agreed* – ideally with the person who will carry out the objective and with anyone who will be affected by the result
- *Realistic* – achievable within the constraints of the situation and in alignment with other objectives
- *Timed* – target time set for achieving objectives.

For example, the aim 'to give accurate information about the service' might be rewritten as a SMART objective as:

> *To give accurate information about the service by producing 1,000 copies of a leaflet, using our team experience to design them and our clerical resources to copy them, so that they are on display for use on 1 September.*

This is now a specific objective: you know how you will measure success, it is realistic, and there is a time limit. However, there is another dimension. Although an objective like this could be put into action and the degree of success could be measured, is it an action worth carrying out? It is very important that objectives lead to a worthwhile result. Effectiveness is not only about doing things well (efficiency) but also about doing the right things.

If we look again at this example of an objective, it would be of little use if the leaflet could not be read or understood by the service users. A draft of the leaflet needs to be tested, perhaps with some willing members of the potential readership. There may be problems with size of print or layout or over the language used: it is easy to make assumptions when you are writing about something that is very familiar to you. There may also be problems about different ways of seeing things – perhaps different values – which might mean that the way in which you present information is less acceptable to particular groups of people. You may even discover in trying out the draft that using leaflets is an unhelpful way of presenting information to some communities and that you have to find an alternative approach. You might then amend your SMART objective to:

> *To give accurate information about the service by producing sufficient copies of a leaflet (or something similar) that fully meets the needs of service users, using our team experience and resources to produce the information ready for use on 1 September.*

Achieving this objective might not be quite as easy to measure, but the emphasis is more on finding out what would meet the needs of service users and then providing the information in an appropriate way. Success will be measured against the criteria that have been identified in terms of what service users need, as well as in terms of both quality and quantity. If it turns out that users want information in leaflets, this objective will be helpful in reminding the manager responsible to pilot drafts of the leaflet to make sure that it fully meets users' needs, and also to find out how many leaflets will be required. If it is found that users of the service would prefer a poster or access to information by telephone, a different approach can be taken and money will not be wasted on leaflets. Whether you can frame your objectives in very precise terms depends on how much you know about the situation or whether you need to allow for more research before deciding exactly what action to take.

ACTIVITY 2.6

Rewrite three of the aims you drafted earlier so that they meet all the SMART criteria and provide a guide for meaningful action.

Long-term and short-term objectives

'The over-emphasis on objectives is possibly the most urgent aspect of the government's reform agenda in need of reassessment. The government seems to equate good management practice in the private sector with the achievement of objectives through clear, precise targets. But this is to ignore the unique features of public sector management. . . . The unrelenting concentration on objectives can distort because the problem of balancing objectives, values and interests is neglected. This balancing act lies at the heart of management in the public sector. Setting objectives is easy, balancing them less so.'

(Hunter, 1999)

If you systematically develop a list of aims and objectives from your and your organisation's perceptions of the needs of your different target groups, your list will probably contain far more objectives than you can hope to achieve in the near future. You will have to establish priorities. One way of doing this is to review your list to identify what has to be done urgently and what can be planned to be achieved later.

You might begin by asking yourself what it is that you want to achieve in the long term, and what you might realistically achieve in the short term. Your long-term objectives are likely to emerge in response to such fundamental questions as 'What is our real purpose?', 'Where are we going?' and 'Where do we want the service to be in five years' time?' Your short-term objectives should be a first step on the way towards achieving your longer-term objectives, and are likely to be identified in response to much more basic questions such as 'To what extent can we reduce our waiting lists over the next twelve months?' or 'In what ways might we improve our services over the next twelve months?' As your thoughts begin to clarify, create two lists – one of objectives to be achieved in the long term (say, over three years) and the other of those to be achieved in the short term (say, over one year).

Having produced separate lists of long- and short-term objectives you might then review each of these in turn, asking yourself which of the objectives are absolutely essential and which are simply desirable.

If determining priorities is an effort involving several people – as it usually is – it is almost inevitable that you will encounter conflicting points of view from time to time. Different people are likely to have different perceptions of what needs to be achieved in the short or long term and to have different views as to what is essential as opposed to desirable. Value judgements are involved. It is up to those concerned to make their views explicit, and for you to ensure that an agreed view is established.

However, these are not the only conflicts that might arise. Whenever a multiplicity of aims or objectives is identified, there is always a possibility of some being in conflict. For example, one of your aims might be 'to provide the best possible conditions for service user or patient care', while another might be 'to maximise service user or patient throughput in order to reduce waiting times'. There may be a conflict between these, and it is up to you and your team to determine an appropriate balance between them. It is sometimes helpful to look at each objective and to ask, 'How will this improve the experience of the service for the patient or service user?' as a way of deciding how to set priorities. There may, for example, be ways in which the conditions for care could be improved quickly (making appointments to reduce the need for long waiting times, providing more chairs, making refreshments available). The other objective of maximising patient throughput might be a longer-term objective needing more research and wider co-operation (including the co-operation of patients or service users) to achieve success.

ACTIVITY 2.7

Think of an example of two conflicting aims or objectives which your own organisation is seeking to fulfil.

What is the nature of the conflict? Is there a possible compromise? How can you, as a manager, help your team to achieve your objectives with as little conflict as possible?

Now that you have some clear objectives, you can set about achieving them.

Achieving your objectives

As a manager, your objectives are not only your own concern: they are also your team's concern. Your objectives probably include some that involve the work of the whole team. If you involve your team in agreeing how these objectives will be achieved, this will help to develop a shared understanding.

Once you have determined your priorities, you should ensure that your key objectives are expressed in terms that ensure that your team can determine for themselves whether or not their contributions to them have been achieved. You will need to work with your team to identify the sequence of activities that needs to be completed to achieve each objective and the measures that will demonstrate that each has been achieved. It is helpful to agree a process for the whole team to review progress. This provides an opportunity to correct things if they are not working as planned. It is particularly helpful if you plan early review dates, so that if things are going wrong there is time to rethink your plans. If review dates are too late to allow plans to be revised, there is often a tendency to look for someone to blame for the lack of success rather than to think positively about how to achieve success in a different way.

It is important to bear in mind the distinction between *key objectives* and *key activities*, since you want to be sure that, at the end of the day, you are measuring what you achieved rather than simply what you did. The key activities might be expressed as sub-objectives, the smaller tasks that have to be completed in order to achieve a key objective. For example, the objective:

> *To give accurate information about the service by producing sufficient copies of a leaflet (or something similar) that fully meets the needs of service users, using our team experience and resources to produce the information ready for use on 1 September.*

could be subdivided down into the tasks:

1 Check what information is most often required by service users.
2 Draft the answers you and your team usually give and agree their accuracy with your team.
3 Research with service users how they prefer to access information.
4 Design a leaflet (or poster or information service) to meet the needs identified.
5 Agree the design of the leaflet (or other approach) with your team.
6 If you are proposing an alternative approach rather than the leaflets that were anticipated, confirm with your manager that this is acceptable.
7 Try out the draft leaflet (or other approach) with a few service users to make sure that it meets their needs.
8 Revise if necessary and secure final agreement from your team (and other managers if necessary).
9 Ensure that there are sufficient resources to go ahead within the time-scale.
10 Ensure that the information is available for use from 1 September.

Each of these tasks needs a time-scale attached to it to ensure that the whole job will be completed by the target date. Each task will also need to be allocated to someone who will take responsibility for completing it on time. You will need to have a way of keeping an eye on overall progress to make sure that it goes to plan. You should also arrange to review the extent to which the leaflet or other approach has achieved its purpose and whether you need to make any changes after a few months.

Setting clear objectives makes it much easier to identify the tasks involved in achieving results and to review progress using both your list of tasks and your key objectives. You can be very busy but find that you achieve very little unless you are clear about what you are aiming to do and when you expect to achieve your outcomes. In addition, of course, the staff who carry out the tasks will need to be motivated and co-ordinated through effective leadership and management.

Now try this Activity, which will enable you to apply these ideas in your workplace.

ACTIVITY 2.8

Prepare up to five draft key objectives for your department or section. Write these in SMART format so that they provide a framework from which key activities could be derived for you and your team.

Discuss them with your line manager to ensure that you have captured the essential aspects of the work expected of you.

Once this has been agreed, discuss the objectives with your team and agree how each will be achieved. This would be a useful team-building exercise, as well as helping to develop clarity of purpose. It is important to recognise that your team might not agree with your proposals and to be ready to listen to their ideas and to accept some of their suggestions. This approach would demonstrate to your team how you intend to be effective as a manager and how you expect them to be able to demonstrate their individual and team effectiveness.

This chapter has focused on one of the most fundamental skills that managers need. We have stressed that if you want to be an effective manager you must be clear about what you want to achieve and how you intend to go about it. In particular, we have stressed the importance of giving careful consideration to:

■ the needs which you and people in other parts of your organisation perceive to be important
■ the priorities to which you intend to respond
■ the key objectives you intend to achieve
■ the key activities through which you will achieve your objectives

■ the key results which will indicate whether or not you have achieved the objectives.

You should now be able to identify the factors upon which managerial effectiveness depends, to clarify your own objectives and to plan means by which your objectives can be effectively achieved.

REFERENCE

Hunter, D. (1999) 'Dangers of target practice', *Health Service Journal*, 24 June, pp. 16–17.

MANAGEMENT AND LEADERSHIP

In this chapter, we consider 'the way that you do it': your style – both your style of leadership and your style of management. This statement implies that there is a distinct difference between leadership and management. However, as we shall find repeatedly in this chapter, the two words are often used interchangeably, so we shall consider whether there is a difference between management and leadership and what the implications might be for managers. We conclude by inviting you to consider what is your preferred management style and the extent to which you can vary it to meet the needs of different situations.

MANAGING AND LEADING

Both managing and leading are practical activities. Managers are now widely expected to take a leadership role. However, it may be rather alarming for a manager to hear that he or she should be demonstrating leadership qualities. We often associate leadership with great charismatic figures of military or political history. This doesn't mean, however, that managers have to show similar characteristics in their leadership roles.

One way of using the word 'leadership' is to describe the way in which senior managers and directors set out a strategy for the work of an organisation. For example, the leaders of political parties are expected to provide the vision and the inspiration, but the party managers look after the day-to-day running of party business. In commerce and industry the same is often true, with many (although not all) top executives taking a high profile and leading the way. From this perspective, managing might appear to be something that supports the leaders of an organisation. Could it be that those people who rise to the top specialise in just a few of the functions of management, such as setting goals and inspiring people to work towards them? The more routine functions of management, such as planning, resourcing and organising, then become the responsibility of managers further down the line.

However, these managers also have to lead their teams – to motivate them and to plan and co-ordinate each area of work. In health and social care it is common to find people who are nominated as team leaders. The qualifications for appointment as a team leader are often connected with expertise and experience, particularly the experience of supervising and developing other people.

Let's look briefly at some of the views of leadership and management that have influenced our expectation that managers should be prepared to adopt a leadership role. Traditional ideas about leaders and leadership are often based on a military model in which the leader decides, directs and commands. However, in a modern organisational setting, few of us are willing to follow a leader with absolute trust that their view of what action should be taken is always right. Most of us want to contribute something from our own perspective and want our experience, knowledge and skills to be acknowledged. Many managers think of the people who work with them as colleagues rather than as followers.

Transformational leadership

Transformational leadership describes leaders who are able to involve staff in willingly transforming themselves and the ways in which they work:

> Transforming leadership occurs when one or more persons engage with others in such a way that leaders and followers raise one another to higher levels of motivation and morality. [Through] leadership the objectives of all team members become fused to address a common purpose. Various names are used for such leadership: elevating, mobilising, inspiring, exalting, uplifting, exhorting, evangelising.
> (Adapted from Peters and Waterman, 1988, and Burns, 1978)

Transformational leadership implies being able to inspire people to lift their attention above everyday affairs (although these must still be carried out efficiently and effectively). It is concerned with sharing values and developing a sense of doing something purposeful. The focus is more on the purpose and excellence of work than the power or personality of the leader. The essence of transformational leadership is that leaders transform the way their staff see themselves and the organisation:

■ They make staff aware of the importance of their role to the success of the organisation, and of how dependent organisational achievements are on their individual achievements.
■ Because the skills of staff are so crucial, they encourage people to manage their own personal development and performance.

■ They motivate staff to work both for their own personal goals and for the goals of the organisation.

These principles are uncontentious, but they have significant implications for the behaviour of leaders. Transformational leadership depends to a considerable extent on the personal power of the leader: he or she is expected to communicate a clear and achievable vision, and to do so with an enthusiasm that inspires staff. If staff are to be encouraged to engage with and 'own' organisational issues, and to use their intellect in group problem solving, the leader must focus on the development of their capabilities. The use of symbols is important – the leader manages meetings, ceremonies and appearances in a way that communicates to staff his or her vision of how the organisation should function, thus 'binding' them into this vision.

A consultation document from the NHS Confederation (1999) said:

Leadership is largely about a relationship between the leader and those who follow . . . [T]ransformational leadership . . . embodies the notion of leaders as having a responsibility to serve those who follow them, to engage their commitment and develop their potential.

This in no way undervalues the contribution of managers. Indeed, at present, 95% of those who lead healthcare organisations as chief executives have a managerial background and it is of the utmost importance that they are developed as individuals to assume these leadership roles effectively. To do so, they also need to be developed in their professional roles as managers . . .

The concept of transformational leadership . . . refers to the process of influencing followers or staff by inspiring them or pulling them towards the vision of some future state. Transformational leaders exhibit some or all of the following four characteristics:

■ *charisma*: provides vision and a sense of mission, instils pride, gains respect and trust
■ *inspiration*: communicates high expectations, expresses important purposes in simple ways
■ *intellectual stimulation*: encourages followers to question basic assumptions, and to consider problems from new and unique perspectives
■ *individual consideration*: gives personal attention, treats each employee individually, coaches, advises . . .

There is research evidence that transformational leaders are more likely to be seen by their colleagues and employees as satisfying and effective leaders.

Many of the values of health and social care are about empowering others. A report to the Local Government Management Board said:

Transformational leadership is not simply the result of performing certain competences, though these are no doubt essential prerequisites for the credibility of a manager. It is also reflected in fundamental personal dispositions. These include empathy, openness to criticism and the ideas of others, a degree of selflessness, and some judicious risk-taking in empowering others.

It is also about enthusiasm, articulating a clear vision and showing a determination to achieve it, and involving others so that they take on ownership of the vision. Transformational leaders are perceived as individuals of high integrity and self-confidence. They not only maintain a close relationship with and accessibility to staff within their organisations, they are also very sensitive to the concerns of elected councillors and develop a wide network of external relationships.

They are highly skilled both in internal organisational politics, and in relating effectively to external politics that impact on their organisation and service. Transformational leaders also have the intellectual capacity to think broadly – even divergently at times – but also to adopt rational modes of analysis and to see some of the detail in an issue or problem.

(Adapted from Alimo-Metcalfe, 1998)

Gone are the days when managers had subordinates whom they could 'command'. Going are the days when people readily accept that the role of a manager in normal circumstances is to 'direct'. The majority of people in the democratic and high-tech world of today are highly educated and highly trained. Commanding them or directing them is unlikely to gain their willing collaboration and their commitment. Managing them in an appropriate style is a much more effective way of influencing them, and this is the modern form of leadership.

Modern leadership

Leadership in the modern context is a reflection of:

■ the way in which managers carry out their managerial functions
■ the way in which they exercise power and authority.

In other words, leadership is not a matter of indefinable attributes or of inspiring followers in the heroic style. Rather, it is a matter of influencing people to do the things that must be done by the way you do things as a manager. It is your management style. As Handy (1989) comments:

> The modern leader lives vicariously, getting kicks out of other people's successes – as teachers have always done. Authority [in new-style organisations] does not come automatically with the title; it has to be earned. The authority you need is not based on being able to do the job better yourself but on your ability to help others do the job better – by developing their skills, by liaising with the rest of the organisation, by helping them to make the most of their resources, by continual encouragement and example. The job of the leader is a mixture of teacher, consultant and trouble-shooter. Some say it is not a job for mere mortals. It isn't, unless you have been trained and developed for it. Then it can be a most exciting way to work.

You can go a long way towards inspiring people and winning their willing commitment if you carry out your managerial functions and exercise your authority in a style that suits the circumstances of your job and your organisation and is acceptable to the people you are managing. If you can find the style to match the circumstances, you will gain respect as a manager, your personal standing will rise, your confidence and authority will increase, and you will be accepted as a leader. By learning to carry out your managerial functions in a competent, professional, understanding, compassionate and appropriate way, you can improve your leadership abilities.

There are, however, limitations. The way in which you prefer to do things (in other words your preferred or natural management style) is primarily a reflection of *you* – your fundamental nature, your values and your beliefs. Some managers prefer to adopt a high profile and to lead from the front assertively. Others prefer to manage quite differently, fulfilling the functions of management in a less forceful way, leading from the side rather than from the front. Yet others prefer to push from the back.

Situation and setting

But the style that you adopt should not only be a reflection of you and your preferences. To be successful, it must be appropriate to the *situation*. In times of crisis and emergency, for example, most people look for a leader who can confidently point the way and inspire people to follow it, and who can act as a focus and rallying point. This decisive – even authoritarian – style of leadership may also be the most appropriate when a member of staff fails to perform to the appropriate quality or safety standards. You might also lead from the front when a decision has been made that is non-negotiable and must be implemented, for example, actions that must conform to legislative, financial or service constraints.

The *setting* is also important. Different organisations, and different departments within them, need different styles to match their particular circumstances. Virtually every organisation, whether it be a railway or an electronics company, a residential home or a general practice, requires its management to fulfil broadly the same functions. The managerial functions – of setting objectives, planning, providing resources, and so on – remain the same. The thing that varies from one to the other is the way in which these managerial functions are carried out. Each organisation, indeed each department within an organisation, is in a different situation and requires a different kind of leadership. Each organisation probably has a different view about the kind of leadership that it needs, and it selects its managers to provide that kind of leadership. Its view about the kind of leadership it needs is influenced by the traditions and experience of the organisation and by the prevailing values of the people running it.

Some kinds of leader could never hope to survive in some kinds of organisation – they would not be tolerated. However, situations change and organisations (and departments) must change with them. What happens to the organisation whose management style is not changing as quickly as the situation? What happens when the organisation's traditions and values cannot tolerate the kind of thrusting, dynamic, entrepreneurial leader who is needed because other factors in the situation require a new and different kind of leadership? They need someone to carry out the same functions of management as before, but they need someone who can carry them out in a different way. They need a different style of management, one in which the leadership element matches the changed circumstances.

Most organisations tend to select and develop managers who are capable of managing in a style that is suited to the culture of the organisation and the circumstances in which it has operated in the past. If the management cannot change its style to provide the leadership that is needed, it may have to be replaced. Successful managers are those who can develop a leadership style that is appropriate to the circumstances.

We shall now consider some of the choices you have about your actions as a manager and a leader.

ACTIVITY 3.1

Go through the checklist below and tick each item that you, as the leader of a group, have done in the past six months. Then go through the list again, this time thinking of yourself as a member of a different group, and tick the items that the leader of the group has done in the past six months.

			You as a leader	You as a member of a group
1	a	Set the task of the team	❐	❐
	b	Put it across with enthusiasm	❐	❐
	c	Remind people of it often	❐	❐
2	a	Plan the work	❐	❐
	b	Pace its progress	❐	❐
	c	Design jobs to encourage the commitment of individuals and teams	❐	❐
3	a	Set individual targets after consultation	❐	❐
	b	Discuss progress with each person regularly	❐	❐
4	a	Delegate decisions to individuals	❐	❐
	b	Consult those affected	❐	❐
5	a	Communicate the importance of each person's job	❐	❐
	b	Explain decisions to help people to implement them	❐	❐
	c	Brief the team regularly on progress	❐	❐
6	a	Train and develop people	❐	❐
	b	Gain support for rules and procedures	❐	❐
	c	Set an example	❐	❐
	d	'Have a go' at those who break the rules	❐	❐
7	a	Care about the well-being of people in the team	❐	❐
	b	Improve working conditions	❐	❐
	c	Deal with grievances	❐	❐
	d	Attend functions	❐	❐
8	a	Monitor action	❐	❐
	b	Learn from successes and mistakes	❐	❐
	c	Regularly walk round each person's place of work, observe, listen and praise	❐	❐

Were you aware of a difference in your experience of leadership when you considered the things that you did yourself as a leader and the way that you felt as team member without the leadership role? Once you have been in a leadership position you might feel frustrated as a team member if the team leader does not carry out most of the actions mentioned above. If you feel that you are achieving something as a team member, you are likely to want to continue to work productively. However, if you feel that your team is not being helped to perform well by its leader, you might be critical of the leadership. This view of leadership sees it as a facilitative role.

Leadership is a facet of management – the facet that reflects the style in which the manager carries out management functions and uses power and authority. You may not be a born leader, but if you ensure that all these functions are fulfilled in a way that satisfies the needs of your team and meets with their approval, the likelihood is that they will willingly accord you the status of leader. They will give you the authority to lead.

MANAGING WITH STYLE

We are taking the view that leadership is a reflection of the way in which you carry out your managerial functions. How, then, can you do this in ways that will provide the kind of leadership that is needed in health and care services? Leadership is mainly concerned with winning and sustaining the enthusiasm and willing commitment of staff to do the work that must be done. It is closely linked with motivating people. It is less concerned with having new and inspiring visions about the future (over which you may have little, if any, control or influence) and more concerned with maintaining the clarity and attractiveness of the current vision and sustaining people's willing commitment to devote their efforts and energies to it. You cannot *direct* people to devote their efforts and energies willingly, but you can *lead* them to do so by managing them in an appropriate style. Within the complex blend of behaviour that makes up management style are five forms of behaviour that are often associated with being an effective leader:

- setting an example
- developing your 'image'
- projecting self-confidence
- influencing others
- establishing personal authority.

Let's look at each of these in turn.

Setting an example

No doubt you expect that the people who work for you will do their work. However, you probably hope for something more from them than that they should merely come to work and do the job in a disgruntled or, at best, an uncommitted way. You probably seek their enthusiasm, energy, effort, commitment, high standards, professionalism and perhaps many other things. Is it likely that your team will provide these very desirable qualities if they fail to detect the same qualities in you? Are you, in carrying out your managerial work, setting the sorts of examples that will influence your team to act in the ways that you want?

We don't suggest that you should pretend to be wildly enthusiastic about everything. There are intermediate points between being artificially enthusiastic and being downright unenthusiastic: you can send out positive signs and signals. If you have deep misgivings about a new issue in the organisation, it is generally better to adopt a neutral position than to set examples of negative attitudes and behaviour which your staff may feel justified in copying. It is often more professional to adopt a neutral position with your staff, while finding out more about the initiative from your own manager and explaining your misgivings and your reasons for concern to him or her.

As a manager, you emit signals continuously that are received and interpreted by your staff. Your style, your manner, your tone, your attitudes and your values are all assessed and determine how your staff react to you as their manager and leader. If they detect in you someone who shows little enthusiasm for the job or the organisation, are they likely to feel enthusiastic themselves? If they do not feel enthusiastic, your job as a manager will be more difficult. Your staff might not follow *you* in the classical sense but, whether you like it or not, they will almost certainly follow *your example*.

Developing your 'image'

Like it or not, you have an image. It is the way that you are viewed by your colleagues. It is what people perceive as being true that represents the truth for them, even if you see things totally differently. It is in your interest, therefore, to work on your image to make it more professional and positive. Some people might find this idea distasteful, but there is nothing wrong with projecting the best image that you can in a conscious, considered way. It is important to take account of what is expected of you as a manager in your organisation. If you present yourself in a way that is very different from the expectations, it may be more difficult for people to respect you and to listen to you as a manager. We constantly suppress our personal feelings to act in ways that are appropriate at work rather than in ways that we might personally prefer. There is an opportunity for you, as a manager, consciously to seek to project an image of yourself that will help you to manage better and to provide the leadership that is needed.

This is precisely what we do in our professional lives, whether we are pharmacists or physicians, finance officers or physiotherapists, social workers or counsellors. We all present ourselves in ways that confirm our professional standing. Experienced professionals probably do it quite unconsciously, but in our early days as professionals we quickly learn that the ways in which we say and do things can enhance or damage our credibility. Precisely the same is true in management.

'I have learned the difference between my own view of myself and that of others. I thought I was perhaps too democratic, whereas others see me as somewhat autocratic. This was quite a shock . . . '

(Comments of a young health service manager, quoted in Stewart, 1989)

You have opportunities to improve your image in everything you do as a manager. You can work energetically, plan enthusiastically, show commitment to your job and your staff, carry out all your managerial duties with the same high standards of thoroughness and attention to detail that you would aim to achieve in your professional duties. You can conceal any potentially negative signals. You need not, for example, reveal it if you are tired and disenchanted with the job. You need not reveal any misgivings about plans that you are responsible for implementing. You might be tired, you might be disenchanted, you might have misgivings but, on balance, it would do more harm than good to reveal it, not only to your image as a manager but to the enthusiasm that your staff bring to their jobs. Don't openly 'knock' the system: your staff see you as part of it. If there are problems in the system, acknowledge the difficulties and try to make improvements. Make a point of congratulating people who do a particularly good job and make sure that your team recognises and shares a sense of success whenever this is appropriate.

It is not just the way you *do* things as a manager, it is also the way you *say* things. You are communicating much of the time, gathering and disseminating information, checking progress, explaining plans and policies, counselling and advising, criticising or praising. The manner in which you do this 'speaks volumes'. Your tone of voice, your way of speaking, can indicate much more clearly than any words whether you are committed to an idea or opposed to it, whether you are energetic or worn out, whether you are treating something seriously and professionally or merely 'going through the motions'.

Unfortunately, it is often when you are feeling most pressed yourself that revealing it to your staff can increase your problems rather than reduce them. However, it can often be helpful to share information about your workload and deadlines and to expect co-operation at particularly busy times. As always, this works both ways and your staff will reasonably expect you to recognise their particularly busy times too.

Projecting self-confidence

There is an unwritten contract that exists between managers and their staff. Your staff expect things from you just as surely as you expect things from them, and they have every right to feel short-changed and disgruntled if you do not provide them. Your staff probably expect you to make clear what they are supposed to be doing. They expect you to provide them with all the resources that they need (if necessary, by going out and fighting the system to get those resources). They expect you to keep a check on the way things are going so that their work runs smoothly and according to plan (nobody enjoys working in a shambles). They expect you to ensure that they are rewarded for their efforts, even if it is only by a pat on the back and a word of thanks. They expect you to ensure that decisions are made, even the difficult and unpopular decisions. They expect you to support them, and fight on their behalf if the need arises, remembering that loyalty works both ways. However, these are merely the functions of management. Your staff also expect you to lead.

Your staff will look to you to point the way, not necessarily to have a new and exciting vision of the future, but rather to make clear – and keep clear – what their objectives are and how they are going to achieve them. It is important to be as clear as you possibly can about the objectives and the way forward (not always an easy task), and to communicate this to your staff plainly, accurately, authoritatively and perhaps repeatedly. This is one way in which you can project your image as the person who knows where the group is going and how it is going to get there.

To achieve this implies that you must project self-confidence. Can you imagine a group placing its confidence in someone who appeared to have little confidence in himself or herself? Your manner, your style, your voice, your appearance, your posture, all send out messages about your self-confidence. You may not feel very confident but you can suppress signals that suggest nervousness and lack of confidence. Better still, you can emphasise signals that imply self-confidence.

We tend to assume that people are self-confident if they speak in a firm, well modulated voice, neither too quickly nor too slowly, and look us in the eye frequently (but bear in mind cultural differences here). Confident posture is relaxed but not slack; gestures appear natural and controlled. The signs that suggest lack of confidence are generally the opposite of these: a strained voice that might sometimes break, delivery that is too rapid or painfully hesitant, a tense, uncomfortable posture, an embarrassed or uncomfortable expression, nervous gestures, very frequent movements and avoidance of eye contact.

It is a long-term undertaking to transform yourself 'on the inside' from being an under-confident person to becoming self-assured. However, to transform yourself 'on the outside' is not so difficult. You can learn to hide any lack of confidence and to project a self-assured image. Many experienced managers would privately admit to suffering from 'butterflies in the tummy', amounting almost to panic, every time that they have to speak at a formal meeting or address a large group. Many of them, however, have learned the techniques of suppressing or hiding the give-away signs. These techniques include consciously standing (or sitting) still, imagining that you are speaking to just one person – a close friend – in the comfort of your home, and holding on to something so that your arms do not wave around or your hands scratch nervously at your nose and ears. Many managers find that learning presentation skills boosts their confidence in other situations.

'You need to learn the art of acting, of appearing confident even if inside you are scared . . . most important is learning to be confident.'

(Manager, quoted in Stewart, 1989)

Influencing others

Your ability to influence others is a crucial management skill. It is particularly important in settings where there are complex power relationships and many different types of teams working together to provide a service. In order to clear the way for action you may need to negotiate or influence, particularly in joint working situations where you have no formal authority other than in your own area of work. *How* you influence others – your staff, your peers and senior managers – is very much a matter of style.

Your staff will develop trust in you if you are consistent and fair. You need to be prepared to explain your decisions to make sure that they understand why you think that they are fair. You might have to reconsider a decision if your staff put a point of view that you had not been aware of. It is usually better not to pretend to know about something that you don't know about, but to be prepared to listen and to explore new ideas with your staff.

You have the opportunity to help others to develop by sharing the new perspectives that you gain as a manager. You have to be careful to keep confidential matters confidential, but there will be many aspects of the information that you receive as a manager that might interest your team and help them to keep abreast of developments and trends. You can be supportive in helping staff to assess their development needs and in providing training. You can support staff to explore tasks and projects that are new to them. You can win trust by making sure that those who have completed difficult tasks or who come up with good ideas are given the credit for doing so. One of the advantages of behaving in these ways yourself is that you can then expect fair and supportive behaviour from your staff. If you demonstrate ways in which you can help each other to perform better, you will be able to be open about how you can help your staff and how they can help each other and you.

Influencing your peers can be more difficult. There is often some rivalry between peers, particularly if senior managers encourage competition. However, there are very few areas of work in health or social care in which a high-quality service can be provided to patients or service users without the co-operation of a number of complementary service areas. Influence is often about identifying reasons to co-operate that allow both parties to benefit. Look for ways in which you can help your peers to achieve their goals and ways in which they can help you to achieve yours. Once you have some ideas about how this might work, discuss them with the people concerned and progress the ideas with those who are receptive by working together to identify and achieve common goals. In this way, it may be possible for all of you to achieve your personal objectives in the process of developing more integrated services to benefit patients and service users.

It is unlikely, however, that it will be quite as easy to do this as it is to describe it. If you do not already have an open relationship with your peers, you may have to be prepared to share some of the problems you face and to be open to discussion of alternative ways of addressing issues. You will also need to listen to the problems others want to discuss and to share your ideas about how they might address problems in their areas of work. Influencing peers is easier if you are ready to share the credit for ideas and actions that lead to success. It is often helpful to have these discussions with your peers and to consider alternative ways forward before discussing the problems with your manager. All managers like people to bring them options for solving problems rather than just a description of a problem and a plea for help to solve it!

Influencing your manager and other senior managers is often called 'managing upwards'. You may think that this is not something for which you should take any responsibility. However, senior managers do not have access to the detailed operations of the organisation in the way that you do as an operational manager or team leader. There may be times when you are aware of something that it would help them to know about or that they should be warned about. You are in a position to provide feedback to them about how their actions and behaviour affect your staff. Even if they don't ask for this, you might ask them if they would like some feedback.

Once again, influencing is often about finding common goals, so that many objectives can be pursued together instead of trying to progress one initiative in competition with others. You may be in a good position to see ways of making progress that are more appropriate than those that your manager has suggested because of your knowledge of your team and what helps it to work well. Remember that your manager and other senior managers have objectives to achieve and will welcome your contribution to furthering them. Senior managers usually welcome suggestions for ways of addressing problems that fit well with their objectives.

Establishing personal authority

Your staff expect you to show authority. Every manager needs to establish and maintain personal authority.

Possibly we need to distinguish between being *an* authority and being *in* authority. Most managers need to be both. It helps to have the facts at your fingertips. This means thorough preparation for meetings, thorough attention to detail, thorough mastery of techniques and procedures, a detailed awareness of what is going on. Some people amass information and detail easily. Others need to work at it. Few managers can afford to be exposed as being ignorant of the facts or unaware of what is going on.

Being *in* authority is rather different. It might be a matter of confidence that helps you to present an authoritative air and style. An appearance of being in authority is often achieved by demonstrating that you take responsibility for wider aspects of the organisation than just for your own area of work. You can make sure that the organisation presents the best image that it can to users of the service and to visitors. You can demonstrate how to be helpful to visitors; you can show that you care about the image of the organisation.

'People have looked to me as a leader so I have had to do things even if I am quaking inside. I always think I look calm on the outside: serene as a swan on the outside, yet underneath I am paddling like hell.'

(Hospital manager, quoted in Stewart, 1989)

One aspect of conveying an image of authority is to seem in control and to be able to cope with situations that arise unexpectedly as well as those that had been anticipated. Managing time is an important aspect of appearing to be calm. The managers who create the best impression and who inspire most confidence in their staff are those who can give the impression of being in control. Inside, they might feel jumpy, anxious, irritable. They might feel snowed under and be wondering to themselves how they are ever going to get through the workload. Yet somehow they manage to suppress the signals that would reveal their anxiety and that might disconcert their staff. One way in which you can give the impression of being in control of yourself and in control of events is by setting aside enough time to see people and discuss their problems in a relaxed way.

We suggested earlier that you need to do things in a style that is acceptable to your staff. This does not mean that you should do everything that they want you to do, nor does it mean that you should seek their approval for everything you do. They expect you to take difficult decisions. They expect you to have to act in ways that will not be universally popular. The important thing is that you do this in a style that makes your decisions and actions acceptable. This usually means that you should be *seen* to be doing things firmly but fairly. Favouritism or bias is a sure way of damaging your authority and losing your acceptability as a leader. However, it is important to show a concern for people and their feelings even if you are a person who, by nature, prefers to remain reserved and distant. Let your staff know that you appreciate their efforts and their concerns. On the other hand, do not become emotionally involved, or try to be 'one of the gang'. Some psychological distance is helpful, and is acceptable, although this is often difficult to establish if you were one of the gang before you became their manager. Managers cannot hope to be accepted as leaders unless they carry out their managerial functions with an appropriate style. Some people can do this naturally. Others, possibly most, need to do it in a conscious, considered way.

YOUR PREFERRED MANAGEMENT STYLE

Like most managers, you probably have a preferred style of management, a preferred way of exercising your power and authority. Some managers are naturally authoritarian. Others prefer not to exert their authority but to let people 'get on with it' in an almost *laissez-faire* style. Others adopt intermediate positions. Some managers prefer to be directive in all things; others prefer a much more consultative or participative style. Your preferred style is the one that you tend to fall into naturally unless you have carefully considered the situation and have consciously or intuitively decided that some other style would be more appropriate.

Your preferred style is influenced by a number of factors. Of prime importance among these are your personal values. Some managers feel that the most important thing is to get the job done – regardless! Others are less concerned with getting the job done than with keeping people happy.

ACTIVITY 3.2

On a scale of 1 (low) to 10 (high) what scores would you give to the following for concern for the task and concern for people?

	Concern for the task	*Concern for people*
Yourself	❐	❐
Your boss	❐	❐
Your boss's boss?	❐	❐
What scores do you think your colleagues would give you?	❐	❐
What scores do you think your boss would give himself or herself?	❐	❐

The scores in Activity 3.2 do not tell you your style: they merely indicate your sense of values as between task and people. Nevertheless, they probably give a hint of the kind of style that you would naturally fall into if you did not give careful thought to the style that is best suited to the particular circumstances in your section or department.

But there are other personal values that also affect the management style you prefer. We each have our own sense of the 'proper' way to behave. Many people feel that a manager has to assume responsibility, and should not share it with those who are more junior. Such an attitude would belong to the directive end of the scale. Others feel exactly the opposite, believing that the leader is the voice of the group, and as such should always consult the members of the group and expect them to participate in decision making. Such beliefs belong to the more consultative end of the scale. Some enjoy telling others what to do, others hate it. None of these attitudes is right or wrong, but they do restrict your range of operation. It is wise to be honest with yourself about your instinctive preference.

Besides your personal values, a number of other factors may influence your style:

- *Your confidence in your staff* – Your staff may be thoroughly competent, but if you are not entirely convinced of their abilities, you are unlikely to let them participate in deciding what to do or how to do it.
- *Your need for certainty* – An open style or approach involves handing over some control to others. There is a positive gain in that, but there is also some risk, as there always is when you relinquish control. If you have a low tolerance for uncertainty, do not like risks or do not think that the situation justifies it, you will prefer to lead in a more directive way.
- *Your personal contribution* – Your need for certainty is affected by your estimate of what you can contribute. If you believe that you know what is the right thing to do, you will not want to treat the problem as an open one, and will tend to want to tell others what to do. Managers who have done every job in their departments tend to be more directive, although this may be inappropriate.
- *Stress* – The pressure of work and events can produce a sense of overload, worry and pressure which, in excess, can lead to stress. Stress usually pushes people to one or other end of the style continuum. They either become very directive, in an attempt to reassert control over the situation, or they abandon control altogether and become apathetic.

ACTIVITY 3.3

Which way does each of these factors tend to push you? Place a cross on the scale below to mark where you are now in your present job. Place a tick where you think you would like to be.

	Directive	*Consultative*
Personal value system		
Confidence in subordinates		
Need for certainty		
Personal contribution		
Stress		

Many people lie further towards the directive end of the scale than they would like to be. This is not to say that it is always wrong to be at that end of the scale: it is not. However, to be locked into that end because of factors in you, rather than because of the situation, is to limit your flexibility and your potential effectiveness as a leader.

You have power because of your position as a manager. Power is necessary to manage resources and to ensure that they are used to meet the goals of the organisation. Some people are frightened to think of themselves as having power because it is sometimes considered that power is corrupting. But power is not good or bad in itself: it is the way in which you use your power that is important. To use your power for personal gain would be abusing the trust that your organisation places in you. However, failing to use your power can mean failing to contribute as fully as you can to the work of your organisation. You are expected to use the power of your position to do your best to achieve the goals of your work area. Using your power does not mean that you have the adopt a directive style so that everyone can see that you have power. You can choose to delegate some tasks and resources to your staff and you can choose to share decision making with them in a consultative style when it is appropriate.

Some managers might feel that a consultative style is expected by their staff and that nothing else would be acceptable. In health and social care, staff are usually highly intelligent, highly qualified and highly motivated people who could usefully contribute to making managerial decisions – if not to decisions about 'what to do', at least to those about 'how to do it'. It is widely believed that staff who participate in decision making will have some 'ownership' of the outcome and will co-operate to take the action that is decided upon. However, it is not always appropriate to adopt a consultative style, even if this is your preferred approach. In emergency situations, or when a decision is needed very quickly, you must take the responsibility. And at the other extreme, your staff would very soon tire of participating if they were involved in making all the repetitive and trivial decisions that are necessary in any work area.

So should you just rely on your preferred style because that is the one which you are most comfortable with? Or should you consciously push yourself to the consultative end of the scale? Or should you become tougher and consciously move towards the directive end? Is there a right style to use?

There is often a need for different management styles within a single managerial job. Consider your job, for example. You may have several different tasks within that job, which will require you to adopt different management styles with the same group of people.

The routine activities may well be suited to a directive style because they are well defined and need to be carefully monitored. You should not need to consult your team about them once they have been defined. Your job is to see that the duties are done.

There are likely to be other aspects of your job that require you to take initiatives or develop new opportunities. Tackling these challenges will probably require a different style of management. You will need the commitment and the creative ideas of your team. When you step into the unknown it is best not to do it alone, although the inspiration, the energy and, ultimately, the responsibility remain with you. A shift

'I know my preferred style. I am a benevolent autocrat at heart. I tend to reach conclusions much more quickly than most people, and I get impatient with their endless discussions in search of the answer. Experience also tells me that my solutions are usually right – so my natural tendency is to impose them if I possibly can. Fortunately, perhaps, I recognise that I must be a pain to work for. So generally I try to curb my natural preferences, and manage in a way that is better suited to the very experienced and well-qualified people who report to me.'

(Confessions of a senior manager)

towards the consultative end of the scale may well be needed for this part of your job.

To be effective in their jobs, let alone between different jobs, all managers need to vary their management styles to suit the particular circumstances. However, this raises the question of whether managers are capable of varying their styles of management. Research shows that few managers are able to change their preferred styles. The reasons for preferring particular styles are as deep-seated as those underlying their very personalities, and nobody can be expected to change personality at the drop of a hat. Fortunately, however, most managers have a range of styles on either side of their preferred style within which they can operate without discomfort and within which they can maintain credibility. For some managers, that range is quite extensive. The effective manager knows that the style that he or she would prefer to adopt is not likely to be appropriate in all circumstances, and that the ability (and willingness) to adjust his or her management style, within the available limits, are a fundamentally important managerial competence.

REFERENCES

Alimo-Metcalfe, B. (1998) *Effective Leadership*, Local Government Management Board.

Burns, J. M. (1978) *Leadership*, Harper and Row.

Handy, C. (1989) *The Age of Unreason*, Hutchinson.

NHS Confederation (1999) *Consultation: The Modern Values of Leadership and Management in the NHS*, NHS Confederation.

Peters, T. J. and Waterman, R. H. (1988) *In Search of Excellence*, Harper and Row.

Stewart, R. (1989) *Leading in the NHS: A Practical Guide*, Macmillan.

VALUES AND VISION

This chapter is designed to help you to identify some of the important values that underpin your work and to consider to what extent your own values are aligned with these. Managers sometime assume that the values of all the members of their team are at one with the prevalent organisational values. In practice, there are often differences that have not been recognised or understood. Assuming that values are held in common may bring difficulties because it implies that there is agreement about ways of doing things that are consistent with these values.

The values held within an organisation have an important influence on its goals and the ways in which it works. An organisation's vision is the picture of its goals – what it is trying to achieve. Vision and values are closely connected because a vision is inevitably coloured by values that view one set of goals as more desirable than another.

VALUES

Values are deep-seated beliefs about what is right or wrong, and what is important and unimportant. An organisation's values are influenced both by values held in the wider world within which it functions, and also by values held by the people who work in it and who use its services. In thinking about values, it is helpful to consider these different levels. A useful mnemonic is SOGI:

- Societal values
- Organisational values
- Group/team values
- Individual values.

The interactions between the levels at which values are held are illustrated in Figure 4.1. The values of a society influence organisations and an organisation's values influence the values of teams and individuals

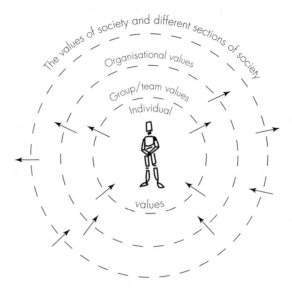

Figure 4.1 Interactions between values held at different levels

within it. But the influence does not only pass downwards: individuals also influence their groups, their organisations and the society in which they live.

Societal values

Values vary enormously in different countries, communities and cultures. In Western cultures, for example, time is thought of as linear and progressing in one direction, whereas in Bali it is thought of as cyclical and in Japan as ephemeral. Darwin proposed that there is competition in the natural world between and within species; the Navaho think of the universe as a mutualism between human beings, nature, spirits, animals and ghosts. Different religions have different explanations for how the world was created, and may have one God or many. Societies are organised in different ways: democracies accept majority rule, whereas Eskimo and Navaho societies are organised without hierarchies (Maruyama, 1981).

Modern industrial societies are complex: they include communities with very different values, living and working together in ways regulated by society as a whole. Frequently there are tensions between different societal values. In the United Kingdom, for example, there is a tension between the extent to which a 'free market' is allowed to shape the ways in which people live and work, and the extent to which public services are funded by taxpayers to provide essential services.

Public services are very much influenced by the values of the government in power. During the 1980s and early 1990s three elements shaped the attitudes of the British Government towards health and social care:

- concern about the cost of public services, their poor quality and their lack of responsiveness
- distrust of a 'nanny state', which the Government saw as creating and perpetuating dependency
- dislike of government intervention, and preference for an increased role in health and social care for the private market and the family.

Attacks on public services for being bureaucratic, over-centralised and dominated by professionals struck strong chords among both the public and progressive professionals (Hadley and Hatch, 1981). There was increasing pressure for more attention to be paid to the views of users of public services. In addition, an increasing body of evidence was emerging that public services too often reflected the discrimination present in the wider society (Williams, 1989).

A number of movements emerged to press for a greater say for people about their lives and the services they used. Disabled people, people with learning difficulties, young people in care, older people and people with mental health problems are among those who developed their own pressure groups, with their own demands, during the 1980s. There was support for this trend from many professionals, particularly those working in social care who wanted to work in different ways, and who were often unhappy about the inflexibility and unaccountability that characterised many of the organisations in which they worked. New kinds of support services emerged that demonstrated different ways of working. For example, women's organisations set up support groups in the form of rape crisis centres, and gay and lesbian organisations set up telephone helplines. These established different relationships between service users and service providers, met needs that had previously been ignored and were often run in more collaborative ways than traditional services.

New philosophies have given greater force and focus to ideas of citizen involvement. The theory of 'normalisation' brought an emphasis on social integration and offered a coherent value base for services. However, it reflected traditional values in many ways, particularly in assuming that there could be an acceptable 'normal' state. More radical perspectives were taken by some groups, for example, disabled people developed a new politics of disability, based on a critique of existing services. They redefined their situation and expressed a desire to create alternative arrangements for support that would be controlled by disabled people themselves.

This involvement and empowerment of patients and service users have been given added force by broader developments in society. They reflect a renewed concern in the late 1980s with the rights and responsibilities that go with membership of a democratic society. People have been encouraged to challenge the biases and limitations they perceive

The proliferation of groups, networks and formally constituted organisations is astonishing. One London primary care group identified more than 300 service user and carer groups in its locality, and the College of Health has more than 2,500 self-help and service user groups on its database . . . There is a real opportunity to be seized – and a real threat to be challenged. For if this movement is not recognised and appropriately valued, then patients, clients and carers will see only tokenism and betrayal – not the 'partnership' that is so often, so rhetorically and so frequently proclaimed.

(Sang, 1999)

in the delivery of public services, echoing the demands of women and members of minority ethnic groups for an equal voice and equal opportunities.

The tensions between professionals, service users and the public were exacerbated by concerns that those who were entrusted with responsibility for public funds were not always putting the interests of the public before their personal interests. Lord Nolan was asked to convene a committee to consider and report on the expectations that the public might reasonably have of those holding public office. The Nolan Committee was particularly concerned with setting principles for those who hold senior and influential positions in public life, but the values expressed in these principles might be considered appropriate for anyone with any level of responsibility in public service.

Selflessness

Holders of public office should act solely in the public interest. They should not gain financial or other material benefits for themselves, their family or their friends.

Integrity

Holders of public office should not place themselves under any financial or other obligation to outside individuals or organisations that might seek to influence them in the performance of their official duties.

Objectivity

Holders of public office should make choices on merit in carrying out public business, including making public appointments, awarding contracts or recommending individuals for rewards and benefits.

Accountability

Holders of public office are accountable to the public for their decisions and actions. They must submit themselves to whatever scrutiny is appropriate to their office.

Openness

Holders of public office should be as open as possible about all the decisions and actions that they take. They should give reasons for their decisions and restrict information only when the wider public interest clearly demands it.

Honesty

Holders of public office have a duty to declare any private interests relating to their public duties and to take steps to resolve any conflicts that may arise in a way that protects the public interest.

Leadership
Holders of public office should promote and support these principles by leadership and example.

(Nolan Committee, 1996)

This statement of principles is helpful in making the notion of a 'public service ethic' more explicit. You may have personal experience of feeling compromised by the expectations of others. For example, you may have been offered a free lunch by a sales representative who hoped to be rewarded by your support for a decision to purchase their drugs or equipment. You may have been offered some benefit for giving some-one preferential treatment or you may have been asked to help someone to jump the queue for a service. It is more difficult to be selfless in a situation like the last one if you see a member of your own family having to queue when in pain and waiting for an operation. If you have been involved in appointing staff or in contracting for services provided by other organisations, you will recognise the importance of objectivity, openness and accountability.

If you are managing in an organisation in the voluntary or private sector, your service users are also likely to expect you and your organisation to demonstrate values similar to those expressed by the Nolan Committee's principles. They will also expect selflessness, integrity, objectivity, accountability, openness, honesty and leadership to be evident. Within society as a whole, people who work in various professions and occupations often have their own sets of values which, though drawing on broader societal values, have their own particular characteristics. These are often expressed in the form of codes of ethics or statements of values or standards. The multi-occupational nature of health and social care means that different sets of values can be seen within a single organisation, or between organisations that are working collaboratively to deliver a coherent service to patients or service users. Here are three examples.

British Association of Social Workers

Basic to the profession of social work is the recognition of the value and dignity of every human being, irrespective of origin, race, status, sex, sexual orientation, age, disability, belief or contribution to society. The profession accepts a responsibility to encourage and facilitate the self-realisation of each individual person with due regard to the interests of others.

Institute of Healthcare Management

In making decisions and taking actions, managers will:

■ respect the dignity of every individual
■ respect and welcome diversity amongst patients, colleagues and the public
■ listen to the views of others
■ respect the confidentiality of all patients and colleagues
■ respect the professional standards to which colleagues owe allegiance
■ use resources responsibly
■ strive for accessible and effective health care according to need
■ use processes which are open
■ promote a climate in which patients, colleagues and the public can register concerns and where discussion is encouraged and valued
■ provide equality of opportunity for personal development
■ communicate with integrity, balance and clarity
■ take personal responsibility
■ be sensitive to the consequences for others of their actions
■ ensure that their own skills, knowledge and experience are continually developed.

General Medical Council

Patients must be able to trust doctors with their lives and well-being. To justify that trust, we as a profession have a duty to maintain a good standard of practice and care and to show respect for human life. In particular as a doctor you must:

■ make the care of your patient your first concern
■ treat every patient politely and considerately
■ respect patients' dignity and privacy
■ listen to patients and respect their views
■ give patients information in a way they can understand
■ respect the right of patients to be fully involved in decisions about their care
■ keep your professional knowledge and skills up to date
■ recognise the limits of your professional competence
■ be honest and trustworthy
■ respect and protect confidential information
■ make sure that your personal beliefs do not prejudice your patients' care
■ act quickly to protect patients from risk if you have good reason to believe that you or a colleague may not be fit to practise
■ avoid abusing your position as a doctor
■ work with colleagues in the ways that best serve patients' interests.

In all these matters you must never discriminate unfairly against your patients or colleagues. And you must always be prepared to justify your actions to them.

ACTIVITY 4.1

If you were the manager of a service in which doctors contribute to its delivery, are there any aspects of doctors' values that could potentially conflict with values held by other members of your team?

There is little in the General Medical Council's statement about efficiency, choice, democracy or universality. It focuses primarily on the relationship of the doctor with the individual patient rather than the relationship with the general public. Thus, for example, keeping to appointment times in clinics may be seen by doctors as less important than taking enough time to give full attention to the patient in front of them. The focus on the individual patient may also sometimes lead to a tension between delivery of a service to one person and delivery of that service to many people.

Organisational values

Organisations in the health and social care sector are guided by values expressed at a national level. Here are some examples drawn from the health service that reflect the influence of government policy.

Values for the National Health Service across the United Kingdom

- to renew the NHS as a genuinely *national* service
- to make the delivery of healthcare against these new national standards a matter of *local* responsibility
- to get the NHS to work in *partnership*
- to drive *efficiency* so that every pound in the NHS is spent to maximise the care for patients
- to shift the focus onto quality of care so that *excellence* is guaranteed to all patients
- to rebuild *public confidence* in the NHS

(Department of Health, 1997)

Values for the National Health Service in Wales

- *fairness*: patients should have access to treatment and services according to their clinical needs
- *effectiveness*: treatment should reflect the most up-to-date scientific evidence and clinical practice
- *efficiency*: NHS Wales should achieve best value in its use of resources

■ *responsiveness*: services should be designed with the individual patient's needs in mind
■ *integration*: NHS Wales and other organisations should work together to deliver integrated packages of care for each patient
■ *accountability*: NHS Wales should be more accountable to people
■ *flexibility*: services should be flexible enough to meet local needs, while also delivering wider improvements in health.

(Department of Health, 1998)

Values for the National Health Service in Scotland

■ to ensure equity of access to services
■ to identify and seek to meet people's needs and wishes
■ to set and aim to achieve the highest standards possible
  – of care and respect for each person
  – of results
■ to improve standards through research, education, monitoring and review whilst enabling those who work in the service
  – to achieve its purpose
  – to share its values
  – to feel valued themselves.

(NHS Scotland, 1998)

ACTIVITY 4.2

The statements of values in the shaded box are taken from government documents outlining proposals for modernising the National Health Service in the United Kingdom in general and in Wales and Scotland. Many of the themes will be familiar to you whether you work in health or social care and whether you work in one of the countries in the examples or elsewhere – the emphasis on modernising public services is international. Some of them will be relevant even if you work in the private or voluntary sectors.

Identify any values from these examples that you recognise as concerns within your area of work.

All the statements have an emphasis on standards and accountability, both of which are concerns in the public, private and voluntary sectors. The values for Scotland are more specific in mentioning both standards in relation to the results achieved by services and standards of care and respect for people, as well as improving standards through research and education. The UK-wide values emphasise the achievement of national standards being a local responsibility and focus on high-quality care that delivers excellence to all patients. The use of the word 'flexibility' in the Welsh values similarly indicates a concern to meet local needs while contributing to wider health improvements.

The UK-wide statement refers to improving public confidence, while the Welsh statement mentions responsiveness to the needs of individual patients. The Scottish values are more explicit about responsiveness, requiring services to identify and seek to meet people's needs and wishes, which could indicate a concern to listen to a wider public voice than that of patients and service users.

The Scottish values bring some different perspectives in their concern for those who work in the service, aiming to enable staff to work purposefully while feeling valued and sharing the values of the service. Managers who work in multi-agency or multiprofessional teams often have to deal with situations in which there are conflicting or competing values. In such situations it may be necessary to reinterpret core values in the new setting. It is helpful to try to establish agreement over a more inclusive set of values, for example by focusing on what the service is aiming to deliver or on broader public service values.

All these themes are related to modernising services in ways that fit more closely with public expectations as well as meeting national and local needs. Although the examples were drawn from health services, the themes that emerge are relevant to all areas of public services and are central to the aim of providing integrated services rather than separate specialist services. People who are working in health services, for example, can expect to work more closely in future with people in social care, housing and education. There is an increasing emphasis on making sure that services are 'joined up' and do not leave patients and service users with their needs only partially met.

The Institute for Public Policy Research (1999) has attempted to identify eight values that provide a national health service with its 'moral base':

- good health – a commitment to improving the nation's health
- efficiency in the use of public resources – treatments should provide high value relative to opportunity costs
- equity – with recognition that this is a major issue given the climate of priority-setting and rationing
- choice – the state should allow some degree of personal choice for individuals
- democracy – public accountability for the quality of service provision
- respect for human dignity – the relationship between the provider and the receiver of health care should reflect this
- public service – includes some of the above but also covers 'altruism rather than profit' and the notion that health service staff should work for the common good
- universality – a service for all, paid for by everyone via taxation, is

essential to provide security and reassurance to the population and to foster social cohesion.

The Institute's report acknowledged that some of these values conflict: for example, patient choice may conflict with efficiency. The public may place a much higher value on access to a local hospital threatened with closure than on (possibly) higher-quality outcomes for a small group of patients with a particular condition.

This list of values relates to a national health service as a whole, but you will probably be able to identify organisational values in relation to the unit or department in which you work. However, within a large organisation like a hospital or a social services department, the extent to which staff are aware of and influenced by organisational values can vary enormously. A junior doctor or social worker may be completely unaware of the hospital's or department's values and may identify far more readily with the values of his or her medical college or professional association. In addition, there is sometimes inconsistency between the values that an organisation tries to uphold and those that it demonstrates in its actions. This is sometimes referred to as the difference between an organisation's *espoused* values and its *enacted* values.

Group/team values

Within health and social care organisations, there is usually a complex array of staff teams comprising people from many occupational areas. Teams that work together regularly often adopt common values that focus on the purpose of their work, and recognise the contribution made by team members who bring particular and different skills. In addition to these teams, as we said earlier, an increasing number of groups within the community have their own sets of values. These groups seek to influence the values of organisations, teams and individuals that are responsible for health and social care. Their values are often expressed in codes of practice directed towards the behaviour they expect of health and social care professionals. Here is an example that focuses on empowering users of services for people with mental illness.

Staff work within constraints imposed by their employers. But within these constraints there are choices. Depending on the choices you make, service users will feel you are on their side, indifferent, or against them. You can contribute towards our recovery or our hopelessness. Here we propose some dos and don'ts for staff wanting to relate to individual service users in ways which are empowering.

This is the user speaking:

1 DO let us know what our rights are. Often we feel we have none, and are treated as if we have none. Let us know about our rights to refuse treatment, leave, make a complaint, or be represented at a mental health tribunal. It helps to be told more than once, and also to be given the information in writing.

2 DON'T hide behind a mask of professionalism. Don't use words we don't understand. Don't pretend you know more than you do. Mental health work is full of uncertainty, confusion, controversy and contra-dictions. Honesty is empowering.

3 DO ask us what we want. You may not be able to provide it. You may disagree. But do ask us. Potentially at least, we are the experts on our own needs.

4 DON'T dismiss our complaints and worries as symptoms of our 'mental illness'. Too often people's physical illnesses have been disregarded, women sexually molested in hospitals and hostels have not been believed, and genuine grievances have not been taken seriously.

5 DO recognise our talents, capabilities and potential. Support us in trying new activities, taking on responsibilities and finding outlets for our creativity.

6 DON'T panic when we express feelings. Often it is useful to sob, shout, scream, shake or shiver. We appreciate being listened to and encouraged. We want space to do that without disturbing other people.

7 DO tell us as much as you can about the drugs we are on, the diagnosis we have and the options open to us.

8 DON'T write us off. We are fed up with being told 'You will have to take these pills for the rest of your life' or 'There's no cure for manic depression'. Throwaway, negative or dismissive remarks may cause great hurt and be a source of pain to us for years. Many of us have overcome the most disabling distress, often despite the pessimistic predictions of so-called experts.

9 DO talk to us. Emotional distress is isolating. Help us break through it. Be friendly and treat us as equals. But don't try to force us to talk when we clearly don't want to.

10 DON'T forget that we live in a multicultural society, in which people have different beliefs and values. Learn all you can about the people who use your service, not least by asking them.

(cited in Spear *et al.*, 1994)

ACTIVITY 4.3

Read through these dos and don'ts again. How might users of the service(s) for which you are responsible feel? Make a note of anything that you could do or influence that might make the service better from the point of view of service users, patients or carers (or the people who use your services if you are in finance, administration, or another supporting or commissioning service).

This perspective might be one that you have not considered before, particularly if the setting in which you work puts more emphasis on the operational side of service delivery than on the experiences of patients and service users. Could this code of practice be applied to any service?

Other managers may be more familiar with the need to consider values in delivery of services. For example, values are recognised as an important element of competence for those who practise in social care. The expectations are explicit in two of the standards set for vocational qualifications in care:

Promote people's equality, diversity and rights.

Develop, maintain and evaluate systems and structures to promote the rights, responsibilities and diversity of clients.

These values place a responsibility on managers in a care setting to do rather more than respect the equality, diversity and rights of other people. There is an explicit expectation that they should be proactive in promoting these values, and in developing systems and structures that demonstrate that these values are underpinning practice.

Many service teams have statements of their guiding principles which, although differing in detail, have much in common. Here are some examples.

Older people's team
To respect the dignity and choice of older people, and to enable them to enjoy the maximum independence possible, whether their choice is to live at home or in residential care.

Mental illness team
Everyone experiences stress at times of crisis. This can sometimes trigger a mental illness. People with a mental illness should be treated with dignity and respect, and be given the chance to make informed choices about their care whenever possible. Support should be offered in the community to enable independent living and to minimise the need for institutional care.

Physical disability team
To base services on the recognition of individual needs; to help and enable people to live a lifestyle of their choice, as fully and as independently as possible, in their community.

Learning difficulties team
To enable people with learning difficulties to secure a normal way of life, living independently wherever possible; to support and consult families and carers about their needs; to enable people to develop their potential to the maximum; to recognise their ambitions and preferences, and to protect their legal and human rights.

(adapted from Williams, 1991)

As public services are encouraged to develop more integrated provision and to work more closely together, the values underlying principles like these need to be more widely discussed and considered from a number of perspectives if they are to be implemented across services.

Individual values

If you are asked what your personal values are, would you find it easy to explain them? The next Activity might help you to clarify some of them.

ACTIVITY 4.4

Imagine that you are discussing your area of work with a close friend. What will you say? Complete the following sentences:

One of my greatest concerns is _____

One thing that I would really like to change is _____

If there was enough money I would _____

I get most angry about _____

I am most proud of _____

Now read through your sentences and try to identify what values underlie each statement. For example, if you said that one of your greatest concerns is the time that some service users have to wait before they can receive an important service, your values might be related to equal opportunities or quality of life.

Our personal values arise from the values of our social background, our religion (if we have one), our ethnic origin or subculture, our upbringing and education, and our experience of life and work. They continue to develop and change throughout our lives as we encounter new and contradictory situations, and as we reflect on our experiences. Our early values are based on the culture in which we grew up, often in the narrow confines of a family or social group. It is not until we experience unfamiliar settings that we encounter views and behaviours that surprise us or, sometimes, offend us. We then have opportunities to consider the values that we hold which cause us to respond as we do. Some people are very aware of their values and how they use them when making judgements, but others make judgements without questioning the value base that underpins them. We are all individuals and we are all different. No wonder that it is sometimes difficult for an individual to fit in with a group or an organisation!

ACTIVITY 4.5

How familiar are you with the values of your organisation or service? You might find statements of values in annual reports, staff handbooks or information leaflets for service users. Think about your personal values – particularly those that influence your choice of the work you do. Make a note of areas in which you are comfortable with the ways that you are able to work in your organisation or service. Then make a note of any aspects of your work that you feel do not fully fit with your personal values.

Individual values fit broadly into two types – those that are about how you think things should be done and those that are about goals. Values about how things should be done include working hard, and being honest, open-minded and forgiving. Values about goals include happiness, prosperity, accomplishments and self-respect. The challenge is to understand your own values and why you hold them, so that you can be more aware of how other people are driven by their values. If you can recognise the differences and tensions that arise from value conflicts, you are more likely to be able to help to resolve them. It is often possible to secure agreement over the core values of service delivery, and to work from that agreement to an understanding of how individuals and teams can contribute to the work of the organisation without feeling that their values are being compromised. If you challenge another person's values, you may appear to be challenging very personal issues – even the other person's identity.

As an individual, have you considered the values you hold with respect to other people's equality, diversity and rights? It is important for you to be aware of them if you are not to be prejudiced when you have to make judgements in delivering any aspect of a service. Prejudice is based on assumptions made about the world. It has no rational basis.

It is often difficult to identify our own prejudices because they are often associated with assumptions that are central to our sense of personal security. When our assumptions are challenged, we feel uncomfortable and have to deal with our feelings as well as with the issues that have been raised. Managers in health and social care work in complex settings in which their personal values are sometimes challenged. The assumptions that they have been able to make in previous settings may no longer be appropriate. It is helpful to develop the ability to listen and to suspend judgement for a while, even to take time to check out an issue with a colleague if it is outside your experience.

ACTIVITY 4.6

O'Hagan (1996) suggested the following list of beliefs that underpin the values that an individual might hold in relation to child care. Tick those with which you agree.

I believe that:

- any child's welfare is of paramount importance ☐
- children should be listened to and respected ☐
- every child is a unique individual ☐
- parents are individuals with their own needs ☐
- parents have rights as well as responsibilities ☐
- children should be raised in families ☐
- child care services should be an expression of social justice and must be anti-discriminatory ☐
- child care workers are individuals who have rights and feelings ☐

Depending on which of these beliefs you have ticked, you might have a problem when there is a conflict between the interests of a child and the interests of the parents. It might then be necessary for you to make judgements about the relevance and relative weighting of each value, and these could change according to the circumstances. If there is a situation in which a child may be at risk because of the behaviour of a parent, there is a tension between assisting the parent to gain control and to improve the quality of his or her life, and taking action to prevent harm to the child. However, there is legislation governing how public services must treat children and, in addition, your organisation may have set out key values to guide practice. These must override your personal values.

Anyone in a management role has to work within the values of their organisation and also has to be aware of their own values, the values held by the various individuals and teams in their area of work, and those held by patients, service users and carers.

VISION

A vision can be created by an individual or by a group of people: it describes a desirable future in a way that conveys meaning and inspiration to others. Vision is therefore closely associated with values. The word 'desirable' carries a multitude of value implications, as each aspect of a desirable future implies a judgement about what is good and what is not. Vision has overtones of seeing something that is not clear to everyone, seeing details that others are not able to see and being able to convey to others a picture of an optimistic future that they have not imagined. One of the characteristics associated with leadership is the ability to identify a vision and convey it to others – the leader does not necessarily have to be the person who creates the vision.

Vision is important because it offers a picture of the future state that an organisation or service wants to achieve. It is a picture of the outcome for which to aim.

In many organisations today, people feel isolated and over-whelmed by complexity; they have no clear sense of the future and cannot, consequently, see the meaning of what they do. These problems can be addressed by a process called *visioning*, in which a picture of the future is created . . . A vision can be described as a living picture of a future, desirable state. It is living because it exists in the thoughts and actions of people, not just in a written document. It is a picture because it is composed not of abstractions but of images. As Bernard Lievegoed noted in his book 'Man on the Threshold', 'Images are more meaningful than abstract definitions. Images always have a thought content, an emotional value and a moral symbolic value.' A vision is thus integrative because it brings these dimensions together.

The focus of a vision is on a desirable future, where circumstances are different and better than current ones. It does not, however, concentrate on how to achieve that future.

A vision orients, and thus steadies, a person. It can be used to organise materials and thereby control complexity. By establishing future goals, it can give meaning to current thoughts and actions. When it is shared by people within an organisation it helps define relationships and overcome alienation. The more it is held as a common picture, the more powerful it can be in helping overcome the inertia of the present state.

(Burnside, 1991)

Holding a vision involves personal commitment. This is sometimes referred to as having a commitment of both 'head and heart'. It implies that you are feeling comfortable with your organisation both on the level of your thinking about its direction and processes, and on the level of your feelings about your work and the setting in which you work. One of the most prized aspects of leadership at all levels of an organisation is the ability to develop – with others – a vision that enables everyone to make a commitment to achieving it. This has been recognised as a feature of successful leadership for a long time.

> Whenever individuals become attached to an organisation or a way of doing things as persons rather than as technicians, the result is a prizing of the device for its own sake. From the stand-point of the committed person, the organisation is changed from an expendable tool into a valued source of personal satisfaction . . . The institutional leader, then, is primarily an expert in the promotion and protection of values.
> (Selznick, 1957, quoted in Peters and Waterman, 1982)

Once there is a clear picture of the outcomes that an organisation is aiming to achieve, it is much easier to plan how the vision can be attained. By clarifying goals, a vision can give more meaning to the day-to-day activities that take the organisation into its future. Since all individuals can contribute to achieving the objectives of the organisation, they can also relate to the organisation's vision, and understand how their actions can help to shape its future.

Some organisations involve all their staff in developing their vision. This is probably the best way to ensure that everyone feels part of the outcome and is committed to the vision. However, it is more usual for the most senior leaders of an organisation to develop and communicate the vision, and for managers at lower levels to be involved in developing the strategies and plans that are needed to work towards achieving it. These managers thus have the opportunity to demonstrate their own leadership skills in interpreting the vision with their teams.

REFERENCES

Burnside, R. M. (1991) 'Visioning: Building pictures of the future' in J. Henry and D. Walker (eds) *Managing Innovation*, pp. 193–9, Sage Publications.

Department of Health (1997) *The New NHS: Modern, Dependable*, The Stationery Office.

Department of Health (1998) *Putting Patients First*, The Stationery Office.

Hadley, R. and Hatch, S. (1981) *Social Welfare and the Failure of the State: Centralised Social Services and Participatory Alternatives*, George Allen and Unwin.

Institute for Public Policy Research (1999) *A Good Enough Service: Values, Trade-offs and the NHS*, IPPR.

Maruyama M. (1981) 'Endogenous research: Rationale', in P. Reason and J. Rowan (eds) *Human Inquiry: A Sourcebook of New Paradigm Research*, pp. 193–9, John Wiley.

NHS Scotland (1998) *Annual Report 1997/8*, The Stationery Office.

Nolan Committee (1996) *First Report of the Committee on Standards in Public Life*, The Stationery Office.

O'Hagan, K. (ed.) (1996) *Competence in Social Work Practice*, Jessica Kingsley Publishers.

Peters, T. J. and Waterman, R. H. (1982) *In Search of Excellence: Lessons from America's Best-run Companies*, Harper and Row.

Sang, B. (1999) 'The customer is sometimes right', *Health Service Journal*, 19 August, pp. 22–3.

Spear, R., Leonetti, A. and Thomas, A. (1994) *Third Sector Care*, Open University/Department of Trade and Industry.

Williams, F. (1989) *Social Policy: A Critical Introduction*, Polity Press.

Williams, K. (1991) *A Practical Approach to Caring*, Pitman Publishing.

MAPPING THE SERVICE ENVIRONMENT

If you are to understand how your service 'sits' in its environment, you need a mental map that shows how the important elements of the environment relate to each other, and to you and your area of work. We begin this chapter by suggesting a way in which you can map the components of your organisation's environment and categorise them. We identify three major parts of this map – the *internal environment*, the *near environment* and the *far environment*.

The remainder of the chapter focuses on the near environment. We discuss how and why organisational boundaries can change in response to changes in relationships with the near environment. We examine the concept of *stakeholders*, and invite you to identify the main stakeholders in your area of work and their interests. We consider some approaches to managing your relationships with your stakeholders and thus influencing your near environment. We complete the chapter by considering the nature of 'needs' and 'demands' and their impact on the environment of health and social care organisations.

COMPONENTS OF THE SERVICE ENVIRONMENT

Organisations exist to provide services or to make products – to meet needs. They can be very large and complex or they can be small enterprises with only one area of work. Both the size of an organisation and its shape – for example, why certain activities are carried out within it and why others are purchased in or contracted out – are determined by environmental factors. Your organisation does not exist in isolation: it is part of a large and complex network of patients, service users and their carers, suppliers, competitors, regulators, and so on. In addition, the economy, social trends and technological innovations have an impact on it. We can represent this complex network in terms of three environments (Figure 5.1).

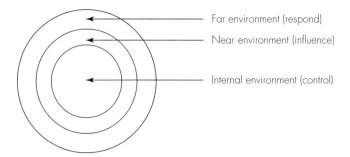

Figure 5.1 The three environments

There is a dynamic relationship between these three environments.

■ The *internal environment* is composed of the staff, resources and facilities within the organisation. These components can be *controlled* – to a large extent, at least – by the organisation's managers. The internal environment is, however, influenced by the near and far environments, which the organisation is unable to control.

■ The *near environment* includes patients, service users and carers, contractors, suppliers and competitors. It also includes local politicians, other organisations that are partners in service delivery and local pressure groups. These components of the environment are all close to the organisation and they interact with it in a variety of ways. They cannot be controlled by the organisation, but they can be *influenced*.

■ The components of the *far environment* are those factors that can neither be controlled nor influenced from within the organisation. They include a wide range of social, technological, economic, environmental and political factors. Every organisation has to *respond* to the impact of these external factors. Some respond more thoughtfully, quickly and successfully than others.

Each organisation and area of work has different components in these three environments. You might have staff teams or groups of volunteers in your internal environment, along with internal administrative services or resources like buildings, facilities and equipment. In your near environment you might have those who use your services, services in other organisations or agencies with which your organisation regularly works, and local people and organisations that have an impact on your organisation in some way. Components of your far environment might include new legislation that requires your service to change and developments that change the nature of the local community (for example, your locality becoming an increasingly popular holiday destination).

The boundaries of an organisation

If a new acquaintance asked you where you work, would you reply giving the name of an organisation like 'I work at Barsetshire Council' or 'I work at the Royal Hospital', or would you say something like 'I work in social care' or 'I work in the health service'? The acquaintance might then ask you to explain a little more, to give some idea of what your work involves and how it relates to other services. This sort of discussion is often about boundaries. It is similar to discussions you might have about your own job, and where the boundaries are between your responsibilities and those of others. Like jobs, organisations have invisible boundaries that define what is 'inside' the organisation; they are part of the way in which an organisation carries out its purpose. They also define what is 'outside' the organisation, but contributes in some way to its work.

Organisations differ in where they draw the boundary between their internal and external environments. There are lots of examples.

- Some residential care organisations carry out all their catering and cleaning activities themselves and others buy in these services from external suppliers.
- Some doctors' practices collaborate to run out-of-hours services whereas others use private deputising services.
- Some local authorities carry out services such as home care with in-house staff whereas others use contractors.

There may sometimes be a special relationship between a contractor and its client organisation, for example where the contractor's staff are people who formerly worked for the client organisation and now sell their specialist service back to it. Other types of special relationships are partnerships or network arrangements (such as the information services run by rail companies) or franchises (such as most fast-food outlets and many hotels).

These examples illustrate that organisations have choices about where they set their boundaries. The activities that are included within the organisational boundary and those bought in from outside may change over time. The main choice is between carrying out activities *in-house* and using contractors (*outsourcing*). If you use outsourcing, you are buying services from what is available externally – from the 'market' – looking for levels of quality and price that meet your organisation's needs. If there are many potential suppliers, you can make choices and demand exactly the service you want. But if there are few suppliers, it might be difficult to buy in the service you want at the price you want to pay.

It can be very frightening for staff who are accustomed to being valued employees of a stable organisation to hear about the possibility that their service area may be outsourced. But there are many advantages and disadvantages of outsourcing that need to be considered.

In-house services are often valued for their 'fit' with the organisation because they are managed within the same policies, structures and culture (although specialist services such as personnel and training often have their own cultural flavour). However, in-house services may have high overhead and management costs, particularly if the volume of service is not large enough to justify the infrastructure required. There may be difficulties in reducing or increasing the volume of the service quickly enough to respond to needs. Also, small in-house services may not be able to keep up to date with developments that enable new ideas and technologies to contribute to improving the quality of service delivery within an organisation in which the core work and investment are focused on other activities. Investment for development can sometimes be found by creating external partnerships – one form of outsourcing.

If organisations become very large and carry out a wide range of different activities, they may become difficult to manage and difficult to change. Skilled staff who perform well may often be the best people to continue to carry out the activities being considered for outsourcing. It may be possible to transfer them so that they can do so under different management arrangements in new organisations. This has become common practice in public services, leading to the creation of many organisations that are able to deliver specific and focused services. Creating these new organisations requires new skills, such as contract management and quality assurance. Communication becomes increasingly important to ensure that they work well together. Integration of services is an important theme in health and social care nowadays, to ensure that service users receive an appropriate set of services to meet their particular needs. If there are different service providers, with parts of services outsourced, effective co-ordination is essential.

The advantages and disadvantages of in-house provision and outsourcing are illustrated in Table 5.1.

Table 5.1 Advantages and disadvantages of in-house provision and outsourcing

	Advantages	Disadvantages
In-house	Control Reliability Flexibility (resources can be reallocated) Accumulated experience Quality control	High overhead and management costs Costs inflexible if requirements change Limited economies of scale Lack of access to new ideas and technologies Lack of specialist skills
Outsourced	Easy to expand/reduce resources Access to specialist suppliers Reduction in in-house fixed costs Overall cost savings	Loss of in-house expertise in key areas Need for contract management skills Possible loss of quality control Possible loss of short-term flexibility

ACTIVITY 5.1

Consider an activity currently carried out inside your organisation that could possibly be outsourced. It might be a catering service or support for a technical function, or perhaps even provision of a professional or specialist service. Make a note of the advantages of the current in-house provision and compare these with the potential advantages of outsourcing.

You may conclude that – at least for the time being – the advantages of keeping the activity in-house outweigh the advantages of outsourcing. There is a tension between keeping all services within the ethos of an organisation, and the potential financial and quality advantages of outsourcing. Many organisations prefer to retain their core services and contract out the facilities that support these. However, as the environment in which your organisation functions continues to change, there will be pressure to keep these options under review, particularly if financial resources are limited. It is important to ensure that the organisation is investing its resources in the services it is required to deliver (its core services) and to focus on how these services could be improved, rather than keeping a support activity in-house if it is performing less well than it could if it were outsourced.

Organisational boundaries are not fixed. They can change in response to political pressures (such as 'compulsory competitive tendering' or 'best value' in the public sector) or pressure on costs or the introduction of new technology. In their efforts to improve the quality of the services they provide, organisations are constantly seeking the best balance between short- and long-term objectives, between operational and strategic considerations, and between the needs of their different stakeholders. It is to the interests of stakeholders that we now turn.

STAKEHOLDERS AND THEIR INTERESTS

In the first half of this century, political meetings throughout Europe would be interrupted by shouts of 'What about the workers?' More recently the shift to a more consumer-oriented society has changed the concern to 'What about the customers?' Employees and customers are both examples of stakeholders – people who have a 'stake' in an organisation in the sense that they have a keen interest in what the organisation does and how it does it. In the voluntary sector, stakeholders include funders, donors and volunteers. In the public sector, they include the general public in their capacities as citizens, taxpayers who fund public services, and beneficiaries of those services as patients and service users.

All organisations have internal stakeholders: employees, managers, directors, trustees, and board and committee members. They also have stakeholders external to the organisation, but strongly linked to or affected by it: patients, service users and other customers, suppliers, funders and possibly competitors. Other external stakeholders are more indirectly affected by the organisation: the local community, the general public, community health councils, pressure groups, local councillors and Members of Parliament. (These three categories correspond to an organisation's three environments.)

It is important for you, as a manager, to be aware of who your stakeholders are because these are the people who can influence the working of your organisation. Some stakeholders' interests are protected by law. Employment legislation and health and safety legislation provide increasing protection for employees. Contractual relationships protect the interests of partners in service provision. The legislation governing services for children regulates most aspects of care involving children.

Different stakeholders have different interests, which may conflict. For example, the interests of employees in security of employment and increased earnings may conflict with those of funding agencies which may be seeking short-term cost reductions. The interests of taxpayers may conflict with the interests of those who depend on public services. A proposal to build a new care home or motorway is often opposed vigorously by local communities. The culture, structure and governance of an organisation will determine how these conflicts are resolved and, in some cases, the interests of one stakeholder group will have a dominant influence. Organisations may have to work hard to ensure that the interests of other stakeholder groups are not compromised.

Your internal stakeholders will include your colleagues, other employees of the organisation and possibly staff in other parts of the organisation who provide services linked with those in your area. Near environment stakeholders include all those who use or purchase your services, and others who come to your organisation for a particular purpose. They might also include those who take an overview of the services provided by your organisation, including external quality assessors and external organisations to which your organisation is accountable. Professional bodies may be part of your near environment because of their concern for the maintenance of professional standards. However, professional bodies could also be considered to be part of the far environment: it depends on how you view the strength of their influence. National bodies, such as the Government and the Department of Health are likely to be part of your far environment.

Analysing stakeholders and their interests is important for two reasons. First, it emphasises that different stakeholder groups have different interests and that managers have to balance these interests when making decisions. Second, it helps you to appreciate the relationship between your organisation and its external environment.

Identifying stakeholder groups in your near environment

If you work in an organisation that provides health or social care services, you will have a number of groups of stakeholders. Some of these are shown in the form of a 'stakeholder map' in Figure 5.2.

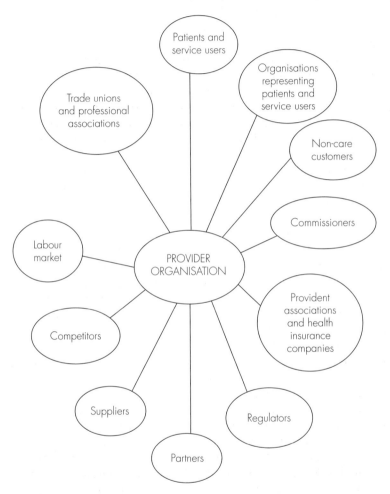

Figure 5.2 A stakeholder map for an organisation providing health or social care services

Here are a few comments about each of these groups of stakeholders.

- *Patients and service users* include their relatives and carers, who may receive services in an indirect way. This group could also be described as your external customers, in the sense that they come from outside your organisation and are consumers of the services you offer.

■ *Organisations representing patients and service users* include voluntary organisations such as MIND and Age Concern, as well as your local Community Health Council.

■ *Non-care customers* are those to which your organisation may sell services (other than care services) to generate income. For example, hospitals may rent space to shops or sell franchises to photographers of newly born babies.

■ *Commissioners* (the word now preferred to 'purchasers') are also customers, since they are paying for the services that you provide. They act as the agents of patients and service users. They include health authorities, health boards in Scotland, primary care groups and trusts, and local authority social services departments. As the emphasis on joint investment and joint commissioning between health and social care increases, local health care commissioners and local social care commissioners will both be important to you, whether you work in health or social care. There will certainly be arrangements for joint consultation. For example, the local social services department is responsible for commissioning social care for your local population: as a manager in an organisation providing health care, your work may have an impact on that responsibility of the local authority – as well as on its housing, education or environmental health departments – and on the police.

■ *Provident associations (such as BUPA) and commercial health insurance companies* are probably the main purchasers of your services if you work in a private hospital, although some patients will be paying directly from their own resources. (In the case of independent health care, which forms only a small part of health services in the United Kingdom, the user and the purchaser are one and the same.) Even if you work for a public-sector provider, you may still have services for private patients, again mainly purchased by insurers.

■ *Regulators* are responsible for ensuring that service provision is of a sufficiently high quality and meets agreed standards. At a local level, some forms of regulation are part of the function of commissioners, but there is an increasing emphasis on the development of national service frameworks to ensure that health and care services are provided equally effectively in all geographical areas. National standards are inspected by regional units. There may also be increasing links with other service areas for example, inspection of playgroups and inspection of child-minders may be linked with inspection of the education service.

■ *Partners* include any other organisations with which your organisation collaborates in delivering services. Partners may work together in order to share expertise across a wider service area, or they may have pooled their resources because they are then better able to deliver co-ordinated services in a geographical area. Partnerships are usually formed because there is a clear advantage for both partners, and they may have varying degrees of formality. When the need to work closely is very strong, organisations may even merge rather than retaining distinct characteristics as in a partnership. At the other extreme, many organisations have loose alliances within which they have mutually beneficial working arrangements.

- *Suppliers* are the firms and organisations from which you buy goods and services – from food to high-tech equipment to domestic services to management consultancy.
- *Competitors* are other organisations (whether in public or private ownership) providing services that commissioners may see as actual or potential alternatives to the services you provide. Although public services no longer operate in such an overtly competitive market as they did in the early 1990s, there is still some competition in the sense that patients and service users can sometimes choose which service provider they use, and commissioners can select service providers that most closely meet their criteria. Organisations which can demonstrate that they attract high numbers of users are likely to attract continuing funding and thus survive more easily than organisations that are not the first choice of service users.
- The *labour market* is made up of individuals who actually or potentially possess the skills and knowledge needed in your organisation. You cannot provide services without sufficient numbers of suitably qualified staff. Your organisation has a reputation within its environment and staff recruitment may be assisted or damaged by its reputation as an employer.
- Some *trade unions* and *professional associations* will have members within your organisation, but you may occasionally find yourself dealing with them as external organisations, perhaps in educational or disciplinary matters or over the recognition of a training post in your organisation.

If you work in a commissioning organisation rather than in an organisation that provides services, the organisations that provide services will be an important group of your stakeholders. Some of the group of stakeholders in Figure 5.2 (such as patients and service users) will be just as important for you as for provider organisations, while others (for example, competitors) will be less significant than they are for provider organisations.

You may have been surprised at how many different groups of stakeholders can be identified, particularly if you have recognised some that you have not previously considered as having a particular interest in what you do and how you do it. If you are considering a change in a service that you offer, each stakeholder group will take a view of the proposed change from their particular perspective. You and your colleagues may see the benefits to be gained by making a change, but some of your stakeholders may feel that the disadvantages outweigh the benefits of the proposal or may want to propose a different way of achieving similar benefits.

The interests of each stakeholder group will vary according to the circumstances. If a proposed change will have immediate consequences for a particular group, it is easy to see that their interests should be taken into account. However, changes often have less obvious repercussions for other groups and it is helpful to think about any proposal from a range of different perspectives in order to consider how each group of stakeholders might perceive it. Your organisation probably has a variety of ways of keeping in touch with its stakeholders' views. However, team leaders and other first-line managers are often closer to the stakeholders who are in direct contact with their services and are in a good position to ensure that the stakeholders' views are understood within the organisation.

INFLUENCING THE NEAR ENVIRONMENT

The near environment consists of people and organisations (stakeholders) with whom, in a loose sense, your organisation has to 'trade'. Either you need things from them, or vice versa, or both.

One way of thinking about the relationships in an organisation's near environment is to consider the choices and constraints that exist because of the availability of the resources that the organisation needs in order to operate effectively. This approach was called *resource dependence* by Pfeffer and Salancik (1978). They took the view that no organisation can be completely independent – all need resources, including money, materials, personnel and information. Organisations acquire these resources by interacting in their environment with others who control the available resources. There is a constant struggle for balance as an organisation confronts difficulties and constraints imposed by these external circumstances. As all organisations experience similar difficulties in obtaining resources, those which work geographically close to each other or which deliver similar services are often interdependent. One organisation may be dependent on another to buy its services, another may be dependent on those that provide it with services or goods. These dependent relationships are more or less important, depending on how critical the resource is.

It can be useful to think about what is the scarcest resource that is critical in enabling you to provide your service effectively. In some cases it is availability of skilled professionals – for example, a serious shortage of nurses and junior doctors in some parts of the country. In other service areas there are shortages of transport, sheltered housing or hospital beds. Some resource shortages might be resolved if more money were available, but many would take a considerable time to develop, even with additional funding. Sometimes the solution may be to find an alternative source (doctors and nurses from overseas) or a substitute for it (physiotherapy aides to do some of physiotherapists' more routine work). In other cases a new process can change the demand for resources – for example, minor surgical operations are now often carried out in GPs' surgeries without the need for patients to be treated in hospitals. Developments like these change the balance of dependency: organisations then have to respond to different levels of demand, and demand for different types of services needing different types of resources. Pfeffer and Salancik suggested that there are four ways in which an organisation might balance its dependencies.

- *Adapt to the conditions*   This could be done by reducing levels of service, restricting use of resources, slowing down the speed of response to demand or influencing the types of demand made on its services. For example, a small hospital might reduce the number of different services offered, and specialise in treating a particular condition or a particular group of people (for example, admitting only older people or only children).
- *Alter the interdependencies*   This could be done by merging with another organisation that controls some of the needed resources. It could be done by growing and providing a wider range of services, so that the organisation is not dependent on providing only one type of service. For example, a small community-based home care service might link with a community health service to provide care for people who need support at home when they leave hospital.
- *Negotiate the environment*   This could be done by creating partnerships with other organisations to deliver services jointly or to share resources. One way in which this is increasingly happening at the present time is by developing links between social services and health services, sometimes including contributions from the voluntary sector.
- *Change the environment by political action*   This could be done by influencing decision makers to change the conditions in which the organisation operates. An example would be lobbying local Members of Parliament in an effort to prevent the closure of a hospital or to try to obtain subsidies or special financial allowances when the demand for a service increases unexpectedly (as often occurs for health and social care organisations in harsh winters).

All organisations have relationships with other organisations and may have to adopt one or more of these strategies to ensure that they are able to access sufficient resources to continue to deliver their services. All these relationships can be – and need to be – managed. Part of the role of management is to manage externally in this sense. Although this may not be a central part of your role as a first-line manager, you do not need to become the chief executive to be involved with this near environment. In the language of systems theory, such managerial roles are part of *adaptive systems* – those whose function is to help fit the organisation into its environment and thereby to ensure its survival.

Despite the impact of environmental pressures, organisations may develop habitual patterns in the ways in which they manage the external environment. Miles and Snow (1978) suggested that there are four different organisational approaches to the environment.

- *Defenders* aim to satisfy a stable and fairly well defined segment of their market or environment. Their emphasis is on efficiency and quality; they are not quick to undertake radical new developments. This approach is not always appropriate if the environment changes rapidly and the organisation is not quick enough to respond. The emphasis in organisations that adopt a defender position is on doing things right, being efficient and managing resources well.
- *Prospectors* are at the opposite end of the spectrum from defenders. They are more concerned with innovation of technology or service or both. The emphasis in these organisations is on doing the right thing rather than doing things right – on being effective rather than efficient. This approach needs a flexible workforce to cope with frequent changes. There is a risk of lack of co-ordination when many different initiatives are evolving independently.
- *Analysers* try to maintain a balance between the defender and prospector positions. This approach has the advantages of both the previous ones, with the potential of minimising risks and maximising performance. It attempts to be both efficient and effective. There may be two different styles of work within the organisation if it has a focus on innovation and fast introduction of new initiatives alongside provision of well established and routine services.
- *Reactors* are outside the scope of the continuum from defender to analyser to prospector. They simply react, perhaps arbitrarily, to pressures as they occur. As a result, their decisions are likely to be inconsistent and perhaps inappropriate. These organisations are in danger of running out of resources or of offering services that people no longer want.

Miles and Snow regarded any of the first three of these approaches as being viable in principle. They did not consider the fourth approach viable for any length of time. Most large organisations providing health and social care services probably either lie on Miles and Snow's continuum between the defender and analyser positions, or else are reactors. Harrison *et al.* (1992) suggested that, until the late 1980s, the strategy of reactors was not only the norm in the health service, but was also the most effective approach when the environment was slow to change. The more recent arrival of an environment for public services that is more focused on customers and quality seems likely, however, to require a move towards the analyser and prospector parts of Miles and Snow's continuum. If the environment is changing rapidly, as it has throughout the 1990s, managers have to devote much of their time and attention to ensuring that the organisation continues to deliver what is wanted by those who fund it and ensuring that staff, skills and capacity are developed so that the organisation is in a position to deliver new services as new opportunities evolve.

We have introduced the idea of creating a map of the environment of your organisation as a first step towards understanding – and thus managing – its relationships with the wider world. Many managers in health and social care are involved in working jointly across traditional boundaries in order to develop service provision. An understanding of the environment of your service and your organisation is helpful in enabling you to think ahead and to be sensitive to the ways in which you and your organisation respond to the influences of the environment while respecting the interests of your many stakeholders. You are in a position to influence the ways in which relationships with your stakeholders develop.

However, managers in health and social care also have to consider the influence of 'needs' and 'demands' on their organisational environment and strive to be responsive to both need and demand.

NEEDS AND DEMANDS

The concept of need is somewhat problematic in health and social care. If you have acute appendicitis, you definitely need a surgical operation, but there are other cases where an alleged need (for example to have your tattoos removed, or for you or your partner to be provided with *in vitro* fertilisation) would be the subject of fierce contention. It is not difficult to make a conceptual distinction between need and demand: *need* is usually thought of as the ability to benefit from a service, while *demand* constitutes people claiming services. However, despite the conceptual clarity with which this distinction can be made, there are real problems in *using* them: people may demand what they don't need and vice versa. If you are a carer, who other than yourself is entitled to say whether you need – will benefit from – periods of respite when alternative care will have to be provided? Demand is not a simple concept either, because it has overtones of the consumer-led market. But in modern public services it can be seen as emphasising an appropriate focus on the service user.

Many people prefer to think in terms of health and care services responding to demand. None the less, variables such as the demographic structure of the population, the known pattern of mortality (death) and morbidity (illness), and the extent to which various services are utilised are often treated as indicators of need when forecasts of future expenditure or plans for future health and social care services are being made. Let's look briefly at each of these variables.

The *demographic structure* of a population is an important determinant of need for health and social care. This occurs in two ways. First, the age structure of a population determines whether more or less of a particular service is needed. For example, if the birth rate falls there will be less need for maternity and child health facilities (as well as for playgroups and infant schools). Second, and more importantly, people of different ages tend to have different patterns of usage of health services, with different cost consequences. In general, very young children and older people are much more expensive to provide for than other age groups. In private health insurance, these differences are reflected in the premiums that subscribers have to pay.

Mortality rates and the causes of death within a population are regarded as important information about a population's needs for health care, as well as about its health in a broader sense. The attraction of mortality as a measure of these needs is that death is both unequivocal (except in the relatively few cases of people in a persistent vegetative state) and it is the subject of statutory recording through death certificates. The causes of death recorded on certificates are, however, a matter of medical opinion (confirmed by post-mortem examination in a minority of cases) and, over longer periods, are susceptible to changes in medical knowledge and perhaps diagnostic trends.

Morbidity is the prevalence of disease in the community. The diagnoses of hospital patients are sometimes used to assess morbidity, but this only reflects illness among people who have *both* approached a doctor (usually a general practitioner) *and* been referred to hospital. To obtain data on illness across the whole population, whether under treatment or not, it is necessary either to undertake special research (something which is normally only feasible in a specific geographic location or among a particular social group) or to rely on answers to questions about health that are included from time to time in data-gathering exercises such as the Census or the General Household Survey. Since such data are self-reported, they cannot provide accurate objective information about needs for health and social care. Nevertheless, they provide useful information, for instance about the prevalence of long-standing disabilities.

Utilisation rates are measures of the extent to which the public use health and social care services. They are sometimes assumed to represent need and they certainly reflect demand. However, it is not always clear how the demand created by professionals interacts with the demand created by patients and service users (for example, you cannot be admitted into hospital without a doctor's agreement).

At this point, it is useful to consider separately how health and social care services each meet needs and demands.

Meeting need and demand in health services

There are many difficulties in bridging the gap between acknowledging that health services and service managers are affected by public need and demand, and knowing what can be done about it. But it is important to recognise that people's health problems are *filtered* by the services that exist. Various studies have demonstrated that the health service deals with only a small proportion of the health problems present in a population at any particular time. Most people do not contact any formal services when they have symptoms of illness. The term 'symptom iceberg' was coined to draw attention to this situation. Consider some of the following evidence.

- A survey of 1,000 adults in London found that only 49 were free of symptoms in a two-week period. Of the remaining 951, only 21 per cent had seen a doctor for their symptoms. The majority had treated themselves with medicines purchased at a pharmacy.
- A group of general practitioners asked a sample of young and middle-aged women in their practice to record symptom episodes in a health diary. When they compared the evidence of the diaries with records of attendance at the surgery, only one in every 37 symptoms had been presented to the doctors.
- Serious illnesses may go untreated. With problems as diverse as hypertension, rheumatoid arthritis, diabetes and psychiatric disorders, the number of cases in which treatment has not been sought may be as high as the number of patients receiving treatment.
- Among those over the age of 85, one-third will not have reported problems of poor hearing, giddiness and heartburn to their GPs and one-quarter will not have reported problems they experience with their feet.
- Social background appears to have a significant influence on whether a doctor is consulted. Among women, the ratio of medical consultations to rates of illness in Social Class I is 2.0 compared with 0.7 in Social Class V. In other words, women from professional backgrounds are more than twice as likely to consult their GPs.

In meeting health care needs it is useful to think of three filters: the individual, the GP and the hospital consultant.

A number of considerations are involved in *individuals'* decisions whether to seek health care in relation to a health problem. For example:

- Are the symptoms worrying?
- How painful/uncomfortable are the symptoms?
- Are the symptoms to be expected?
- Do the symptoms disrupt daily life?
- Is it appropriate to seek care for this particular problem?
- Can the doctor do anything for the problem?
- Would it be embarrassing to take this problem to the doctor?
- What are the costs of consulting the doctor in terms of time and inconvenience?

Perhaps symptoms such as headaches or changes in energy may be considered trivial or to be expected as part of everyday life. On the other hand, a sore throat may be considered a problem for which the doctor can prescribe treatment, and a pain in the chest may be considered life-threatening. From a medical point of view, many of these perceptions may not be well founded, but they are powerful influences over behaviour in relation to illness. They can change over time as health services change. Suppose that a general practice began to provide and promote awareness about migraine clinics. Consultations for headaches might increase as people became aware of the availability of services.

General practitioners manage virtually all health problems initially and refer patients to hospital care only when primary care is insufficient. They may filter patients' problems in at least two ways.

First, there is considerable research evidence that GPs may not be aware of many of their patients' problems:

■ Half of patients' disabilities may not be known to their GPs.
■ Two-thirds of patients' mental disorders may not be recognised by their GPs.
■ GPs may have no record of 77 per cent of adult patients' smoking behaviour and 41 per cent of blood pressure measures.

This kind of evidence suggests possible shortcomings or limitations in primary care that can lead to undesirable filtering of health problems.

The second way in which GPs can act as a filter is in their decisions to refer. Some of the most puzzling data for the health service can be found when the rates at which GPs refer their patients to hospital are calculated. In one study, GPs with the highest referral rates were found to send patients to hospital four times more frequently than GPs with the lowest rates. The differences could not be explained in terms of patients' demands. Also, when GPs do refer their patients to hospital, their goals and expectations may be different both from those of the patients who are referred and from those of the hospital doctors. One study examined whether the primary purpose of the referral was diagnosis, treatment, investigation or reassurance: the GP, consultant and patient all agreed in only one-third of the referrals.

Once patients reach hospital, *consultants* decide whether and how to treat them, what X-rays and pathology tests to request, whether to admit them as inpatients, and when to discharge them. Just as there are substantial variations in GPs' practice, there are also substantial variations in consultants' practice. For instance, rates of tonsillectomy vary between different parts of the country by as much as four to one.

The management of public need and demand therefore involves a complex mixture of internal variables (for example, the doctors) and external variables (the public).

Meeting need and demand in social care

In providing or commissioning social care services for adults, the 1990 NHS and Community Care Act requires local authorities to separate the process of assessing people's needs from decisions about what services should be provided and how and by whom they should be delivered. Assessments of need cover a range of issues, including people's housing circumstances, the financial resources available to them, their physical and mental incapacities, their family and social environments including the needs of informal carers, and the transport available to them. The type and cost of services supplied vary according to the needs identified, the preferences of the people concerned and the resources available to the local authority. Thus a person who requires help with washing, dressing, going to the toilet and cooking is deemed only to need help with these activities. This is rather different from describing people as 'needing' a particular service, such as residential care or day care.

The financing of social care services is very different from the financing of health services. Some social services have always been available for private purchase. Some services are available from local authorities, but are subject to charges. Local authorities are not required by law to provide or commission a service on behalf of service users at no cost to them, although they may do so. Pressure on resources has increasingly led to higher charges for services such as care in the home, coupled with raising the threshold (or eligibility) criteria – the level of need required before a service will be provided. Evidence of this can be seen in residential care homes. Thirty years ago most residents would have been able to wash and dress themselves, and those with greater care needs would have been in a hospital or nursing home. Now most residents of care homes require more intensive personal care. This has led to considerable changes in the types of accommodations and care services available, both in the public and independent sectors.

Unlike most health care services, social care services are often required for life (for example by those with learning difficulties, physical disabilities, mental health problems or frailty in old age). They are also required to provide for the whole person – not just for physical care, but also for the emotional and social aspects of life. This has major implications both for the long-term cost of services and for the range of services that are required.

A challenge for local authority social services departments, in identifying needs and in commissioning services, is to keep in mind the needs of people who are excluded from services by eligibility criteria. As the severity of the needs of those who receive care rises, more people with mild or moderate needs are excluded from receiving social services unless they can afford to pay for them themselves. The preventive effect of providing low levels of care to help with everyday needs is gradually lost, thus increasing the number of people with higher levels of need. Similar processes apply in the provision of services for children and families.

WORKING WITH YOUR ENVIRONMENTAL MAP

You should now have a better understanding of how your service 'sits' in its environment and of how the important elements of the environment relate to each other, and to you and your area of work. You should be able to 'map' the main implications for your organisation of the *internal environment*, the *near environment* and the *far environment*. As an operational manager, your work will probably be most affected by the internal environment, but your understanding of the issues arising from the near and far environments will help you respond to their impact of the different pressures as they change over time.

You should also be able to identify the main stakeholders in your area of work and their particular interests. You have many opportunities to influence your near environment through the ways in which you manage relationships with your stakeholders.

We completed this chapter by considering the nature of 'needs' and 'demands' and their impact on the environment of health and care organisations. It is often difficult to respond positively to everyone's needs and demands when your resources are limited. Every manager of health and social care services may expect to be involved in contributing to the improvement of services as they change to address newly identified needs and demands.

REFERENCES

Harrison, S., Hunter, D. J., Marnoch, G. and Pollitt, C. J. (1992) *Just Managing: Power and Culture in the National Health Service*, Macmillan.

Miles, R. E. and Snow, C. C. (1978) *Organisational Strategy: Structure and Process*, McGraw-Hill.

Pfeffer, J. and Salancik, G. R. (1978) *The External Control of Organisations: A Resource Dependence Perspective*, Harper and Row.

DEVELOPING EFFECTIVE PERFORMANCE

A large part of your work as a manager probably involves collaborating with others in groups or teams. Although the terms are often used interchangeably, it is useful to distinguish between them.

A *group* is any collection of people who interact with one another because they perceive themselves to have a similar purpose or similar interests.

A *team* is something more. It is a group with a sense of a common goal or task, the pursuit of which requires collaboration and the co-ordination of the activities of its members, who have regular and frequent interactions with one another.

However, the distinction is not a clear-cut one. It is a matter of degree – a group becomes a team when a similar purpose becomes a common goal and when interaction becomes collaboration and co-ordination.

Most people find that working in a group or team has a significant effect on their behaviour. People in a group may reach decisions and take actions which, as individuals, they would not have had the confidence or aspiration to do. If you consider people only as individuals, you are ignoring some of the most significant and powerful influences that determine how effectively they will work. Managing groups and teams – supervising and organising their work so that their talents and resources are deployed efficiently and effectively – is essential to the delivery of health and social care services.

Groups and teams vary greatly in size and complexity. Some managers are responsible for only two or three people. Others are responsible for the work of several hundred or even several thousand. Yet others have no line management responsibility for staff but still need to exert influence in the teams of which they are members.

TEAM WORKING IN HEALTH AND SOCIAL CARE

Health and social care teams often have to struggle with issues that dramatically affect people's lives, often at some personal cost to members of the teams. They are usually part of very large organisations which require labour to be organised and controlled, as well as huge sums of money to be accounted for. Teams often work with ambiguous – even contradictory – objectives (for example, 'meet demand and give the best possible care . . . but stay within budget'). They are often organised around a specific task and composed of people from different areas of work who have different concerns and interests (for example, a team of people collaborating to address teenage pregnancy might include social workers, teachers, GPs, health visitors, health promotion specialists and parents).

In some parts of the health and social care sector, developments in information technology have had a significant impact on how groups and teams interact. Where there are electronic communication links within or between organisations, there are more and more 'virtual groups'. Their interaction patterns are interestingly different from those of groups that communicate face-to-face: the culture of communication on electronic nets is free and easy.

Managing teams and groups of diverse composition and size requires considerable skills. These include both the conceptual skills of being able to analyse what is going on in the group and the practical skills of dealing with many 'people' issues at once, such as communication skills and influencing skills.

There are a number of reasons why people prefer to work in groups, including for affiliation, to gain a sense of identity, to help each other to make sense of the world, to protect their own interests and to get things done. Many managers say that they get satisfaction from being in a well led work team. Working in such a team, for many, seems to model the sort of inclusive and consultative approach that health and social care services should reflect, and embodies the way they feel they should interact with service users.

However, Casey (1985) suggests that genuine team working requires:

> enormous effort, and quite a large act of faith, on the part of any management group and its leader. It requires a huge effort to . . . say what you mean, express your feelings openly, engage in open warfare, trust your colleagues, speak your mind . . . Most British managers have spent their working lives learning the exquisite skills of doing the exact opposite!

He argues that the only justification for that sort of effort is if it leads to the task being done better. He categorises tasks into three types (Table 6.1), and proposes that the nature of the task is a key determinant of whether a team is needed at all.

Table 6.1 Types of tasks

Simple puzzles	Complex puzzles	Genuine problems
Solution exists, and can be found by an individual with the right skills.	Solution exists, but requires more diverse skills to analyse and collate the information required to find it.	So difficult that no one knows the answer – sometimes even the problem cannot be understood with clarity.

Casey does not see the need for any special team skills – other than basic social skills – to solve simple puzzles. 'Typical simple puzzles', he says, 'are technical and inside one member's own technical function – others may need to know but no real sharing is necessary. Often these puzzles arise at a full meeting and then are quickly and properly delegated to the individuals concerned.'

Complex puzzles, on the other hand, involve 'work which no individual can do on their own . . . there is a need to share, but only at a level which enables the work to carry on, not at a level of baring of souls. . . . When a group is working well in this mode, members recognise the need for give-and-take, co-operation, negotiation, seeing the other person's point of view and sharing information on a need-to-know basis. . . . We are not talking of teamwork, at least not in the ideal, open, sharing model of teamwork advocated by team builders.'

It is in the case of genuine problems, Casey says, that real teamwork is called for, because 'nobody knows what to do; no-one round the table has the appropriate expertise because nobody knows what expertise is appropriate.' In order to address this sort of problem, people 'need to share deeply and personally, because dealing with uncertainty is fearful and you can't do it unless you feel safe. Any suggestions you might make are fragile and tentative and that would leave you vulnerable; you won't do that until you feel supported, liked and valued as a person.' Casey suggests that this is why many groups shy away from addressing genuine problems. Genuine teamwork requires high-level interpersonal skills, especially from the leader, and some real incentive to go through the uncertainty of team building.

Casey's analysis has its merits, in particular in identifying simple puzzles which can often be more quickly and efficiently solved by a single person with the necessary expertise. We are all familiar with situations in which a group wastes time and energy trying to deal with issues like this – often unproductively.

However, some people would say that Casey oversimplifies matters, particularly in seeking to make a distinction between complex puzzles and genuine problems. For example, improving the arrangements for discharging older people from hospital is a matter of improving co-ordination between the professionals involved – doctors, nurses, social workers, and managers of home care services and residential homes. Casey would say that this is therefore only a complex puzzle.

Yet such a problem can be quite intractable (a genuine problem) from the perspective of any one of the professionals or managers involved, since he or she is responsible for only one of the services that need to be co-ordinated.

Conversely, the following case study suggests that genuine problems can sometimes be reframed as everyday complex puzzles, with the objective of improving collaboration and co-ordination.

A psychotherapist contacted one of us on behalf of a multidisciplinary child guidance team based in a hospital. The team comprised psychotherapists, consultant psychiatrists, a social worker, an occupational therapist, a psychologist and two administrators. They were having difficulty working together as a team and had obtained funding for an 'away day' in which to try to sort out their differences with the aid of a facilitator.

The facilitator had difficulty agreeing achievable goals for the day with them, not least because every time he wrote or telephoned he found himself dealing with a different person. He asked every team member to write him a letter explaining what they saw their difficulties to be. When he had read these letters, he wondered what on earth they could do about it all in a few hours.

On the day, he asked them for examples of what they regarded as teams. They said a football team, or the team in an operating theatre. He pointed out all the ways in which they were not like these teams: there was no goal that they were all shooting at; they worked with their clients only singly or in pairs, never all together; they were in different professions with different values and conventions; they all had different bosses; one member, the social worker, was in a different organisation from the rest of them. He asked why they didn't forget about being a team and regard themselves simply as colleagues who met periodically to discuss and co-ordinate their work with children.

The mood shifted during the day. They had seen themselves as failures, unable to live up to their ideal of team working. Now they began to see themselves as achieving a modest but useful level of collaboration in the face of massive obstacles. What is more, they were working together very effectively at that moment, listening to each other, making inventive suggestions and ignoring differences in status.

(McCaughan and Palmer, 1994)

Multidisciplinary and multi-agency teams

An increasingly important aspect of health and social care today is managing teams which include different professions or representatives of different organisations. Bringing together a range of specialisms and expertise offers opportunities to create services that are more effectively integrated for the benefit of patients and service users. Gorman (1998) identifies four features of such teams that require particular attention: their members have different professional perspectives and lines of accountability, work within different legal and statutory frameworks, and carry out work that is funded from different budgets. Let's look briefly at the implications of each of these.

Different *professional perspectives* are based on different sets of values that lead to different interpretations of problems. For example, the medical perspective differs from the social, the managerial from the clinical, the financial from the service providers. Different professions also bring different experiences: for example, doctors have been through education processes that are didactic and hierarchical in nature; social workers through processes that emphasise the importance of ownership and self-determination of issues by service users and carers. Power relationships may differ, too: a hospital consultant may assume that the influence he or she has in the workplace will be transferred to working in the group, whereas a junior doctor will not have the same expectations.

The whole point of multidisciplinary teams is to bring together a range of different perspectives on the care of people. This purpose needs to be made explicit in the team's objectives and the differences between its members' perspectives need to be explored, not hidden. This necessitates a thorough sharing of background and experience and identifying people's legitimate roles within the group. Gorman says: 'It is your task as a manager to lead your team through the development so that they understand and respect the differences and these differences become a source of strength not a source of weakness.' This is something to which you can contribute even if you are only a member, rather than the leader, of the team.

Many people working in health and social care have dual *lines of accountability*. For example, an occupational therapist may be accountable to the leader of a therapy team, as well as to a senior occupational therapy professional. When someone is part of a multidisciplinary team, lines of accountability become even more complicated. A nurse on the board of a primary care group, for instance, will be expected by the primary care nurses in the area to represent their interests; he or she will also be expected to act corporately, as a member of the management team. The nurse may also be responsible for a particular aspect of the board's work, for example as chair of a working group on a particular aspect of health improvement. In addition to all this, the nurse will also have a 'day job', perhaps as the leader of a team of health visitors that has particular interests for which he or she has responsibilities.

Gorman says that, in a situation like this, 'It is important to be as clear as you can so that everyone – you, the staff and your colleagues – are clear what the areas of accountability are and where the boundaries fall between them.' He also argues that it is worthwhile putting in a lot of effort to try to ensure that the people who are engaged in the work of the team have the power to 'own' and implement decisions:

The White Paper *Modernising Social Services* (Department of Health, 1998) describes the ideal make-up of inspection teams for residential care:

'The workforce will consist of people with skills and qualifications from both social care and health care, including nurses. The benefits of combining these two sets of skills and backgrounds will best be realised if there is true integrated working, allowing – for instance – nurses to be involved in inspections of children's homes, and social care professionals to be involved in inspecting social aspects of nursing homes.'

'Although it can take longer in the short term, sometimes a lot longer, the investment of getting all the right people in the room is usually rewarded in the long run. It means that you can ensure that the decision is clear, individual roles are clear and that people will actually deliver on their commitments.'

The health and social care sector operates within a complex array of *legal and statutory frameworks*, and most people have an understanding only of the parts of the law which immediately affect them. In addition to the legal frameworks that govern the professions, the health service has always had a centralised, top-down system of control, with national 'guidance' on practice and procedures issued frequently by the National Health Service Executive. In addition, each trust has its own frameworks setting out what can and cannot be done by individuals, for example, on issues about sharing information. By contrast, until recently, each local authority had its own local system of accountability, with local politics having a considerable impact on day-to-day decision making about social care. In the past decade or so, however, social services departments have became increasingly subject to 'control by government circular'.

Gorman points out that, to work effectively within these frameworks, it is necessary to understand them and the impact they have on your colleagues. You need to set feasible objectives in the light of the things you cannot change.

'There is a new acronym developing around here – a development of NIMBY (Not In My Back Yard). It's NIMBA – Not In My Budget Allocation.'

(Manager of a Mental Health Acute Admissions Unit)

Any cross-boundary activity that involves spending money can raise issues for those with *budgetary responsibilities*. People are usually subject to rules that constrain how their budgets can be spent. Gorman accepts that there may be little that you can do in the short term to change budgetary rules. However, taking advice from someone who thoroughly understands the rules (such as a management accountant or finance director) may give you a clearer idea of the extent to which they are capable of 'interpretation'. You can also make those who set the rules aware of any constraints they may be placing on service improvements, in the hope that this may lead to changes being made – at least in the longer term.

In all these situations, the time available for team working is a mundane but practical issue for most multidisciplinary and multi-agency teams. It is not easy to work around the busy lives of health and social care professionals to gain the level of commitment that others, with different priorities, expect. The apparently simple task of getting everyone in the same room at the same time can absorb disproportionate amounts of effort. There needs to be a commitment to continuity: multi-agency work can often be undermined by frequent changes in the faces sitting around the table. Even when the same people can meet consistently, decisions often need to be referred back for the agreement of the home agency of each team member. With good planning, however, these challenges can be overcome by anticipating them. The effort is worthwhile if it brings benefits for patients and service users.

Here is an example of effective multi-agency working.

A health service trust and a social services department decided to plan and deliver their community care training programme jointly. To plan the programme, they invited 50 of the key local players with an interest in community care to a one-day conference. Each of the major agencies made a presentation about new initiatives they were planning for the year and the issues they wanted the joint programme to address. This enabled the conference to develop a picture of how community care was likely to change in the coming year and the demands that would be made on staff. The second half of the day was spent identifying and agreeing the main topics that the joint training programme should address. A small inter-agency steering group was formed, with representatives from each of the main players, and given the task of developing the detail of the main topics and agreeing and organising the delivery of the programme. The programme was so successful that the agencies agreed to repeat the process the following year.

(Adapted from Gorman, 1998)

And here is one where things didn't go so well.

Early on in my experience as a chair of child protection conferences, I had closed a meeting and people were departing. I thought I had concluded the business of collecting evidence of alleged harm or injury to a child, that we had reached consensus about the degree of risk and the actions to be taken, and that we had allocated tasks. But then one of the people involved in the meeting came up to me and gave me some additional information – something she hadn't liked to say in the meeting because she wasn't sure if it was relevant. She related an incident that she had observed between the stepfather and the child which was of very great potential significance. I had to reconvene the meeting. I had learned the hard way that one of the skills I needed as chair of such meetings was to conduct a very formal meeting in order to ensure accuracy of information and objectivity, but that this was only achievable within an atmosphere of trust and with sufficient informality to encourage participation.

ACTIVITY 6.1

Think about a group of which you are a member which includes people from different professions or agencies.

1   How effectively does this group handle issues of different professional perspectives, different lines of accountability, different legal and statutory frameworks and/or different budgets?

2   Is there any special behaviour or support that you – or someone else – could provide that may be helpful to the group?

Groups at work – whether they are formal or informal – can have considerable influence over the way people value what they and others do, and thus their behaviour.

If the present rate of change in health and social care continues, the creation of new groups that work together effectively will continue to be important. Getting people with different perspectives and values to work in collaborative groups will continue to tax the skills of managers. You are now more likely than ever before to work in several teams, in roles that may not be clearly defined. You may be expected to play different roles in different teams, and to contribute to working out what these roles should be. This demands considerable insight into your own style and flexibility, and into that of others.

PLANNING SYSTEMATICALLY TO MEET TRAINING AND DEVELOPMENT NEEDS

Working effectively in groups requires considerable skills, effort and time. However, the potential payback is almost limitless, in terms of improving outcomes for patients and service users. People need training and development to enable them to learn and practise new ways of working – even those who have had extensive professional training prior to taking up posts need support to develop as conditions and requirements change.

Training and development should focus on developing the skills and knowledge that an individual needs to perform effectively in his or her job, as well as on his or her needs for personal growth and career development. It is often categorised into three types:

■ *Job-specific training* helps people to acquire and develop the necessary skills and knowledge to do their current jobs effectively and safely, for example, induction of new staff, or preparation of staff to enable them to take on delegated tasks or new projects. Staff may also need training to prepare for changes arising from new national requirements (such as new health and safety legislation) or new organisation-wide policies or plans (such as the introduction of a new equal opportunities policy).
■ *Continuing professional development* (CPD) is about helping people to keep up to date with the latest research, approaches and techniques within their particular field. This is important for all professionals working in health and social care and is of particular importance in clinical fields where technological developments are

continually providing opportunities for improving care. Some professional bodies require individuals to provide formal evidence of CPD for continuing membership and registration to practise.

■ *Personal development* provides people with the opportunity to develop a successful career within the organisation and to prepare for a possible career outside. It also recognises that the personal growth of the individual is important in maintaining his or her motivation.

Training needs analysis

An important outcome of appraisal is the identification of training and development needs of all these types for the individuals within your team. This is one source of information for a *training needs analysis*, which pulls together all the individual needs into a summary of the collective training and development needs of the team. But appraisal is not the only source of information for a training needs analysis. You may also wish to gather information from:

■ staff questionnaires
■ customer surveys
■ talking to staff individually or in small groups
■ recruitment and induction interviews
■ evaluation of training and development events.

ACTIVITY 6.2

Read the case study that follows. It describes how a community health-care trust completed a training needs analysis for the organisation. You may be able to use some of their experiences to develop a process that would work within your department. As you read it, you might like to use a highlighting pen to mark any points that might be useful in undertaking a similar exercise within your own department.

A total training initiative within a community healthcare trust

The aim of our 'total training initiative' was to identify current and future training and development priorities and to make plans to address these. Not untypically, prior to this initiative the trust had no overall approach to link staff training and development to business requirements: it had previously taken a piecemeal approach, dealing with the needs of each professional group separately. The initiative was developed in response to growing demands placed on trusts and their human resource managers to be mindful of cost efficiency and effectiveness at a time when training and development were becoming increasingly important. All the resources directed towards training had to be justified in terms of the trust's service and business needs and priorities. The initiative involved an analysis of all present and future training and development needs to inform the creation of a trust-wide training and development strategy.

We developed a project plan for the work with four key stages.

Stage 1:   Work with the senior management team to identify current and future service and business priorities. These were validated with staff at all levels in the organisation during stages 2 and 3.

Stage 2:   Work with both the senior management team and service directorate teams to identify organisational and management development priorities to meet the service/business priorities.

Stage 3:   Work with the service directorates to identify professional and technical training and development needs.

Stage 4:   Work with the trust's Director of Human Resources to review the outcome of stages 1–3 and to produce a five-year training and development strategy.

Stages 2 and 3 involved all staff at all levels in the trust in the training needs analysis in two ways:

■   There were two-hour facilitated workshops with groups of staff from all levels and departments in the trust. A SWOT analysis (strengths, weaknesses, opportunities, threats) was completed in small teams followed by a full discussion of all the SWOTs with the full workshop group.

■   We conducted one-to-one interviews with members of the trust staff drawn from all service directorates and departments. These interviews focused on the individuals' experiences of training within the trust and on current and future training and development needs.

Additional information was provided from the business plans of directorates and departments, job descriptions, personal development plans and reports of exit interviews.

Within the time and resources available, it was not possible to involve every member of staff directly. The training needs analysis involved staff from each directorate and department, ensuring a cross-representation of professional disciplines and roles, level/status, length of service within the trust, age, gender, ethnic origin, shift patterns and perceived capability. The information collected from stages 1–3 was analysed to identify training and development needs within each directorate and department, common needs across the organisation and needs specific to staff groups. The data were also analysed according to training topics. The training needs analysis enabled the organisation:

- to identify training and development priorities for the next twelve months
- to produce a timetabled training plan which set out the options available to meet the identified needs, their resource implications, and the advantages and disadvantages of each.

The key factors in the success of this total training initiative were:

- the establishment of current and future service and business priorities
- the involvement of all staff in the process of identifying needs
- ensuring all existing information was used (for example, customer surveys, objectives and personal development plans agreed through the appraisal process, staff opinion surveys)
- the production of a five-year training and development strategy and plan that will receive full support from the senior management team
- a realistic and achievable action plan
- offering opportunities fairly and equitably to all staff
- a review and evaluation mechanism to monitor implementation.

The Project Team kept staff regularly informed of progress through written communication and regular meetings. The process was highly participative, with staff involved in shaping the outcomes through workshops and interviews. When the training plan and programme were published, staff were able to make decisions with their managers about the most effective ways of meeting their individual needs. The senior management team has also used the information gathered by the training needs analysis to help them to develop a range of skills-training packages and to review the appraisal system.

(Sally Cray)

Developing a training plan

As in the case study, a training needs analysis should lead to the development of a training plan to meet all the identified training and development needs of your team. The plan should identify:

- needs that are common to more than one member of the team
- needs that are unique to individual members of the team
- how you intend to meet each identified need
- a timetable for all the training and development activities to be undertaken by the team
- the resource required to support each training and development activity (time, internal or external expertise, money)
- arrangements for the release of staff, where appropriate
- arrangements for ensuring that the learning that individuals and the team acquire is brought back to and used in the workplace

■ proposals for monitoring and evaluating all training and development activities

■ proposals for building both the training plan and the outcomes of training and development into your organisation's business planning cycle

■ a way of maintaining records of training and development that individuals have completed, and how this has met identified needs.

The process of developing your training plan is one in which you should involve your whole team. The collective knowledge of the team about development needs will help you to draw up a plan that develops the whole team as well as the individuals within it. You could also involve the team in researching opportunities to meet their needs that exist within and outside the organisation. If you share with the team the process of making decisions about how best to meet identified needs within limited resources, training and development are more likely to be effective in improving performance. Members of the team can help to find ways of sharing their learning with the team, rather than keeping it to themselves.

The work that your team and your department do is likely to change: nothing stands still for very long in the world of health and social care. Your training plan will therefore need to be regularly reviewed and updated to reflect changing work demands and priorities. Even if the team's development needs do not change significantly in the short term, the way in which you choose to meet them may change. For instance, new work demands may create new opportunities for projects to help individuals gain experience in new areas and thus develop their skills. Longer term, as the demands on the team change, new training and development needs will arise to prepare the team to meet new challenges.

Reviewing and evaluating progress

You are likely to spend time and money in training and developing your staff. As a manager, you are responsible for ensuring that this is a worthwhile investment for your organisation. You need to be able to demonstrate tangible benefits as a result of spending that time and money.

Some trainers use course evaluation sheets, but these have become commonly known as 'happy sheets' because they tend to measure how much individuals enjoyed a course rather than tangible benefits. They do not measure the effectiveness of the course in increasing skills and knowledge, or the impact of learning in the workplace. These can only be measured weeks or months after the learning event, when the individual has had an opportunity to put what he or she has learned into practice.

If you are going to be able to measure tangible benefits after a learning event, you must be clear beforehand about the outcomes that you expect from your investment. These may be outcomes for the individual or for your department or both. Here is an example.

Training and development activity

A member of staff will be attending a two-day course on health and safety.

Expected outcomes

The individual will acquire sufficient knowledge and understanding of current health and safety legislation and good practice to develop a health and safety policy for the department.
   The outcomes will be measured by:

■ meeting with the individual two days after the course and asking him or her to tell me what has been learned
■ setting the individual the objective of developing a health and safety policy for the department within six months
■ reviewing progress towards this objective at monthly intervals.

ACTIVITY 6.3

1   Think about a training or development activity that one of your staff is due to attend. Identify one or two outcomes that you would like to see as a result of that activity. (These could be outcomes for the individual or for your department or both.)
2   How could you measure the success of the activity in terms of these outcomes?

You can play an active role in helping each member of your team to think about ways of applying and further developing his or her newly acquired skills or knowledge within the workplace. Both during and after the learning activity, you should allocate time to talk to the individual about what he or she has learned and to identify how the learning can be used to improve the individual's own performance and the performance of the department. Your discussions might focus on:

■ what has been learned

- whether the learning experience has met the identified development needs
- how this learning can be applied in the workplace to achieve improvements
- objectives for the individual that will encourage use of the newly acquired knowledge or skills
- how the individual can share his or her learning with the rest of the team, so that the team can benefit from the investment in developing the individual.

An equal opportunities perspective

There may be questions to be resolved about who receives development opportunities and who does not. The problem is often one of having to set priorities: the time and money available just will not stretch to everyone. Decisions therefore have to be made about who should be included and for what reasons.

Employers are required by law not to discriminate on the grounds of gender, marital status, race or disability when making decisions about training opportunities. It is also good practice not to discriminate on the grounds of age.

Policies on training and development should reflect a desire to maximise the potential of all staff. If a minority group is under-represented in a certain grade or post, or if they have had career opportunities denied to them in the past, it may be possible to design development opportunities with the express purpose of changing this. This is one step that can be taken to promote equal opportunities for minority groups, but all training and development should take special needs into account so that neither direct nor indirect discrimination occurs.

Training and development activities can play several roles in promoting equal opportunities:

- The overall staff development process should address how all members of staff can be developed to their full potential, regardless of gender, race, age or disability.
- The equal opportunities dimension should be addressed during in-house or externally arranged courses or workshops on a wide range of topics: decision making, change programmes, personnel selection and interviewing, assertiveness, disciplinary procedures, appraisal interviewing, redundancy, and so on.
- Courses or workshops should provide opportunities for everyone – not just people with equal opportunities concerns – to talk through their views, discuss the practical implications of particular objectives and how implementation difficulties may be overcome, and examine their own practices and prejudices.
- External courses and workshops may provide opportunities for

those from disadvantaged groups, who may feel isolated and exposed within their organisation, to support each other, share experiences and pick up new ideas.

■ Targeted development opportunities can help individuals who belong to cultural or ethnic groups that are under-represented at particular levels in the organisation to achieve the positions they may aspire to and should rightly hold.

DEALING WITH POOR PERFORMANCE

The ideal way to deal with poor performance is not to let it happen in the first place! However, that is dependent on getting a lot of things right. Motivation theory tells us we have to put many things in place: clear objectives, the resources required, the right skills, clear outcomes and linked rewards, and so on.

In practice, all of us have performed poorly at some stage in our working lives. There is often a fairly stressful period when we first come into a job, while we work out what is wanted from us, and then a further period before we learn how to be effective in the job. Detecting poor performance is not always easy to do for ourselves, let alone for others.

Poor performance is far easier to spot in some jobs than in others. In jobs for which there are clear and objective standards for performance, underperformance is much more easily detected. As we said earlier in this session, the aims should be to develop explicit, clear and mutually agreed objectives, to agree appropriate ways of monitoring performance against these objectives, and to address any barriers to effective performance.

In some jobs, however, such as those with job titles including liaison, co-ordination or facilitation, standards of performance often depend to a large extent on the perceptions of other people. It is then necessary to negotiate a shared perspective of what constitutes 'good' and 'not-so-good' performance, and the involvement of other stakeholders may be helpful. Mechanisms such as 360-degree assessment of performance may be helpful both to the stakeholders and to the person in the job.

If you suspect that an individual is underperforming, it is worth asking yourself some questions.

'I find my role very difficult. I have a fairly clear idea of what I ought to do, but my managing group has a mix of different ideas. The trouble is that there isn't any accepted idea of what the job should look like: it's a relatively new role and it's being worked out in all sorts of different ways across the country. I'm not really sure whether I'm doing the right things, and I find it hard to persuade myself at the end of the day that I've done a good job. It requires a degree of arrogance almost – that I'm the best judge of my performance.'

(Clinical audit co-ordinator)

ACTIVITY 6.4

Think of a situation in which you have been or are concerned about the performance of a member of your team or another colleague, and make notes in response to the following questions.

1   Exactly what is it that I am concerned about? If I had to describe this to an outsider, what specific examples or evidence would I present?
2   Do I understand the context in which this is happening? Am I aware of any factors that may be affecting the situation, such as inadequate equipment, stress or incompatible priorities?
3   How important is this problem? What is its impact on patients or service users? Does it harm our collective effectiveness as a team?
4   Are my concerns important enough or legitimate enough to merit intervention? Am I concerned about isolated incidents or small behavioural quirks that may not be important to others?
5   Would another colleague/manager see the problem in the same light? Is there any indication that my concerns are shared (or not shared) by others?
6   Would it be helpful to share my perceptions with the person involved? Would it help him or her to understand how he or she is being seen, and provide an opportunity to clarify some mutual expectations?

'Our performance problems can be categorised into three: don't understand cooking, can't cook, won't cook. The first is a managerial problem and relates either to poor induction or to poor clarification of role by the manager, the second is a capability problem, the last a disciplinary one.'

(Personnel Director)

The reasons for poor performance usually fit into one of three categories:

- a person doesn't understand what he or she has to do
- he or she is not capable of doing it consistently
- he or she is knowingly not doing what is required.

The first two of these reasons for performance are often described as issues of *capability*. The third, because of the element of 'knowingness', may lead to the need to invoke *disciplinary* procedures if the person is challenging (openly or otherwise) the nature of his or her job. Let's look at each of these two situations separately.

Capability issues

The root of a capability problem may not lie with the individual, but with others in the organisation. Perhaps the person was appointed to an inappropriate job in the first place, or perhaps the content or context of the post has changed over time. Perhaps the person's objectives have not been adequately clarified – or perhaps objectives have not been set at all. Perhaps appropriate training has not been provided – either at the stage of induction into the job or at a later stage.

But there may be other factors that *do* lie within the individual. Perhaps the person cannot sustain the necessary level of performance because of physical or mental ill-health. Some health problems, such as stress or substance abuse, may not be immediately obvious.

Dealing with inadequate capability needs to be approached in constructive and supportive ways, with the aim of returning the person to a satisfactory standard of performance. However difficult, it is your responsibility to tackle the problem.

Your first steps in dealing with capability issues will probably be at an informal level, unless the breach of standards of performance is so potentially hazardous as to merit immediate formal action (and if this is the case, you will need to record the details of events as precisely as possible, and involve your personnel department and/or senior management). You should share your concerns about performance, as specifically as possible, with the individual concerned, and encourage the person to state his or her point of view and raise issues that may have a bearing on performance. It is important to be sure that he or she is very clear about the performance standards required in the job and you may find it helpful to refer to job descriptions and appraisal records.

When you have clarified the problem, you will need to establish how best to help the individual, agree the details of that, and set a date for reviewing progress. You should also point out the consequences of not making satisfactory progress: he or she may not be sufficiently aware of the seriousness of the issue – especially if you are being supportive! It is worth making a written record of what has been agreed, so that arrangements are explicit to both parties and you can justify your actions if you need to pursue the issues later.

If you suspect that the person has problems that he or she is unwilling to share with you, it may be beneficial to involve a third party, such as a personnel specialist or counsellor. If you think that health problems may be involved, you may need to refer to sickness and absence records and involve specialist advisers such as occupational health practitioners.

Should your informal intervention fail to produce results, you will need to involve other people, and fully document your concerns and the action you have taken. Your organisation may have a set of procedures for dealing with capability issues.

Disciplinary procedures

Most organisations have rules that govern the behaviour of employees in the workplace. They set out organisational expectations on issues such as:

- time-keeping
- absence
- health and safety
- use of the organisation's facilities
- discrimination
- disclosure of confidential information
- compliance with instructions
- claiming expenses

- accepting gifts or hospitality
- contact with the media.

If these rules are broken, managers may have to take disciplinary action. This may amount to no more than an informal warning: 'I heard you on local radio last night talking about the proposed closure of the resource unit. You must be aware that you are not allowed to make contact with the media to talk about your work without getting approval in advance from me, as your manager. You did not do so. I'm prepared to overlook this breach of the rules this time, but it must not happen again. If it does, I may have to invoke the formal disciplinary procedure.' However, there are some circumstances in which a breach of the rules, such as accepting a bribe, could amount to 'gross misconduct' and result in immediate dismissal.

An organisation's disciplinary rules must be widely known and understood. Employment law places a legal obligation on any employer with 20 or more employees to include, within written terms and conditions of employment, details of:

- any disciplinary rules which apply to the employee
- the name of the person whom the employee should notify if dissatisfied with any disciplinary decision.

The standard of work produced by an employee can also be a disciplinary matter, rather than an issue of capability, if there is an element of 'knowingness' about non-conformance with performance standards – if the person is familiar with the standards and behaviour expected, but for some reason does not wish to comply.

Failure on the part of an employee to comply with acceptable standards of work performance is often the most difficult area to handle. The key lies in being clear at the outset about what is expected. The Advisory, Conciliation and Arbitration Service booklet *Discipline at Work: The ACAS Advisory Handbook* is a very useful reference for managers, and essential reading for anyone charged with drawing up or managing disciplinary rules and procedures. It suggests that the following principles should be observed when employment commences:

- The standard of work required should be explained to employees clearly so that there is no misunderstanding.
- Job descriptions should accurately convey the main purpose and scope of the job (though the absence of a job description does not preclude disciplinary action if it can be proved that the employee knew what was expected).
- Employees should be made aware of the conditions attached to any probationary period.
- The consequences of not meeting the required standard of work should be explained.
- Where an employee is promoted, the consequences of failing to reach the new standards of performance should be explained.

A disciplinary procedure describes the process by which breaches of the disciplinary rules, or other disciplinary matters, should be dealt with. Its purpose is to ensure that an employee who has breached the required standards of behaviour or work performance, but not grossly so, is given a fair opportunity to improve. Although it may eventually lead to the dismissal of the employee, this is not its main purpose. One of the main areas to come under scrutiny, should a case eventually end up at an industrial tribunal, will be the disciplinary procedure itself: whether it was followed properly, and whether the employer's actions and penalties were fair and reasonable.

As a manager, you should know what your organisation's disciplinary procedure is and ensure that you comply with it. However, especially in the health service, the position is complicated by the fact that, in addition to a trust having its own disciplinary procedures, some groups of staff, such as doctors, dentists and nurses, may be governed by their national terms and conditions of service regarding disciplinary matters, so you may need to take advice from expert practitioners in this area. Your human resources department may have experts or, if not, will probably be able to advise you whom to talk to.

Grievance procedures

Grievance procedures exist to deal with problems arising in the workplace which could adversely affect a member of staff's mental or physical well-being, or his or her ability to perform to the standard of work expected. They provide a formal mechanism through which employees – individually or collectively – can bring their concerns or complaints to the attention of their employer and have them addressed. Employment law requires any employer with 20 or more employees to include in written terms and conditions of employment:

■ the name of the person to whom an employee can take a grievance
■ the way in which a grievance will be handled.

An employee can take out a grievance if treated in a way that he or she feels breaks the rules of law, contract, or the 'accepted custom and practice' of the way things are done, and that works to his or her disadvantage.

Fortunately, most managers are rarely involved in formal disciplinary or grievance procedures. In most cases, people wish to perform well and your role is to support them by helping them to improve their performance.

However, there are occasions when staff do not perform well either because – despite training – they are incapable of doing the job, or because they are not willing to do so. Dealing with situations like this is one of the least enjoyable parts of a managerial job, and one that it is very tempting to shirk. However, it is part of your role as a manager, and 'carrying' someone who is not pulling their weight in the team can have substantial costs, both in terms of its effects on patients or service users and in the stresses and strains it places on colleagues. You may then need to invoke the procedures we have described, and it is important:

■ to have a thorough knowledge of the agreed procedures in your organisation
■ to investigate the problem thoroughly
■ to keep comprehensive and accurate records.

It is also important to consider all reasonable courses of action at each stage in the process and to seek help from a more experienced manager or personnel professional if you are not confident about how to manage the process in a way that is fair to all of those involved.

REFERENCES

The Advisory, Concilation and Arbitration Service, *Discipline at Work: The ACAS Advisory Handbook*, ACAS Reader Ltd.

Casey, D. (1985) 'When is a team not a team?', *Personnel Management*, January, pp. 3–7.

Department of Health (1998) *Modernising Social Services*, The Stationery Office.

Gorman, P. (1998) *Managing Multi-disciplinary Teams in the NHS*, Kogan Page.

McCaughan, N. and Palmer, B. (1994) *Systems Thinking for Harassed Managers*, Karnac Books.

MANAGING CHANGE

Twenty years ago, it may have been sufficient for managers to accept what they found, to keep the organisation moving on its existing tracks, to handle occasional deviations, and eventually, when they moved on, to leave things pretty well as they found them. Today, despite tight resources and ever-increasing demands, the primary task for managers of health and social care, at all levels, is to improve the services they provide to patients and service users. Management is no longer about maintaining the *status quo* (if it ever was); it is about stimulating and implementing change, and encouraging innovation, in order to make improvements.

You may have the task of making a change handed down to you from above, as a result of a decision at a higher level of management. Or you may yourself have identified the need for a change. In either case, taking the lead in bringing about change requires a wide range of management competences. You also need a fair degree of intuition – and some luck. If you can establish an open culture in which you and your colleagues challenge assumptions, test new ideas and share experience, you will be able to learn from your successes – and from the inevitable mistakes. This may be especially important if the change involves working with partners in other organisations, and therefore involves understanding different cultures, structures and patterns of working.

Because management is very much a practical art, the best way of learning from the ideas in this chapter is by experience, in a real situation. Sometimes we suggest that you apply the ideas to a change project of your own, preferably with help from colleagues, especially those who are prepared both to challenge and support you.

ACTIVITY 7.1

Identify an important change that you would like to make at work. You are probably already busy, so don't add unnecessarily to your workload. Choose a project that you need to tackle in any case – one which matters to you, your manager and your service and is in line with your organisation's aims. It could arise from one of your formal objectives.

You will need to strike a balance between selecting a project in which there is a fair chance of success and one which exposes you to new, stretching demands from which you can learn; between playing to your strengths and seeking opportunities for personal development.

Decide on who else you will involve. How will you include the rest of your team? Is there someone that you can use as a sounding board to test out ideas and as an adviser when things go astray? This could be your manager or your mentor. It could be a more experienced colleague or even a friend with appropriate experience from outside your organisation.

1   Describe the issue, problem or opportunity as you currently see it. Use the simplest language possible. If you can express it in a single sentence, so much the better. (You may come to see it differently as the work proceeds and you understand more about it: this often happens.)
2   Write down the objective(s) of your planned change as precisely as you can. How will you measure whether you have been successful?
3   Who will be most affected by the change? When will you involve them?

There is an element of risk in taking the lead in bringing about change. You can never be entirely sure in advance what will be required. Change often brings unexpected results – hence the need to be as clear as possible about your objectives from the outset.

DIAGNOSIS

The first step in making a change is diagnosis – answering the question 'What is the issue that requires a change to be made?' or 'What changes are needed in my organisation/department/section to make it function more effectively?' This may seem self-evident. Yet how often do we see changes being made that are unnecessary? And how often do we realise, after a change has been made, that it has failed to address the real issue?

We begin with a diagnostic model, a way of looking at each of the separate elements of an organisation – or part of an organisation – and how they relate to one another, to help you to understand the current situation and what changes may be needed. We then apply the model to a case study in diagnosis.

Implementing your change project will take time and effort. Another aspect of diagnosis is therefore to consider the resources you will need to carry it out. The last part of this section invites you to think about what you personally bring to the change process.

Don't forget the manager's motto:

Give me strength to change the things that can be changed, the tolerance to accept those that can't and the wisdom to distinguish between them.

A diagnostic model

Driving into work one day, thinking of the tedious job he had been engaged on for the past three days, Roger suddenly saw the obvious solution. In future, he would not spend the best part of a week every February negotiating the holiday dates with the staff for whom he was responsible. He would simply pin up a chart with a set of rules (no more than two people absent at any one time, no one away in May, the peak season and no one to split their holidays into more than two sessions) and let them mark in their own holidays.

Unfortunately the logic of his reasoning was not obvious to his staff. 'He's evading his responsibilities.' 'It's his job to decide who is needed when.' 'He's stirring up conflict between us.' 'What happens if I'm away when the list goes up?' 'It's the only time I ever got to talk to him about my own affairs – he's keeping me away from him.'

The next morning Roger's manager wanted to see him. 'I've had a deputation calling on me from your staff,' said the manager. 'They are furious with what they call your uncaring arrogance. What happened?' Roger told her. The manager smiled. 'You'll have to learn', she said, 'that what seems logical to one person often seems devious to someone else. If you are going to try to change a system, make sure that they understand that there's a problem before you give them your solution.'

The diagnostic model in Figure 7.1 is based on the work of Nadler and Tushman (1977). In this model, the organisation is seen as if it were contained by a semi-permeable membrane. Inside the membrane lies the organisation. Outside the membrane, in the environment, there are other systems, which influence the organisation and are in turn influenced by it: a process of continuous demand and response.

The internal organisation can be thought of as having four components: the tasks, the formal organisational arrangements, the informal culture and the individuals.

Figure 7.1 The Nadler and Tushman diagnostic model
(Source: Hackman, J. (1983) *Perspectives of Behaviour*, McGraw-Hill, with
permission of McGraw-Hill Companies)

- The *tasks* are the primary part of the system. They consist of the jobs
  to be done, the characteristics of the work itself, and the quantity
  and quality of the service provided.

- The *formal organisational arrangements* include lines of accountability, information systems, monitoring and control mechanisms,
  job definitions, formal pay and reward arrangements, meeting
  structures, operating policies, and so on. These features of the
  organisation are relatively easily described, but often become out
  of date as they fail to keep up with the changing world.

- The *informal culture* is less tangible and more difficult to alter,
  but often drives the organisation. It is about 'the way we do things
  around here', the values, the rites and rituals, the power bases,
  allegiances, tribalism, beliefs, norms, informal rewards and punishments, the networks, and so on.

- The *individuals* bring different skills, knowledge and experience,
  different personalities, values, attitudes and behaviour. They
  make choices about what they do and how they do it. Matching
  individuals and their needs to the organisation's formal and
  info rmal arrangements is particularly critical at times of rapid
  change.

The two remaining elements of the model are:

- The *shared vision* – a description of a better future that is owned
  by the organisation and provides a focus for its energy – the engine-
  room for any change project

- *Leadership* – the activities that keep the organisation moving
  purposefully towards that vision, for example, listening, coaching,
  championing, stirring, and so on.

As well as using the model to structure thoughts about each of the
seven separate elements, it is important to consider how well the
elements fit together. For example, if the task is very static, a formal
organisation that is inherently bureaucratic will make sense. On the

other hand, an organisation that has a mix of cultures will work best if managers can adapt their style to suit the different cultures.

The four internal elements of an organisation are in a state of dynamic equilibrium with each other and with their environment. If an organisation is to remain healthy, as one element changes so the others must shift to accommodate.

The way in which the various elements respond to change is often somewhat predictable. For example, the political networks, which are part of the informal culture, respond as they feel their power base shift under them. They will take negative or positive positions depending on how they perceive the change will affect their capacity to make their influence felt.

Those responsible for the formal organisational arrangements will look for more control; bureaucrats become more bureaucratic and call for more of yesterday's information (which, as it was designed for a system which no longer exists, tells them very little). As organisational arrangements as well as tasks and people shift, it becomes increasingly difficult for managers to exercise the necessary degree of control.

Individuals usually fear the unknown. They have established patterns of behaviour for handling and coping with the current arrangements and will be reluctant to develop new ones. For an individual, the change process can be akin to grieving: denial of the change, acceptance of reality and then accommodation to it. Some people pass through these stages in minutes; some never do and suffer increasingly from problems of stress as a result.

When thinking about your change project, Nadler and Tushman's model can be used to help you understand the current situation and how it might respond to your intervention. The model can also be used more proactively, to help you decide on what intervention to make. For example, replacing a conservative, conformist key individual with one who has grown up in, is part of and acceptable to the culture, yet has revolutionary tendencies, can have a powerful effect on the outcome of your project.

A case study in diagnosis

A nurse manager from the Marsh Community NHS Trust wanted to provide an efficient, effective, integrated service for the people in the village of Dunford. She wanted a service which brought together the services of nursing and therapy staff (currently employed by the Trust), the Dunford GPs and the Fenland Local Authority social workers. Her primary concern was about duplication and waste. To help her understand what changes might be needed to the present arrangements, she spent some time talking to some of the people involved. Here are the notes she made of her conversations.

It proved very difficult to make an appointment with any of the three GPs in the village practice. The senior partner found five minutes to explain that co-ordinated primary care was close to his heart. He holds regular monthly meetings with his practice nurse and his health visitor and these enable them to sort out any problem patients. The meetings usually take about half an hour, but they haven't had one for a while: 'We are all rather busy and nobody had anything to put on the agenda.'

I eventually got together with the other two partners over lunch. Most of the time was spent bemoaning the general underfunding of the service, in particular the problems of meeting the ever-increasing demands of an ageing population. The conversation then turned to the proposals for servicing a new home for physically disabled and mentally ill older people which Marsh Health Authority has commissioned, in collaboration with the primary care group and a local housing association. The GPs are worried that this could add significantly to their workload. It was a short step from this to the difficulties of budgeting for older patients and we were soon back into the issues of shortage of cash. They know little about the concept of primary care teams and showed no interest. I also got the impression that they are not keen to be too involved with the primary care group and are very concerned about the enthusiasm of some of their colleagues to establish a primary care trust.

The health visitor who covers the Dunford practice also works in the Marshborough area, which includes a health centre with four GPs as well as one single-handed practice, both in the same primary care group as the Dunford practice. Her office is in the Marshborough health centre. She shares it with a school nurse, two district nurses, a second health visitor and, occasionally, a community physician employed by the Trust, who has a special responsibility for older people. As well as her normal duties, she and the community physician are members of a team which is implementing the transfer of the first patients from the local continuing-care ward to the new nursing home. The four Marshborough GPs, the health visitor, the district nurses and the social worker meet for an hour on the last Friday of the month and, as they work in the same building, there is also a lot of informal contact. However, the health visitor feels that the Marshborough GPs are enthusiasts for team working only if 'they are in charge'. She is supportive of the idea of establishing primary care teams and is interested in what she described as 'better interagency working'. She has reservations about new work with the Dunford practice because:

- she is already overloaded
- she doesn't rate the chance of success very highly until the senior partner retires – in her view he is one of the old school who just wants the nurses to be at his beck and call
- along with the other health visitors, she has just been involved in devising a health visitor database – this is producing a lot of paperwork and she can ill afford to spend any more time at meetings.

The social worker made time for a meeting with me, although he expressed some concern that it would probably be more appropriate for me to talk to his area manager. He is normally responsible for the industrial areas of Bindhaven and the market town of Marshborough. In addition, he is currently covering Dunford because his department is understaffed. He knows Dunford well, having worked here before the last reorganisation. He talked about the benefits of integrating the efforts of the three services – health, housing and social services. He would prefer to wait until a full-time worker has been recruited and trained, but this could take a year and he agrees that this is unacceptable, given the national pressure to develop a local charter for people in long-term care. He declined to comment on the people involved in delivering health care in Dunford: he said he doesn't really know any of them well enough to make a sensible judgement. He suggested that I should talk to his area manager, who is apparently one of the lead managers working on the charter for long-term care.

I have yet to meet the district nurse. I know that she is committed to team work, and will also be a mine of information.

We can develop a preliminary diagnosis of the Dunford situation using the Nadler and Tushman model.

First, the *environment*. Restructuring and funding loom large in the minds of the Dunford GPs. What is really worrying them? Can the new arrangements be used in any way to further the cause? What about the shift in emphasis to interagency working and the charter for long-term care? Is the new home an opportunity to progress teamwork? The Marshborough GPs seem to be further down the road towards interprofessional collaboration. Are there any ways in which their experience can be translated for Dunford? What links are there between the practices? How effective is the board of the local primary care group? To whom, if anyone, do the Dunford GPs listen?

The housing association could be an important new player. What is its philosophy? Why is it working with the health authority and the primary care group? Are there some allies within its ranks?

The customers – service users and their carers – have not been mentioned once. What do they think about the current services? What worries them most? Have they been consulted about their needs and how they would like them to be met?

Next, the *tasks*. No one has spoken about the outcomes – benefits or otherwise – for service users. Facts are conspicuous by their absence. Are there any data about the social, health and physical needs of Dunford residents, or about the quality, quantity and cost of the services provided, or about the effective use of resources? What are the pressing problems? What might be achieved for the customers if the various professionals were to work more as a team – if there was real inter-agency collaboration? What is there that is currently good and might be put at risk? What do they need to be better at, and what should they stop doing, in order to improve the services they provide?

How big an issue is the new home? Could it be the vehicle for practising a greater degree of teamwork or some interagency working? What is involved in the charter for long-term care?

ACTIVITY 7.2

Now continue the diagnosis under the remaining five headings:

- formal organisational arrangements
- informal culture
- individuals
- shared vision
- leadership.

One way of doing this is to go through the above report, identifying individual issues and writing each on a card. You can then sort the cards into piles which relate to each element of the model in Figure 7.1. Look not only for what is said but also for what may be implied. What is omitted can be very revealing.

How do your conclusions compare with the following?

Formal organisational arrangements

The three services – housing, social services and health – have separate management arrangements and, at the operational level, the staff cover different geographical areas. Housing embraces both the local authority and the independent sector. Health includes the health authority, the primary care group, the general practices and the trusts.

Are there any systems in place which bring the three services together? Bearing in mind the power of information, do the three services share any monitoring and control processes? How much work has been done locally on the performance assessment frameworks for both social services and the health service? To what extent, if at all, do these link together?

Informal culture

Is there one culture, or is there the problem of several separate ones? The GPs seem isolated, and other aspects of the health services seem bureaucratic. Do the social workers have their own culture?

Everyone sounds inordinately busy. Why is that? Is there just too much work? Do they need to be better organised? Are they busy because they need to be in order to prove something to themselves or to their colleagues? Or are they busy because of the amount of change as a result of the aspirations of national Government? Is the busyness a result of reacting against the changes or of working to implement them?

Some of the cultures appear highly 'tribal'. The health visitors have just set up a new database. Did they do this entirely within their profession or did they link in with the monitoring requirements of the performance assessment frameworks? The older GP preaches a team approach but it doesn't sound as if he practises it. The social worker has worked in the district for a long time but says he doesn't know the other professionals well. Is this really so, or is it part of his stance on confidentiality?

Individuals

Most people seem to be making their own assumptions about the needs of older people, which could well be challenged in any attempt to bring about change. Does the nurse manager herself really understand the pressure from Government for all agencies to work together in the interests of the customers of their services? Do the doctors see themselves as the rightful team leaders? There is a flavour of an historical resentment of this by the health visitor. Does she dislike being seen as the doctor's handmaiden – in the GP's words, being 'his' health visitor? The senior partner thinks in terms of sorting out 'problem patients' rather than in terms of quality or 'best value'.

Are any of the group experienced team/interagency workers? Do they possess the appropriate competences to work collaboratively?

Why is the social worker so cautious? Is it connected in some way with a previous reorganisation?

Shared vision

There is no evidence of a shared vision. Why is change wanted or needed? The nurse manager's reasons seem primarily about eliminating waste. Is there factual evidence of what is being wasted? Are primary care teams the answer because locally they are still the flavour of the month, or is there an underlying purpose, as yet unstated, which the potential team might share? Should there be a greater focus on shared outcomes focused on the needs of service users and their carers?

Leadership

Is there anyone who can perform the change leadership role? Is it the problem owner, the nurse manager? The community physician is well placed organisationally, but does he have sufficient respect from his colleagues?

Summary

One word, fragmentation, summarises much of the problem. The key task would seem to be integration based on some mutually agreed outcomes.

We will return to this case study to follow the next steps taken by the nurse manager.

Another way of representing the relationships identified by the diagnosis is in the form of Tony Buzan's (1989) 'mind maps'. Figure 7.2 shows the Dunford diagnosis represented in this way.

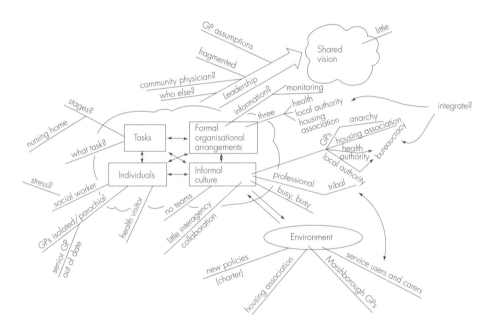

Figure 7.2 Another representation of the Dunford diagnosis

ACTIVITY 7.3

Use the Nadler and Tushman model on your own project:

- to improve your understanding of what you already know about the situation
- to identify what you need to know more about
- to plan how you will collect the additional information you need
- to identify those areas where the components of the model do not fit with each other and to consider what needs to be done to bring about change.

You may wish to carry out this Activity by making notes under the seven headings of the model (environment, tasks, formal organisational arrangements, informal culture, individuals, shared vision and leadership) or you may prefer to annotate Figure 7.1 as a 'mind map', as in Figure 7.2.

You may feel the need to extend this Activity by collecting more information to add to your knowledge of the situation. How you set about this is up to you, but bear in mind that the way in which you tackle it will almost certainly be obvious to those involved. You will send out messages: make sure they are the ones you want to send. Diagnosis is your first intervention in the system. First moves are often remembered.

There is a fairly limited number of ways of collecting diagnostic data: perusal of documents and records, the use of surveys or questionnaires, carrying out interviews, making direct observations and holding diagnostic meetings. All have their advantages and disadvantages.

What you bring to the change process

You stand a better chance of managing change effectively if you understand your own attitude towards change. You will not be able to manage other people through a change if you are unable to handle the emotional and intellectual impact it has on you. Here are some things to think about.

- Keeping in touch with developments in your environment ensures that you and your department or area of work maintain the capacity to make changes when necessary.
- In an era of rapid change, people have to learn new skills in order to cope with changing roles in changing circumstances. How active a learner are you?
- How does change affect you emotionally? How does it feel to be involved in change? Change inevitably produces emotional reactions in those involved. It is therefore important to understand how it affects you, in order to understand better how to help others.

ACTIVITY 7.4

How do you rate your capability to manage your change project? Here are some of the advantages and disadvantages that you might have. Which of them broadly applies to you?

Possible advantages   Yes   No

You understand your organisation (who has power,
how the networks operate, where the barriers are)   ☐   ☐
You speak your organisation's language (its special
jargon, in-jokes, etc.)   ☐   ☐
You understand the local culture and can act in
accordance with its rules   ☐   ☐
Your mental and/or material well-being depends on your
organisation providing effective services   ☐   ☐
You are a familiar and non-threatening figure to
colleagues   ☐   ☐

Possible disadvantages

You are too involved with one part of the organisation
to see it as a whole or without bias   ☐   ☐
Your other duties leave you insufficient time and energy
to devote to the change role   ☐   ☐
Your power base is not secure enough to guard you
against challenges from your managers or others   ☐   ☐
Your past successes or failures may prejudice people
against you   ☐   ☐
Other people's expectations of you in your other roles
conflict with your efforts to work with them on the
change   ☐   ☐

What implications does this analysis have for your role in your project?

Being aware of the factors that may work to your advantage and those that may work to your disadvantage is an important first step. This will enable you to recognise what kind of support you are going to need and whether you have any urgent development needs.

An organic view of the change process

Every change programme involves three states – the current state, the transition state and the desirable future state. All three require managing, and all three compete for resources. It is important is to ensure that you have enough resources to cope with the work of managing all three states, or that you have access to someone who can provide them. However, things are not always that simple.

A more organic – less linear – model of the change process is shown in Figure 7.3. It suggests that the origins of change can often be traced either to experiments, or to 'ice-breaking', or to both.

The innovative organisation builds in change as a norm, by encouraging individuals to experiment, to have a go; within reason, it allows a little anarchy. Budgets are not so tightly constrained that the organisation is in a straitjacket. Successful innovations are publicly rewarded, mistakes privately forgotten.

Ice-breaking may occur when an event, often external, and often unplanned, unfreezes the situation: for example, a White Paper is published, there is a change of Government, or an institutional horror story breaks.

Out of a number of separate, experimental activities – and possibly one or more ice-breaking events – comes successes, whether small or large. If these can be drawn together and shared, it may be possible to bring together a coherent strategy for change. This strategy can then be transformed into action, providing opportunities to do things in ways which are congruent with the emerging future rather than the past. From action comes learning, which in turn informs the development of strategy and thus further action. There are things to be

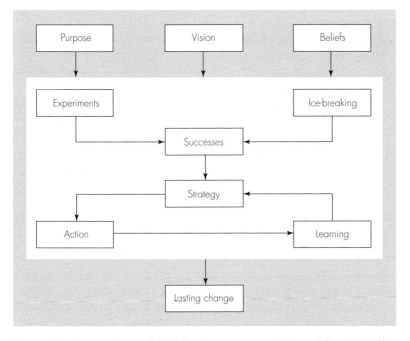

Figure 7.3 An organic model of the change process (adapted from Turrill, 1986)

avoided: fragmentation, duplication of effort, too slow a pace, a pace that is unsustainable, fear and rejection of change, and too prescriptive an approach. The things you need to ensure are:

- engagement and commitment from key groups
- a clear plan with time deadlines for delivery
- a programme with clear 'milestones' for review
- managers and staff feeling that transition is being 'managed'
- a pace which is sustainable
- recognition of success to build confidence
- a clear communications strategy to ensure that internal messages override those which come from outside
- a cost-effective use of time and resources.

An example of significant change drawing on small experiments and successes occurred in the physiotherapy outpatient department of a general hospital.

One of the physiotherapists found that, in addition to giving instructions verbally, it was helpful to write down instructions for those patients who required a cervical collar. A second physiotherapist had begun to collect a small library of booklets for patients to borrow, such as those produced by the Arthritis and Rheumatism Council. Meanwhile, the receptionist had taken another initiative. A friend had given her a poster for a local support group for arthritis sufferers, which she pinned on the wall in the waiting area.

The senior physiotherapist in charge of outpatients encouraged these staff to share their ideas with each other and with the rest of the staff. A strategy began to be developed to improve the provision of information to patients. Action and learning led to the production of a series of instruction sheets describing exercise regimes. These sheets included titles of relevant booklets which patients could borrow from the departmental library and contact addresses for relevant support groups.

There is much discussion among the staff of ways of improving this information.

The organic approach to change involves the affected people at all times. It builds on a number of small successes, rather than presenting major hurdles which have to be jumped and which induce resistance. The complexity and freedom of the process, however, require overall direction to ensure that the sum of all this jumble of activity is purposeful. An organisation which operates successfully in this way invariably has three binding forces:

- clarity about its overall purpose
- a widely shared vision of a better future
- a set of beliefs, values and principles which governs the way it operates.

One final thought: it is possible to make mountains out of molehills, to create hurdles when none really exist. The simplest way of bringing about change is just to do it. You may be surprised. Occasionally people will say, 'About time too!' and get on with it. Intuition is a much underrated commodity when judging whether this is possible. But intuition backed by rationality is safer, if less exciting, than intuition alone.

PLANNING FOR CHANGE

Each of the two tools we describe in this section has two functions:

- to better understand the present situation
- to plan the next steps you will need to take.

The first tool, *force field analysis*, identifies the forces that are helping to drive your change and those that are opposing it. Having identified the forces, you can then decide which positive forces you can take advantage of and which negative ones you can try to reduce. It is a useful tool to apply to any change project, whether the proposed change is major or minor.

Few change programmes can be successfully implemented by one person. One person rarely understands an organisation well enough to produce an accurate analysis, and is unlikely to have access to all the levers of power. A mix of skills, experiences, personalities and perceptions is usually required to manage a change. Nor is it possible to institutionalise a change – and it is very easy to overturn it – when the ownership is vested in only one person. Successful management of change recognises this by building a network of supporters. These are sometimes referred to as a 'critical mass', borrowing a term from nuclear physics to indicate that their combined energy can be explosive. The second tool described, *commitment planning*, will help you assess the work to be done in building this critical mass of supporters.

Force field analysis

Force field analysis is a tool developed by Kurt Lewin (1947). It is extraordinary how its relevance has stood the test of time. It assumes that in any change situation there are two sets of forces, those driving the change and those which oppose or restrain it. These forces can be

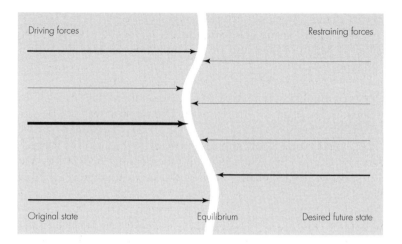

Figure 7.4 Driving and restraining forces

written on a chart using arrows to indicate their directions and relative strengths (Figure 7.4). It is important to recognise that they are forces as perceived by the people involved in the change. For example, there may be no intention to make staff redundant, but if the staff believe that the change will make them redundant, the restraining force exists.

If the driving forces for change are stronger than the restraining forces, progress will be made. The list of forces can be developed by brainstorming or by the use of diagnostic tools like the Nadler and Tushman model. It can sometimes be useful to cluster them under different headings and to use these headings to prompt ideas. Typical clusters would include:

- *personal* (for example, fear of redundancy, loss of competence or loss of pride)
- *interpersonal* (for example, A does not talk to B)
- *intergroup* (for example, home care assistants resent loss of status *vis-à-vis* home care organisers, or surgeons and physicians compete for money to buy new equipment)
- *organisational* (for example, there is an overall shortage of resources or new management structures are being introduced)
- *technological* (for example, records have been computerised or a body scanner has been installed)
- *environmental* (for example, there are more older people or the law on mental health is amended).

Having produced the force field diagram, the first task is to examine it to determine what can be done to reduce the restraining forces rather than increase the driving ones. This seems to be against our natural instincts of pushing change through. However, experience shows that increasing the driving forces produces a quasi-Newtonian effect: for every new force that is introduced, an equal and opposite force tends to arise. If the magnitude of a driving force is increased, the restraining forces often also increase. Some of the restraining forces may even owe their existence to previous attempts to push through change and, paradoxically, the elimination of the appropriate driving force will be helpful overall. You may, however, judge that it is important to maintain some particular driving force and perhaps, with care, increase others.

Completion of the force field analysis may lead to an onset of realism. Once you have a clear view of the forces in play you may decide that your planned change is impossible. Resources are finite. Now may be the time to question whether your resources would be better deployed where there is more chance of a return on their investment.

We left the Dunford case study at the point where the nurse manager was about to complete the diagnosis. In the final interviews she discovered the following additional information.

The nursing home is a 100-place unit that will be run by the housing association, which will employ some trained nursing staff as managers and nurses. The housing association's managers are entrepreneurs, severely antipathetic to the merest whiff of bureaucracy.

It is expected that most of the residents will be quite severely disabled and all will require continuing care and support from a range of services. The medical care will no longer be the responsibility of the hospital consultants. The residents will as far as possible be treated as normal members of the community and routine medical care will therefore fall largely on the home's nurses, the therapists employed by the community trust and the Dunford GPs. There may be a role for other community nurses employed by the Trust. The community physician carries considerable weight with the health authority, the board of the primary care group and the staff of the housing association, because of his excellent work in establishing the home.

The district nurse is a mine of information. She says that the social worker is somewhat embittered, having unsuccessfully applied for the deputy director's post at the time of the last reorganisation. The new deputy director has offered him early retirement but, as his wife has recently died, he wishes to keep working to avoid loneliness. He says he is interested in interagency working, but in reality he has little energy or motivation for reform.

His line manager, the team leader for the geographical area which includes Dunford, is new to the local authority. She has come from another county where a local charter for long-term care has been in place for some time. She is an enthusiast for interagency working.

The Dunford GPs have little contact with their colleagues in Marshborough and even less respect for them. The local medical committee is low key and is now being increasingly overshadowed by the primary care group. The

Dunford GPs rarely attend medical committee meetings and are critical of the primary care group. The primary care group's new management team includes an ex-health authority administrator with an enthusiasm for the concept of integrated primary care.

Both the chair and the secretary of the community health council are keen on the implications of the charter to involve service users and carers.

The nurse manager drew up the force field analysis in Figure 7.5.

ACTIVITY 7.5

In the Dunford force field, which restraining forces might usefully be worked on? How might the nurse manager set about reducing them?

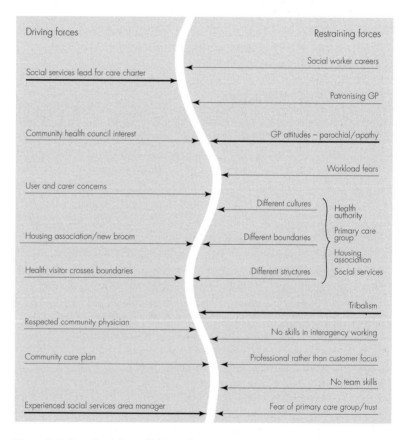

Figure 7.5 Dunford force field analysis

There are many possible answers to this Activity. However, you can test your conclusions against the following points.

- The nurse manager's original idea seems to be along the right lines but may have been for the wrong reasons. Her proposals were not supported by facts.
- She could usefully pay more attention to the wider national and local political context.
- She could reflect on the components that would be uniting rather than fragmenting.
- She could redefine and simplify the task.
- She could reflect on how the project might help to reduce existing fears and worries.

The principles behind reducing the effects of restraining forces are:

- looking for common ground (for example, common values and common desired outcomes)
- ascertaining who has influence and respect
- seeking to show how achievement of the change will add value elsewhere or help overcome an anxiety or fear.

Commitment planning

The aim of commitment planning is to examine how you can build a critical mass of supporters, ready to explode into action. A commitment plan is a chart (Table 7.1) in which the key people or groups are listed down one side of a sheet of paper. Across the top are four headings which indicate levels of commitment:

Not committed	Likely to oppose the change
Let	Will not oppose the initiative but will not actively support it
Help	Will support the change with time and other resources, provided someone else will take the lead
Make	Will lead the change process and make it happen.

Each individual is marked on the chart with an 'O' to indicate his or her current position and an 'X' to indicate the extent of commitment needed. The difference between the two is a crude measure of the work to be done in order to build the critical mass. Sometimes it may be appropriate for the level of commitment to be reduced: perhaps the leadership should move from one person to another, or perhaps one person's enthusiasm is preventing others from joining in.

Table 7.1 A commitment plan for Dunford

Key players	Not committed (oppose)	Let	Help	Make
Community trust chief executive		o →	x	
GP senior partner		x ←		o
Junior GP 1	o ———————			→ x
Junior GP 2	o ———————		→ x	
Community physician		o ———	→ x	
Social worker	o ———————		→ x	
Social services area manager				ox
Chair of community health council		ox		
Board of primary care group	o ———————		→ x	
Health visitor		o →	x	
District nurse			ox	
Therapies manager			o →	x
Housing association managers		o ———————		→ x
Nurse manager				ox

As an illustration, if we return to Dunford, the key players could well be:

- the chief executive of the community trust
- the GPs
- the community physician
- the social worker
- the social services area manager
- the chair of the community health council
- the board of the primary care group
- the health visitor
- the district nurse
- the therapies manager
- managers from the housing association (including the manager of the nursing home)
- the nurse manager herself.

> The nurse manager realises that her project needs redefinition in the light of what she has found out about the work being done in Fenland on a local charter for long-term care. She also realises that the work that needs to be done on the charter is potentially enormous and that some realistic boundaries have to be set if she is to achieve any change. Following a useful meeting with the social services team leader, a joint action plan is agreed.

The nurse manager aims to redefine the project and to link it into the national and local agendas associated with both the charter for long-term care and the new home. She is going to present it as a pilot project to the supportive key players – the community physician, the therapies manager, the social services area manager and the manager of the new home – with a proposal that they form the core of the project management team. They are to be asked what needs to be done to gain the active support from their chief executives and an action plan can then be drawn up.

In consultation with the community physician, the nurse manager decides to seek to involve one of the younger GPs. She recognises that motivating any of them to become seriously involved is likely to be a major problem because the senior partner's somewhat patronising attitude is hindering the process of change. If he can be persuaded to leave this work to one of the junior partners, there will be more chance of getting the support of the rest of the practice staff. Hence he moves from 'make' to 'let' on the commitment chart.

For the majority of the participants, a substantial amount of work will have to be done to increase their commitment to the project if it is to stand any chance of success. This has more to do with the scale of culture change implied by the charter for long-term care than with any fundamental opposition to the principles and values underpinning the national initiative.

The next stage will be to plan the involvement of service users and carers. The aim of the pilot project will be to demonstrate joint working based on clear outcomes. These will reflect local circumstances and the pilot will enable learning to be transferred to a wider base of service provision.

Once you have identified whose commitment is needed, there are a number of ways of gaining it. Here are some suggestions:

- *Use power*   Reward desirable behaviour; ignore or punish inappropriate actions.
- *Treat hurting systems*   Find out what aspects of the current state are hurting the person whose commitment you need, then treat his or her problems. A variation on this is to help people solve problems themselves.
- *Expose the issues*   Find out more about the problems in ways which do not threaten people or force them to adopt stances. For example, hold a private unstructured meeting to talk about a problem, with no minutes taken and with no outcomes other than a better understanding of the issues.
- *Educate and develop*   Use the neutrality of a learning situation to encourage open cross-boundary debates.
- *Role model*   Practise what you preach. As the leader, behave in ways that are in keeping with the desired change.

- *Use peer pressure* Use the influence of respected colleagues. This can be particularly helpful in professional cultures.
- *Encourage sharing* Expose people to others' successes in ways which enable them to copy useful ideas.
- *Encourage discussion* Demonstrate that there are different views of the situation and the potential opportunities and that people involved see the change in different ways.
- *Horse trade* 'Do this for me, and I will do that for you.'

A number of methods can be used to understand the issues and identify the work to be done in bringing about change. Two important ideas have been demonstrated:

- There is a balance of forces in a change situation and reducing constraints is frequently more effective than increasing pressure.
- Change requires a critical mass of supporters and it is important to build this commitment.

You should now be able to use the diagnostic model and the tools of force field analysis and commitment planning to help you to manage change in your own area of work.

REFERENCES

Buzan, T. (1989) *Use Your Head* (rev. edn), BBC Books.

Lewin, K. (1947) 'Frontiers in group dynamics: Concept, method and reality in social science; social equilibria and social change', *Human Relations*, 1: 5–41.

Nadler, D. and Tushman, M. L. (1977) *Perspectives of Behavior*, McGraw-Hill.

Turrill, T. (1986) *Change and Innovation: A Challenge for the NHS*, Institute of Health Services Management.

WHAT DO YOUR CUSTOMERS AND SERVICE USERS WANT?

Almost everyone who works in health and social care is, at one level or another, aware that their function is to deliver – or to support the delivery of – services to patients or service users. However, there are a number of other types of customer in health and social care services. For example, if you work in a home care service in the voluntary or private sector, the local social services or social work department is, in a rather different sense, also your customer. If you work in an out-patient physiotherapy department, local general practitioners (GPs) are also your customers. If you work in a payroll department, all the staff whose pay-slips you prepare are your customers. As a manager, you might also view the staff in your team as your customers.

So, given the size and complexity of many of the organisations that provide health and social care, among the critical issues for you as a manager are:

- identifying who your customers are
- understanding what it is that they require
- knowing how effectively you are meeting their requirements.

The aim of this chapter is to help you improve the responsiveness of your services to the needs, wants and expectations of your customers.

The terms used to describe people who are the recipients of health and social care services have been and continue to be the basis of much discussion – and changing fashions. 'Patient' is still commonly used in the health service, 'client' was until recently the favourite word in social care and 'service user' is regarded by many as a more neutral term in both. Another important term in common use is 'carer', meaning someone who provides a significant level of support to a person in need of health or social care (often a relative or partner, though not necessarily living with the person being cared for). Carers may also require services, and many have needs and views that differ from those of other service users.

For the moment, however, we are going to use the term 'customer' to describe all those who receive services from health and social care organisations – including service users and carers, and also including those who commission services on their behalf and those within organisations who receive, for example, financial, training and information management services. We are using the term 'customer' to emphasise a particular kind of relationship between those who provide a service and those who use it. Instead of seeing users as patients or clients – people whose requirements are assessed by the provider and who are then offered a service that the provider defines and controls – we need to see them as people who have an understanding of their requirements and who can make choices about the nature of the service most capable of meeting these requirements.

DIFFERENT KINDS OF CUSTOMER

We are all customers: every day we buy and receive services from many different providers – banks, shops, transport operators, and so on. The success of each of these providers depends on them delivering what we, as customers, want, such as a reliable, convenient and friendly service and value for money. Satisfying customer requirements is a key element of providing a quality service.

As customers we are often not particularly concerned with *how* our requirements are met. The fact that buying a can of beans involves a complex network of suppliers is of little interest to us. However, managing that network is a critically important task for providers. They need to ensure that all the goods and services that allow them to provide what their customers require are available to the correct level of quality, where and when they are required.

The plethora of agencies involved with commissioning and providing health and social care creates a complex web of customer–supplier relationships. Even within a single organisation like a hospital, there is a network of providers and customers. The pharmacy provides the barium meal for the radiologist-customer who provides the X-ray for the surgeon-customer who needs to perform a bowel operation on the patient-customer because the gastroenterologist-customer's diagnosis, requested by the local referring GP-customer, has proved correct. The subsequent successful operation is of great interest to the health authority-customer which has invested extra cash to help deal with waiting lists.

A helpful way of simplifying the complexity is to stick to the fundamental point: service users are the ultimate customers. They are at the centre of defining and delivering health and social care services. They are the reason that the services exist: the complex interlocking network of health and social care services is constructed to meet their needs. As a manager within a large organisation, however, it is easy to lose sight of what the job is really about and how you can ensure that the efforts of your department or service are contributing effectively.

How easy it is to keep in touch with these things probably depends on your function and that of your team.

If you are part of a team that has direct contact with service users, it will be clear that they are your customers. If, however, you are providing a service that supports those who have direct contact with service users, you and your staff may rarely come into contact with them. Your role might be ensuring the delivery of catering services, the maintenance of essential equipment or the payment of bills. In these circumstances, knowing how much you contribute to meeting the needs of service users is more difficult to assess because of your remoteness from them.

Whatever your job within health or social care, your most important customer is always the service user, though there will always be other departments or agencies inside or outside your organisation who are also your customers. If your situation is one without a high level of contact with service users, you are more likely to think of your customers as those you serve directly, before the service user can receive the appropriate treatment or care. You may offer services directly to other departments within your organisation, for example, clinical departments or social work teams or other support departments. These are your *internal customers*.

ACTIVITY 8.1

Describe in a few words two services that you and your team provide and note the customer(s) for each. Keep your list – you will need it later.

A hospital provides services for the health authority on behalf of the patients in the district, referred to the hospital by local GPs. Who is the hospital's customer – the health authority, the patient or the GP? A community meals service provides services for a local authority's social services department on behalf of older and disabled people living at home who have been referred to the service by social workers and others. Who is this service's customer – the social services department, the person who receives the meals or the social worker? The answer in both cases is all three, but each one will have a different interest in the services being provided. Your customers may be various and, to meet the variety of their requirements, you have to be clear about what exactly each is seeking. What is needed is a way of thinking about the array of customers of (and in) health and social care. Let's look at two ways of approaching this – through the notions of *customer roles* and *customer chains*.

Customer roles

To introduce the concept of customer roles, have a look at the following account of a service and try to identify the customers.

A 'clubhouse' for Bromley

After observing the success in the United States of 'clubhouses' (a new model of day care for people with long-term mental health problems), Bromley Health Authority, in conjunction with the local authority and voluntary groups, decided to include a clubhouse as part of the mental health services that the regional office of the NHS Executive requires it to provide. The clubhouse concept is that people attending are club members rather than patients or clients – with lifelong membership of the clubhouse. Members and staff work together to run all aspects of the clubhouse, such as meals and administration. Transitional employment is offered, giving members the opportunity to use their newly acquired or recovered skills with security, resulting in a gain of personal confidence. This sometimes enables members to go on to obtain employment on the open market. The day is structured carefully into work time and leisure time, which offers members both self-esteem and the opportunity to socialise with family and friends.

In the clubhouse project, the ultimate customers are the members who benefit from the service. So the first major customer role is that of *beneficiary*. However, there are a number of other 'customers' without whom the clubhouse would not exist. The regional office of the NHS Executive requires the health authority to make provision for the care of the long-term mentally ill, and in response Bromley Health Authority specifies the clubhouse project as part of its strategy. It is assisted in its role of *specifier* by the local authority and by voluntary groups. The costs of running the clubhouse fall to the health authority and thence to the NHS Executive, who thus fulfil the role of *payer*. Day to day, however, the running of the clubhouse is carried out by its staff, including volunteers, and also by the members themselves. The members, then, as well as beneficiaries, play another customer role, that of *participants*. Figure 8.1 is a diagram of the players and their roles in the Bromley clubhouse example.

To explore these roles further, you can try applying them to your own situation in the following Activity.

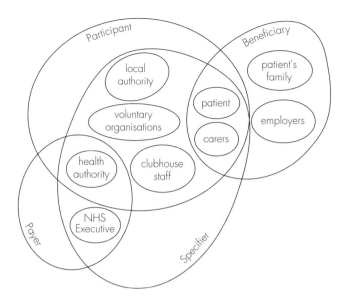

Figure 8.1 Players and their roles in the Bromley clubhouse project

ACTIVITY 8.2

For one of the services you identified in your own area of work, either write down or illustrate with a diagram like Figure 8.1:

- who benefits from the service
- who specifies what is required
- who pays for that service
- who participates in the delivery of the service.

Although the four customer roles of beneficiary, specifier, payer and participant are distinct, you may have found that:

- One of the roles is played by more than one customer (for Bromley, there were several specifiers)
- One customer plays more than one role (Bromley Health Authority played both specifier and payer and even, arguably, beneficiary)
- One of the roles is not played at all (this is not the case in the Bromley example, but some voluntary services do not have a formal payer)
- Some roles are played by customers outside the system (in Bromley, members' families and employers have benefited from the clubhouse project, and some services – such as cervical screening – may be specified by national initiatives quite remote from local circumstances).

Despite these complications, identifying the four separate customer roles can be helpful. It may begin to suggest to you what influences or controls the delivery of the services for which you are responsible, and where you might want to intervene to make improvements.

However, if you have different people or agencies taking different customer roles, there are three reasons why you may have quite a challenging job on your hands:

■ Where there are several different customers, the volume of work in keeping them all happy may be a test of your time-management and organisational skills.
■ Tensions may arise from serving several customers with different roles at the same time. Many managers will appreciate what it is like 'changing gear' between service users, their representatives (such as a community health council or voluntary organisations) and the commissioners of the service, not to mention their own line management.
■ There may be potential for conflict in the different interests of the players of a single customer role. Conflicts are most likely around the specifier role: for example, clinical staff might want the most up-to-date treatment services which require expensive equipment, the health authority might want the most economic services, and patient representatives might want the services that give patients the most say in their own treatment. But other customer roles are also not without the potential for conflict: for example, the payer role for home care services is usually shared between a local authority social services department and service users, and the scale of the charges may be unacceptable to some service users.

In situations of potential conflict, your communication and negotiating skills will be tested: there are often no easy solutions to clashes of priorities between customers. Making judgements about the relative significance of conflicting requirements is part of your job as a manager and requires you to be:

■ clear in your objectives
■ consistent in setting priorities
■ forthright in communication
■ imaginative and flexible in planning.

Keeping the four customer roles in your mind as a framework should help you to define the relationship between your services and their various customers, and to set priorities between their requirements and your services.

In the case of a community meals service, for example, all the specifiers need some involvement in deciding what the purpose of the service is. Is it to do the following:

- enable people to continue to live at home?
- improve their quality of life?
- provide regular contact with the person delivering the food?
- keep the price of meals down to a level that is easily afforded by an older person on a state pension?
- facilitate the discharge of older people from hospital?
- avoid the costs of more expensive residential care?
- allow carers who normally provide hot meals to take a break?

The priority given to each of these purposes will determine what service is provided, how it is provided, and by whom. Arriving at a 'best fit' will involve resolving conflicts between the priorities of the different customers. For instance, improvements in food technology present a stark choice between delivering frozen meals in bulk or offering the regular daily contact of a person who delivers a hot meal.

Customer chains

We have highlighted some of the management complexities that derive from the variety of your customers and the various roles they play in the delivery of your services.

However, your services form only part of the complex network of health and social care. For the benefit of service users, the ultimate customers, all these services have to work in concert.

The key to coming to grips with sorting out relationships with customers is the notion of chains. A simple example is the manufacture of taxis. The taxi cab is a culmination of a series of activities that all contribute in one way or another to the car we finally ride in.

The taxi

The person who grinds the valves on the engine can feel that he or she is making an essential contribution to the finished product. The car will not work without properly ground valves. The immediate beneficiary of the valve grinder's job is the engine assembler. The valve grinder's customer is the engine assembly company.

The engine assembly company sells the completed engines to the motor manufacturer which may be a separate company or a distinct part of the same organisation. The manufacturer benefits from receiving assembled engines. The motor manufacturer is therefore the engine assembly company's customer.

The motor manufacturer sells complete taxis to its customers – the distributors. The distributors sell the taxis to their customers – the purchasers of the taxis. The purchaser of the taxi is the customer of the final product, but is not be the final beneficiary. Ultimately the taxi passengers will be the customers who benefit and will pay to finance the whole chain of activities involved in producing the taxi.

In this example there is a clear chain of benefit passed from one customer to the next along the chain. Hence, the ultimate customers – the passengers – are the customers of the valve grinder, even though the valve grinder never encounters them and is part of a totally separate organisation. There is also a clear chain of payment which gets passed up the chain (Figure 8.2).

The chain of benefit

Just as the taxi passenger receives the benefit that results from a chain of activities culminating in a taxi journey, so does the service user in the delivery of health or social care. The example we used at the beginning of this chapter illustrated how a chain of service providers lies behind a patient's bowel operation. The pharmacy contributes the barium meal, the radiographer provides the X-ray picture, the surgeon performs the operation. There are other chains too: the works department maintains the physical condition of the ward, which is managed day to day by the ward sister, whose style is reflected in the standard of care delivered by the nurses. After the operation, the patient will be unable to eat normally and will need feeding intravenously. The recipe for the parenteral nutrition will be made up by the pharmacist with the advice of the surgeon and nursing staff, and will depend on the patient's metabolism and needs, information on which will come from the pathology laboratory.

So chains of service, from the point of view of service users, are not single lines, but more like a tree or river system. Although the complete network of customer chains may be complex, each strand is a simple

Figure 8.2 Customer chains

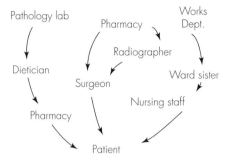

Figure 8.3 A chain of benefit

linear sequence: the benefits flow along each strand towards the service user. The benefit chain for our example is shown in Figure 8.3.

ACTIVITY 8.3

Map the chain of customers who benefit from one of your services.

Wherever you started your chain, you should have the service user as one of the beneficiaries near the end of your chain. If you work directly with service users, your chain may be quite short. Most managers, however, will have several links in the chain.

The specification chain

Returning to the taxi manufacturing example, taxi purchasers will decide which colour and model they want to buy. This will put demands on the distributor, which will have to specify what it wants from the manufacturer. These specifications will then be translated into require-ments for components from their suppliers, so the engine assembly company will receive a specification for engines that will include a requirement for valves to be ground by the valve grinder. There is thus a chain of customers playing the specifying role which percolates through each element of the chain right back to the valve grinder. In taxi manufacturing, specification follows the benefit chain in the reverse direction. In health and social care, however, the chain of specifying customers is often somewhat different from the chain of benefiting customers.

ACTIVITY 8.4

Map the chain that results in the specification of services that you or your department provide.

Your chain of specifying customers is unlikely to follow your chain of benefiting customers. It will probably have additional links for third parties making specifications on behalf of their customers. If you work in the health service, you are likely to have a GP in the chain, acting as an agent for the patient, and the health authority may have something to say about the quantity and quality of service. There may also be professional bodies offering advice on specifications – the British Thoracic Society, for example, provides guidelines on the management of asthma. If you work in children's services, the local authority's social services committee will be part of the chain of specification, as may be voluntary organisations that take an advocacy role in relation to children at risk. National government will also have a part to play, for example through the requirements laid down in the 1989 Children Act, the Quality Protects programme in England, and the Children's Services Strategic Framework in Scotland. This plethora of specifiers may occasionally gives rise to conflict if there are different priorities and interests.

By drawing these diagrams you will see that your department is at one end of the customer chains and the service user is at the other end. Broadly, these chains transmit the benefits in one direction and the specifications for what is required in the other. The payment for the services provided may arrive through another, quite different, chain of customer links.

Although we have examined the chains for each of the customer roles separately, some would suggest that, when the different roles are combined, the chains meet at the ends to form a closed loop. Those who ultimately benefit from the services (the service users) also ultimately pay for them as taxpayers. This apparent closure, however, is a simplification, as many service users are not taxpayers and many taxpayers are not service users. By separating out the different roles that customers play, the relationships between your services and each of the players can be made clearer.

The complete chain is not likely to end with you or your department. It almost certainly extends backwards to other people, departments or agencies, either internal or external to your organisation. Your department is their customer because you either specify, participate in, pay for or benefit from the goods and services that they provide for you. Hence you are a customer as well.

We are building up a picture of chains of service in which you are receiving services from your suppliers so that you can provide effective services to your customers. Like all chains, the ability of the customer chain to do its job is only as strong as its weakest link. The effectiveness of the relationships between the linked customers provides the chain's strength and improves its chances of reaching its ultimate goal without breaking.

As a manager, this means that, as well as having responsibilities as a provider, you also have responsibilities as a customer. If you play several customer roles in relation to a particular supplier, you will have a lot of influence in enabling the chain to operate smoothly. If you play only one or two roles, you will be less in control of what you receive (though there may be organisational benefits from specialist people or agencies performing the different roles).

SERVICE USERS' REQUIREMENTS

Having reached your service, a patient or service user becomes involved in a process of explanation and negotiation as a result of which a specification for treatment or care is established. Let's explore some of the elements in a service user's requirements by considering the following episode.

Jim Matthews' back

Jim, who worked in the local furniture factory, had been suffering from back pain. Initially he felt confident that it was only muscle strain which would be better within a week or so, but after two weeks of severe pain he decided to see his doctor.

He made an appointment and saw Dr Smith. She asked him questions, examined him and decided he needed an X-ray before she could complete her diagnosis. In the meantime, she prescribed pain-killers and they agreed that Jim should come back to see her a week after the X-ray, by which time she should have received the results. She filled in the necessary forms and advised him where he could get his X-ray taken.

Two days later, Jim went to the radiography department of his local hospital for the X-ray and he made an appointment to see Dr Smith a week later.

At the second meeting, Dr Smith informed Jim that he had compaction of one of his vertebral discs and she suggested a range of treatments. After discussing the implications of these, they agreed on a course of treatment involving pain-killers, bed rest and physiotherapy. Dr Smith advised Jim to make another appointment with her if there was no improvement after a month.

We'll use this example to examine four aspects of service users' requirements – whether they are defined in terms of outcomes or means of achieving them, how tightly they are defined, how far the service user is involved in defining them, and what the service user's expectations are.

Outcomes and means

The first point to pull out of this episode is that service users have wants and needs that they express in different ways. At Jim Matthews's initial visit to his doctor he knew what he wanted. He wanted outcomes – he wanted to find out what was wrong with his back and he wanted it to be better. However, he didn't know what was necessary to achieve these outcomes. At the initial consultation, Jim's need was simply to see the doctor: it was Dr Smith who specified the means by diagnosing the problem. When Jim visited the X-ray department he knew his requirement: he needed an X-ray of his back. Later on, Dr Smith prescribed a suitable course of treatment: further means to match Jim's second required outcome.

In our example, Jim Matthews is able to explain his situation. With some service users, alternative methods of communication are needed. For example, Manchester Children's Hospital uses pandas with smiling or crying faces to help children to express their experience of pain.

To generalise this point, some customers may express what they want as the overall outcome required from the service. Expressing the outcome they want is equivalent to stating their objective in using the service. Some service users are happy to leave the decision about how the required outcome can be achieved to professional judgement. Other service users may express their requirements in terms of means – which treatments, protocols, procedures or processes they wish to be used.

How does this distinction between outcomes and means map on to your experience? Does the service for which you are responsible more readily satisfy those who are interested only in outcomes or those who wish to specify means? If your customers define the outcomes and not the means, there is scope for interpreting their requirements and then choosing the means by which the outcomes can be achieved. If your customers also define the means, you will have less scope for flexibility or for choosing between alternatives. The more specialist your services, the more likely it is that service users' requirements will be expressed in terms of means rather than outcomes. Particularly in chains of internal customers, the further away you are from the end-user, the more precisely defined the means are likely to be.

PAIN SCORE

10 NO CONTROL

9 EXCRUCIATING WORST EVER

8 STOPS NORMAL ACTIVITIES

7 VERY BAD SEVERE

6 SEVERE DIFFICULTIES STOPS SOME THINGS

5 QUITE BAD

4 MODERATE

3 FEW PROBLEMS CAN DO MOST THINGS

2 MILD STINGING

1 NORMAL ACTIVITIES

0 NO PAIN AT ALL

PRESENTATION CATEGORY
RED ☐   ORANGE ☐
YELLOW ☐   GREEN ☐

PLANNED RE-ASSESSMENT EVERY
15 MINS ☐   30 MINS ☐   1 HOUR ☐

NAMED NURSE

Tightness of definition of requirements

Jim Matthews's initial requirement of Dr Smith was a few minutes of her time and expertise. This requirement was defined only in terms of when it was going to happen and not what was going to happen. Dr Smith had little idea in advance of what resources would be required to deliver this initial service. The requirement of the X-ray department was quite the reverse. The radiographer didn't know when the service would be required until Jim had made his booking, but she knew exactly what was involved in delivering the service – it was specified on the form that Jim took with him.

ACTIVITY 8.5

For one of your customers who defines the means by which your service should be provided (whether a service user or an internal customer), use the following questions to explore how tightly the requirements are defined.

How closely does your customer define each of the following?

1   How the service should be delivered (who delivers it, what procedures should be used, what equipment should be used)
2   When the service is to be delivered
3   Where the service is to be delivered

Make a note of how the tightness with which the requirements are defined will influence the way you deliver the service to your customer.

The more tightly your customers define their requirements, the more precisely you know what you have to do. Precise instructions can make life easier, but they can also put pressure on your service to deliver exactly what is required. For your customers to be able to define their requirements so tightly, they must know fairly accurately what they are. If you are concerned that their definition is too tight, it might be worth checking that they really do know their requirements so exactly. Perhaps you can negotiate a looser definition that is in both your interests.

Service user involvement

A third point in Jim's episode with his doctor is the way he participated in deciding what was required. In the first visit, he was involved in the diagnosis of his complaint. In the second visit, he was involved in agreeing a treatment: he was presented with some options and made an informed choice from what was on offer. Guided by Dr Smith, his selection was based on considering what was appropriate for his condition, what was available and what was acceptable to him. By contrast, Jim had no involvement in agreeing what was required of the radiographer. She simply had to respond to the requirement established by Dr Smith.

Stepping outside health and social care for a moment, experience shows that involving suppliers at an early stage in new developments leads to better utilisation of resources by both suppliers and their customers. Collaboration between customers in the chain in specifying requirements can make it easier to meet the requirements.

Service user expectations

Before deciding to see Dr Smith, Jim Matthews expected his bad back to be better in a couple of weeks. After seeing Dr Smith, his expectation had been modified. Dr Smith could not provide a service that would match his expectations.

We all have expectations of what is necessary for a reasonable life, including good health and social well-being. Expectations arise from comparisons with our families, friends and colleagues, from previous experience, from what we are used to, and from information about services and treatments. For example, we have a number of expectations of the health service. We may expect:

- our illnesses to be accurately diagnosed
- that most conditions will be treated successfully
- a friendly and courteous service
- to be able to take advantage of the latest diagnostic and therapeutic technologies
- to be treated with respect and dignity.

However, there are often problems with expectations, leading sometimes to disappointment:

- Expectations are not always explicit, so the supplier may not know what, in their heart of hearts, customers are expecting.
- Expectations are not always reasonable, so the supplier cannot match extremely high hopes.

This second problem is a particularly difficult one. Managers have to be very careful about their definitions of 'reasonable'. There is a danger of trying to shape service users' expectations to fit what you perceive is available from your service. There is also a danger of failing to acknowledge that service users may be right, even if your service is not able to meet their expectations.

It is, however, conceivable that expectations that are impossible to meet might need modifying as part of the process of specifying requirements. There may be evidence from a variety of sources – research, clinical audit and reviews conducted by the Social Services Inspectorate and the Audit Commission or the National Institute for Clinical Excellence in England and the Clinical Standards Board for Scotland – indicating that particular treatments or interventions are more effective than others. Being alert to developments in practice is important, especially in these days when information is available both to health and social care professionals and to service users from a wide range of sources, including the Internet.

ACTIVITY 8.6

		Yes	No
1	Are all your customers explicit about their expectations when they express their requirements?	☐	☐
2	Do you ask them what they expect?	☐	☐
3	Do you consciously modify their expectations as part of agreeing their requirements?	☐	☐
4	What about your suppliers? Do they give you the opportunity to express your expectations of them?	☐	☐

Matching the expectations of the customer to what can be delivered is essential if a quality service is to be provided. In the process of working towards an agreement about what customers require, you need to ensure that:

■ you know whether or not the means of achieving the outcomes are included in the customer's requirements
■ it is clear how tightly the requirements are defined
■ customers are involved in setting the requirements at the earliest stage possible
■ customer expectations of the service are addressed.

GETTING FEEDBACK FROM SERVICE USERS

There are a number of ways in which you can seek to develop a picture of how service users view your service. Here are two examples.

Are you being served?

Ellen May was a regular patient at the Edinburgh Royal Infirmary for 12 years following a triple heart bypass operation in 1987. Its bad points, she says, are that there is 'no lock on the toilet doors and inadequate space in the women's toilets'. The best bit of her stays in hospital is always 'the young man who brought papers, drinks and sweets to the ward on a trolley'.

In 1999, Ellen May was one of 200 people asked to record their experience of life at the other end of the stethoscope in three Edinburgh hospitals. Most were interviewed by staff. Ten were given cameras to take pictures as they went along. Lothian University Hospitals Trust allocated 80 staff for a day to interview patients and their families, capturing their experience of life on the wards at Western General, the Royal Hospital for Sick Children and the Royal Infirmary. A full-scale survey of 5,000 patients followed, in what the Trust believed to be the most ambitious attempt ever conducted in the NHS to view patient care through patients' eyes.

Bruce Dickie, planning manager for women's and children's services, was one of the questioners. He says: 'The main concerns patients have are some of the simplest to achieve. They want to be called by their first name, they want to know who is treating them and what is going to happen to them. They want to know the name of the nurse treating them and they want to have the same nurse or nurses treating them. Many of these patients come in regularly for treatment and they would prefer to build on an existing relationship with someone they had seen before than to be continually having to tell people their name, what their problem is, what are their likes and dislikes. Even knowing that nursing and medical staff are quite happy to talk to their relatives about what is happening was an area of concern. At least half of these changes are simple procedural changes, which can be implemented immediately.'

Medical Director Dr Charles Swainson argues that the concerns voiced by patients about toilet doors and newspapers bear out his own views. 'People seldom have concerns about the quality of their treatment in terms of the operation they have, or the medical care they receive', he says. 'What they are often concerned about are the simple issues such as knowing their doctor's name, what treatment they are being given, and the amount of information they receive. They want to be involved in their care and there is a whole range of simple things we can do to ensure that they feel more involved in their treatment. This is about raising staff awareness of what patients feel about their treatment, and trying to give them what they want rather than what we think they want.'

(Adapted from Wright, 1999)

What do users and carers want from domiciliary care?

The fieldwork for this study was carried out in three sites: Hertfordshire, Westminster and Wolverhampton. Six focus groups were held with users of domiciliary care services. We talked to a total of 46 people in these groups: 37 women and nine men. A small number of users were accompanied by a carer or a friend. Members of the groups ranged in age from around 40 to 90, with the majority over 70. Sixteen users were in wheelchairs: others had communication difficulties, some being deaf, blind or disabled following a stroke. Many of the users only ventured out of the house with great difficulty or not at all. All received home care, with levels of support ranging from an hour a week to intensive packages of home care alongside day and respite care. Some lived in sheltered housing.

We also held 16 interviews with service users in their own homes, both with people who received care arranged by the local authority and with people who purchased care privately. Their ages ranged from 31 to 93, but almost all were over 70. Over half lived alone and a quarter had help during the night. We found few differences between those with care arranged by the local authority and those who purchased care privately. The main difference was that private purchasers tended to arrange longer periods of care (of an hour or more) rather than shorter visits. The views of users interviewed individually echoed those of the users in the focus groups.

In the City of Westminster we found that black elders expressed views about personal care services that were very similar to the views of other people, focusing on reliability, honesty and trustworthiness. They were, however, more likely to emphasise gender concerns (black female users were more likely to prefer female care workers), requests for more appropriate food, and concerns about discriminatory practices and racist comments. They appeared to have a low level of confidence in accessing systems to make complaints, and expressed interest in greater access to advocacy, and to information and advice about services.

(Nuffield Institute, 1997)

We are not suggesting that you should initiate large-scale studies like these. But more explicit public consultation and involvement are now considered an important element within health and social care services. How much you are directly involved in getting feedback from service users will depend on your job, the service you manage and the policies and practices of your organisation. However, getting involved in the process of consultation or getting access to its outcomes can provide useful information about who your potential service users are and what they require.

The next Activity should help you to be clearer about the kind of information you need and encourages you to think about how you might obtain it. Gathering this information is not a one-off project: it is a long-term process that you need to keep in the forefront of your work as a manager.

ACTIVITY 8.7

Make notes in response to each of the questions below (drawn from Local Government Training Board, 1987). For each question consider:

- whether you know the answer
- if not, how you could set about getting the answer.

1 What do people want from your services?
2 Why are people satisfied or dissatisfied with your services?
3 Does the local community (existing and potential service users and carers) know what you and your staff can offer?
4 What are the image and reputation of your services locally? For example, do people think you are accessible, efficient, caring and responsive?
5 What services would people like to see increased or improved?
6 If cuts in services had to be made, where would people prefer them to fall?

Some of these questions can be answered by making use of the feedback your staff receive from service users day by day. Staff who work directly with service users often receive expressions of gratitude and thanks, sometimes with detailed comments about what worked particularly well. Managers rarely receive this feedback directly. All feedback from service users provides information about how they view the service that they have received. You can learn a great deal by developing systems to gather feedback about day-to-day service delivery that works well (or badly). You need to analyse and interpret this *ad hoc* feedback to decide what implications it has for the delivery of your services. Some feedback will confirm that things are running smoothly. Some will suggest minor improvements and adjustments. Some will indicate that there has been a serious failure.

If, in addition to making use of day-to-day feedback, you decide to use a more systematic approach to gathering information, the Northern and Yorkshire Regional Office of the NHS Executive (1999) offer the following tips for success:

- Ensure that all those involved are clear about the purpose of involving service users.
- Acknowledge that real involvement and partnership between health and social care organisations and the community may take time to achieve.
- Make sure that the method you choose for involving the community is suitable for the task in hand (for example, is the objective to secure

support for a change in services or is it to assemble information to guide planning?).

- Work collaboratively with other local health and social care organisations and share information with them.
- Recognise that well informed service users can encourage services to change.
- Use language carefully – avoid health or social care jargon.

HANDLING COMPLAINTS

When things go wrong in health and social care settings, they can go very wrong. Mistakes can sometimes result in unnecessary pain and distress and even in the early death of a patient or service user. However, many people who complain are not seeking revenge or even financial compensation: a mother whose young son died following what should have been a routine operation, and who subsequently took legal action, said: 'I wanted three things – an explanation, an apology, and to know that the doctor was unhappy and distressed by the result of his mistake' (BBC Radio 4, 6 October 1999). When she met the doctor concerned and understood his distress, she was helped in dealing with her own grief.

Most health and social care organisations have an established complaints procedure: many are required by legislation or Government guidance to do so. Some complaints procedures require adherence to a strict timetable. The aims of a complaints procedure should be:

- to resolve complaints as quickly as possible
- to ensure that the individuals involved and the organisation as a whole benefit from the experience
- to learn from any mistakes made and make adjustments to the service to reduce the likelihood of them happening again.

A typical complaints procedure

Complaints procedures typically have three stages (Essex and Wide, 1996).

Stage 1 – local resolution

The first stage is an attempt to resolve the complaint informally and as close as possible to the point of contact between the service and the complainant. It may be appropriate for the complaint to be settled between the member of staff concerned and the complainant, but it is wise to ensure that you, as the service manager, are aware of the complaint, and it may be necessary for you to become directly involved, even at this early stage. If the complainant wishes to have the support of an advocate or friend, this is generally something to be encouraged.

Stage 2 – the formal stage

If resolution at Stage 1 proves to be impossible, a complainant can request that the complaint be formally investigated. The significance of Stage 2 is that other people are involved in the consideration, discussion and, possibly, investigation of the complaint. At this stage it is usual to appoint an 'investigating officer', who may be a manager from within the organisation who is not directly involved in the complaint and whose tasks are to establish the facts and to explore what can be done to resolve the complaint. During the course of the investigation the investigating officer may interview the complainant, his or her advocate, staff, managers, and even legal and insurance advisers. In addition, case records may be examined. At the end of the investigation, the investigating officer writes a report detailing the complaint, the method of investigation and the findings, and makes recommendations on any actions that should be taken by the organisation.

Stage 3 – the review panel

If a complainant is not satisfied with the results of the Stage 2 investigation, he or she may ask for the complaint to be reviewed by a panel chaired by an independent person. In some complaints procedures, the Stage 3 panel can reinvestigate the complaint from scratch. In others, the review panel's function is more limited – to check that the complaint and the process have been handled correctly.

As a manager, it is the first of these stages in which you are most likely to be involved. However, you might be required to provide evidence if a complaint against your service reaches the second or third stage. You might also be appointed as the investigating officer for a second-stage complaint.

At Stage 1, your responsibilities are to ensure that:

- the complaint is properly acknowledged
- it is properly investigated
- it is referred to a senior manager if it has wider implications
- an appropriate response is provided to the complainant
- careful records are kept of the complaint and how it has been handled.

The last point is important for two reasons. First, you will need to have a proper record if the complaint reaches Stage 2 or Stage 3. Second, complaints – whether or not they are well founded – are an opportunity to learn: they can provide a valuable source of information about users' perceptions of your service and so may provide ideas for service improvements.

Ways in which complaints are resolved

Essex and Wide (1996) identify a number of ways in which complaints are resolved. In some cases, more than one of these processes may be at work simultaneously.

1   The people involved reach a new understanding of the situation. Complainants might say: 'Maybe I was being a bit unfair.' Staff might say: 'Perhaps we could have handled that differently.'
2   The people involved get over the original hurt or anger they felt at the time. Complainants or staff might say: 'It doesn't bother me any more. It's in the past.'
3   The people involved feel that they have been heard and understood. The complainants receive an apology or explanation and feel that they were justified in complaining. They might say: 'I got a full apology.'
4   The organisation offers a remedy and the focus shifts from the complaint to the solution. Complainants might say: 'I got what I wanted.' Staff might say: 'We can now see how we could deal with a situation like that differently in the future.'
5   The people involved accept the judgement of a trusted arbiter. Complainants or staff might say: 'I lost' (or 'I won') or 'I was right' (or 'I was wrong').
6   The people involved accept that they will get no further with the complaint. Complainants might say: 'I've stopped banging my head against a brick wall.' Staff might say: 'I don't agree but I suppose I'll have to get on with the job.'

To be the subject of a complaint, or to be a complainant, is often a painful experience. The situation needs to be handled with openness and sensitivity. Unnecessarily defensive behaviour on the part of the service can be frustrating for the complainant and reduce the likelihood of resolution. It is important to keep the focus of attention on the lessons to be learned both by the individuals involved and by the organisation, and to look for possible service improvements.

As a manager, you may need to take a lead in establishing the facts of a case. You will have to balance the perceptions and expectations of those making a complaint with those who may be the subject of the complaint. The members of staff involved may be under considerable stress and in need of support to deal with their feelings. You may have to suggest ways to resolve the situation for all parties in an environment where resources are limited but expectations about the level and quality of services may be increasing.

In this chapter we have focused on understanding what users require from your services. We have looked at who your customers are, how service users define their requirements, how you can get feedback from service users, and at the stages involved in handling complaints. No-one likes receiving complaints, but one positive way to respond is to try to learn from them.

REFERENCES

Essex, S. and Wide, M. (1996) *A Matter for Investigation*, Educational Broadcasting Services Trust.

Local Government Training Board (1987) *Getting Closer to the Public*, LGTB.

NHS Executive (Northern and Yorkshire Region) (1999) *Primary Care Groups Public Engagement Toolkit* (http://www.doh.gov.uk/nyro/pcgtoolk.htm accessed 15 March 2000).

Nuffield Institute (1997) *What Do Users and Carers Want from Domiciliary Care? (Update*, Issue 4), Nuffield Foundation.

Wright, C. (1999) 'Are you being served?' *Health Service Journal*, 2 September, pp. 12–13.

MANAGING OUTCOMES FOR SERVICE USERS

This chapter begins by emphasising the importance of being clear about the purposes of the services for which you are responsible, and of identifying their intended outcomes in ways that enable you to measure the extent to which you are achieving them. This may seem self-evident, but it is not always easy to achieve the intended outcomes in health and social care, where many services have multiple purposes, with outcomes that are difficult to define and measure.

We then discuss the different ways in which service users can participate in identifying the outcomes that they require from health and social care services and in designing services to meet these requirements. Over recent years, there has been an increasing emphasis on involving service users more in the design of services – from informing them, to consulting them, to engaging in partnership with them, to delegating control to them.

Finally, we explore the importance of providing health and social care services that are effectively integrated. Many patients and service users require a range of services from different parts of the same organisation or from different organisations. In order to ensure that a complex array of services is provided in an integrated way to each individual patient or service user, managers need to focus their attention on the boundaries between their services and other related services.

PURPOSE AND OUTCOMES

The purposes of health and social care services as defined today have often evolved over many years. Many services now provided by statutory organisations started with a voluntary organisation recognising a need of a particular group of people and raising money to meet that need. For example, the Women's Royal Voluntary Service played a significant part in identifying that older people living alone are often unable to prepare a hot meal for themselves. They prepared hot meals in central kitchens, which they delivered to people in their homes.

People not only liked the hot meal, but also the contact with the person who delivered it. Community meals services now serve a wider variety of purposes, including, for example, enabling the earlier discharge of people from hospital.

A variety of powerful influences determines the purposes of services. National government has a major role in deciding what services will be provided and for what purposes, both through legislation (for example the various NHS Acts, the Children Act and the Mental Health Act) and through policy guidance (for example, in the form of national service frameworks). Local commissioning authorities (health authorities, primary care groups or trusts, and local authority social services and social work departments) have developed sophisticated methods of determining local needs, identifying gaps in services and determining priorities. All these players control substantial funds, which they use to commission services from statutory and independent service providers, and thus determine the purposes, quantity and quality of the services that are provided.

But even though the statutory framework for provision of a service may largely determine its purpose, there is often scope for individual managers to influence this, and they certainly have influence over the way in which it is delivered. How front-line managers interpret a service's purposes can have a significant effect on its outputs and outcomes.

It is important to distinguish between outputs and outcomes. In health and social care, *outputs* are usually procedures and processes completed – for example, numbers of patients treated or numbers of care plans prepared – and they are generally fairly easy to measure. *Outcomes* tend to happen outside the service, back in the patient or service user's own home, and are only partly within the control of those who specify and provide services. In a health and social care context, outcomes include crucial events such as healthy births, quality of life, and protection from harm. The desired outcomes of a service are not always easy to define, and are often difficult to measure. For the recipient of health or social care, the outcome should be better than what would have occurred if no service had been provided: 'This is the acid test of effectiveness, and in a world of finite resources we need to think about how to apply this acid test' (Riley and Riley, 1998).

A statement of a service's purpose should specify clearly who the service is for and the nature of the service provided, and it should be possible to relate this statement to specific and measurable outcomes. However, in health and social care it is not always easy to write an explicit statement of purpose and it is even more difficult to link the purpose to measurable outcomes.

For example, the National Service Framework for Mental Health (Department of Health, 1999) includes the following statement:

> Any individual with a common mental health problem should be able to make contact round the clock with the local services necessary to meet their needs and receive adequate care.

It goes on to say that achievement of this standard should be assessed in terms of 'evidence that services respond to mental health needs quickly, effectively and consistently 24 hours a day, 365 days a year'.

This raises a number of different kinds of questions. First, there are questions of interpretation, for example:

- What does 'making contact round the clock' mean?
- Does it mean that every possible type of service should be available round the clock?
- What does that imply for the skill mix of the personnel required?
- Is every service expected to be accessible to everyone in its catchment area?
- What constitutes an effective response to a mental health need?

Second, there are questions about making people aware of the service, for example:

- How do people know that the service exists?
- If they know that it exists, do they have the means to access it?
- Is it perceived as credible and helpful by all the people who might use it?

Third, there are questions about outcomes, for example:

- Is such a service likely to reduce the incidence of suicide?
- If the incidence of suicide reduced following the introduction of the service, how would you know what contribution the round-the-clock service had made to that reduction?

These last two questions – about identifying outcomes and finding a way of measuring whether they have been achieved – are particularly challenging ones.

Let's look at two examples of service outcomes and how they are measured.

Example 1

The Calman–Hine Report (Department of Health, 1995) drew on available sources of information about the outcomes of treatments for cancer and the care of cancer patients to provide the basis for a radical revision of the way cancer services are delivered in England and Wales.

Among the evidence it drew on was an audit of breast cancer care which identified, through peer review, surgeons who had specialist skills in the management of this disease. It was found that the patients of these skilled surgeons had significantly improved survival rates: an 8.9 per cent better chance of surviving five years after treatment and a 7.6 per cent better chance of surviving ten years after treatment (Gillis *et al.*, 1996).

In this study, the outcomes of treatment were measured in terms of the length of time patients survived after surgery – a straightforward measure. However, there are many other possible measures of the outcomes of cancer treatment and care, for example, in terms of the quality of life experienced by the patients and the economic costs to the health service and the community.

Example 2

The national objectives for social services (Department of Health and Department of the Environment, Transport and the the Regions, 1999) state explicit outcomes for children's services:

1   Children are securely attached to carers capable of providing safe and effective care for the duration of childhood
2   Children are protected from significant harm in terms of emotional, physical and sexual abuse or neglect
3   Children in need gain maximum life chance benefits from educational opportunities, health care and social care
4   Children looked after by local authorities gain maximum life chance benefits from educational opportunities, health care and social care
5   Young people leaving care, as they enter adulthood, are not isolated and participate socially and economically as citizens
6   Children with specific social needs arising out of disability or a health condition are living in families or other appropriate settings in the community where their assessed needs are adequately met and reviewed.

These statements make it clear what care services should set out to achieve for the children concerned – the outcomes – but finding appropriate ways of measuring whether they have been achieved is not easy. Some of the performance measures identified for these outcomes by the Department of Health are:

A   long-term stability of placements for children looked after by local authorities
B   length of time on the child protection register

C proportion of children looked after by local authorities
D spending on children in need
E educational attainment of children looked after by local authorities
F cautions and convictions for children looked after by local authorities
G number of children looked after by local authorities who are excluded from school
H employment, education and training for young people leaving care.

ACTIVITY 9.1

Which of these performance measures (A–H) would you regard as appropriate for each of the outcomes 1–6 above? (For example, you might regard performance measure A as relevant to outcome 1.)

We would say that the most straightforward 'matches', in addition to the example we gave in the Activity, are B for outcome 2, E, F and G for outcome 4, and H for outcome 5. However, there are other – though perhaps less clear – relationships: for example, D is a measure that arguably relates to all six outcomes. But none of the performance measures – alone or in combination – fully provides the means of assessing any of the outcomes.

ACTIVITY 9.2

Choose one of the services that you have some responsibility for. Review any existing statements of its purpose(s) and outcomes that you can find. (You might, for example, look at Government guidelines, national service frameworks, professional guidelines, your local Health Improvement Plan, or reports from the Social Services Inspectorate or the Audit Commission.)

1 Encapsulate, as clearly and briefly as you can, the purpose(s) of this service.
2 Specify two intended outcomes of this service.
3 Identify one performance measure for each outcome.

SERVICE USER PARTICIPATION

What part should service users play in determining the outcomes they seek from health and social care services and the means for achieving them? In the 1980s and early 1990s, there was a trend towards a 'consumerist' view of services, in which the providers of services offer options which service users choose between. More recently, there has been an increasing emphasis on what is sometimes described as the 'democratic' view, through which service users participate, to a greater or lesser extent, in the process of designing the options.

However, it is perhaps unhelpful to view this as a polarity, and the extent to which service users participate in the design of services is more usefully described as a continuum, as shown in Figure 9.1. At one end of the continuum, the relationship between the service user and the service provider centres on the communication and sharing of information. The relationship then progresses through the consultative stage to full partnership (which involves sharing decision making) and ultimately to delegated control.

Each stage involves different ways of working (Living Options in Practice, 1992):

- *Information* – gathering information about service users and carers, ensuring that relevant information reaches them, and sharing ideas and plans about services with them (for example, by means of surveys, leaflets about services and discussion groups)
- *Consultation* – asking people's views and advice on plans, policies and services (for example, by means of advisory groups and public meetings)
- *Partnership* – working as equals to set objectives, make plans and decide funding priorities (for example, through service users being members of planning, review and evaluation committees and groups)
- *Delegated control* – giving authority and money to service users, carers and the wider community to plan and implement services (so that services are actually run by service users and by the community of which they are part).

The consumerist model is located at the information/consultation end of this continuum. It is essentially provider-led: power and influence remain with the provider. The democratic model is located at the partnership/delegated control end, emphasising that services are

Figure 9.1 The service user participation continuum

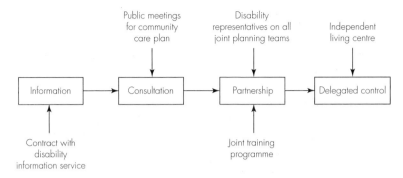

Figure 9.2 Examples of services for people with disabilities

accountable to the public, and that service users and their carers are also citizens.

Although many health and social care services are making considerable progress at the information/consultation end of the continuum, full partnership and delegated control of services are still relatively rare. Figure 9.2 shows examples of services for people with disabilities mapped on to the user-participation continuum.

ACTIVITY 9.3

Where do the services you are responsible for lie on the user-participation continuum at present? Following the example in Figure 9.2, map them on to the continuum.

Thinking about your services in this way may have shown that not all your services involve service users and carers to the same extent. This may be because it is sometimes more appropriate to provide or gather information than to consult, enter into partnership or delegate control. Your strategy for involving service users and carers does not have to be an 'all or nothing' approach. Service users will appreciate it if you are honest and clear about what you are aiming to do. For example, if delegated control is not on your agenda, don't disguise the fact: it will be evident from the way you work with service users, and fudging the issue is likely to end in cynicism and a withdrawal of interest.

Mapping relationships

Another way of thinking about service user participation is to consider the relationships between those who pay for, design and deliver services, on the one hand, and the service users and carers who benefit from them on the other. We are now going to map the relationships between these 'key players' by using four circles depicting those who pay for services, those who design them, those who deliver them and those who benefit from them.

Figure 9.3 shows the relationships in what we might call the *bureaucratic* model of health and social care services. There are close relationships between those who pay for, design and deliver a service. Those who commission a service are involved in both paying for it and designing it. Staff are involved in both designing and delivering it, with managers functioning at the interface of payment, design and delivery. The service is then delivered to the service users and carers who benefit from it.

The *responsive* model is illustrated in Figure 9.4. The aim here is to develop and sustain a dialogue between, on the one hand, those who pay for, design and deliver the service and, on the other, those who benefit from it. However, although the beneficiaries' views and wishes

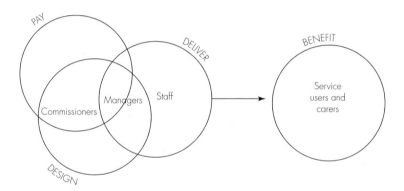

Figure 9.3 A bureaucratic service

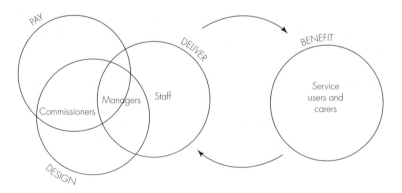

Figure 9.4 A responsive service

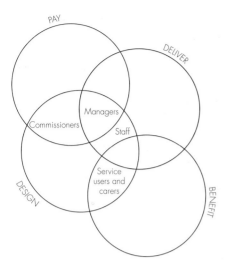

Figure 9.5 An empowering service

are gathered and acted on, they are still excluded from decision making and do not have any power in planning and designing the service.

Figure 9.5 represents one version of an *empowering* service model. The 'design' circle in Figure 9.5 includes the specification of services and the way in which they are planned, and is the crucial element in this model. In contrast with Figures 9.3 and 9.4, almost all the key players, including service users, are now included within the design circle, whatever other circles they may also be part of. This suggests that the power relationships between service users and the other players will be worked out in the design circle: it is here that the amount of influence or power each key player has over service design will be resolved. Service users and carers can only be said to be empowered if they have direct influence in this sphere. Working with the inevitable difficulties this creates – in a situation where a clash of interests is certainly possible – is the central challenge for managers in developing modern health and social care services.

Interestingly, there has also been a shift from the bureaucratic to the responsive model in the relationships between key players *within* health and social care organisations. Ideas have changed about how different departments – and different levels within departments – should relate to one another. Similar diagrams can therefore be drawn for support services, showing the relationships between different parts of an organisation. A crucial move, in the interests of developing a service that empowers staff as well as service users, is to bring those who deliver the service and those who benefit from it inside the design circle.

ACTIVITY 9.4

1   Which of the three models described in this section most closely describes the main service for which you are responsible?
2   Using this model as a starting point, map the relationships between the key players in this service. (Don't forget to identify yourself in the diagram!)
3   How would you like to see these relationships change over the next two or three years?

One of the immediate effects of empowering service users and carers – or internal customers if you work in a support service – is that relationships and roles become more complex. Understanding and clarifying roles and relationships are important both to you and your team and to those who use your services. Changing the roles and relationships may crucially affect the nature of the outcomes that are required of your service by those commissioning it and by those using it – as well as the means of achieving them.

WORKING ACROSS BOUNDARIES

In this section, we explore a number of the issues involved in working together to provide integrated care for patients, service users and carers. The great majority of health and social care services are provided in environments of complex interdependent working arrangements designed to facilitate co-operation between professionals working for the same patient or service user. Some teams and services are specifically set up and designed to work jointly – for example, community mental health services and (in England) area child protection committees. As a manager in any part of the complex health and social care system, you need to be aware of the interfaces – the boundaries where the work you do needs to be integrated with the work of others.

Boundaries may be marked by geography, professional differences, different sources of funding, organisational structures, or differences in values and priorities. Service users will often not understand these boundaries. They – and you – may see them only as a hindrance. None the less, it is frequently at the boundaries between services that crucial decisions are made about the care of a service user.

Conflicts may arise because you do not fully understand how those on the other side of boundaries work and what their priorities and concerns are. The same may also be true of their understanding of your work. If some of the boundaries are unclear – and they often are – you may need to clarify where your responsibilities begin and end.

We are going to present a case study that highlights some of the issues related to working across boundaries. It is written from the point of view of the family of Mr Jones, who is terminally ill. We want you to try to understand their perspective on their experiences and also to look at the events described from the point of view of a manager who may be in a position to take action or to make recommendations to improve the processes involved. We have chosen a case study about a person who is terminally ill because, in one sense, there can be only one outcome – in clinical terms, at least. However, there are many other possible intermediate outcomes of the health and social care services provided to both the patient and his family in a situation like this.

Moving outside health and social care for a moment, Berry *et al.* (1985) conducted extensive in-depth interviews with a wide variety of customer groups in the service sector. In analysing their data, the researchers were able to identify a number of dimensions on which customers assessed the quality of the services they received. These are listed in the left-hand column of Table 9.1, with good and bad examples in the other two columns. As you read through Table 9.1, you may conclude that not all these dimensions of quality are relevant to the

Table 9.1 Customer assessment of quality

Dimensions of quality	Good examples	Bad examples
Reliability	Punctual arrival of train	Failure to phone customer back as agreed
Responsiveness	Maintenance staff who service equipment at short notice	Long queues
Competence	Staff carry out task with skill and competence	Bank fails to cancel standing order, then charges fee for resulting overdraft
Access	Easy to find one's way Easy to get to	Poor signing Limited car parking
Courtesy	Polite and helpful staff	Senior staff patronising and condescending
Communication	Medical staff who explain the diagnosis and alternative forms of treatment without using jargon	Lack of information, when a train is delayed, about the cause and duration of the delay
Credibility	A solicitor you feel you can trust and depend on	A salesman who uses hard-sell tactics
Security	A feeling of personal safety and confidentiality	Unlit access at night
Understanding/knowing the customer	Staff who make an effort to meet a customer's individual requirements	Staff who don't recognise a regular customer
Tangibles	Pleasing physical appearance of facilities	Poor or out-of-date equipment being used for the service

(Source: Berry *et al.*, (1985) A Practical Approach to Quality, Joiner Associates Inc. © Oriel Incorporated, formerly Joiner Associates, reprinted with permission)

services for which you are responsible, but it is likely that you will be able to make at least some connections with your experience at work.

When asked about the issues that they regarded as most important to their situation, the Jones family identified the following:

- whether Mr Jones and his family felt psychologically safe
- whether Mr Jones was physically safe
- the accessibility and responsiveness of the health and social care services involved
- who was empowered to make what decisions
- the effectiveness of the communication between all those involved
- the effectiveness of the integration of the various services involved.

You will notice that these concerns correspond quite closely to a number of Berry's dimensions of quality. Apart from the fact that some of Berry's dimensions are not included at all, there are three other differences. First, the Jones family distinguished between two aspects of what Berry calls 'security' – psychological safety and physical safety. Second, they combined two of Berry's dimensions in their concern for accessibility and responsiveness of services. Third, they focused on who was empowered to make decisions and on the issue of integration of services, which do not feature on Berry's list, although both might be related to Berry's dimension of 'understanding/knowing the customer'.

ACTIVITY 9.5

Read the case study below. It is divided into six phases. Pause after you read each of these and, from the perspective of the Jones family, make a brief note of how you think they may have felt at this point about the first three of the issues listed earlier: psychological safety, physical safety and accessibility/responsiveness of services.

The story of Mr and Mrs Jones

Phase 1

Mr Jones was 83 and suffering from terminal cancer. He was gradually getting weaker, and was confined to bed most of the time. He wanted to die at home, although neither he nor his wife were sure how the illness and his care needs would progress. Since the diagnosis had been confirmed three months before by a scan, his treatment plan was in the hands of his GP, who visited weekly. The GP's treatment plan was minimalist – not intervening with drugs unless absolutely necessary and choosing a time to allow the inevitable infections to take their course – a plan with which the family had no disagreement, given Mr Jones's age.

Co-ordination of practical care was in the hands of the district nurse. Auxiliary nurses were helping with washing Mr Jones, but for the rest of the time his wife (also aged 83) was his carer, looking after everything to do with finances, cooking, shopping, washing, etc. with a little help from neighbours who provided transport and other bits of practical help.

The local social services department had been contacted and had supplied information, but had not carried out an assessment.

No one had suggested that Mr Jones was entitled to an attendance allowance from the Benefits Agency, but fortunately his daughter knew about the fast-track arrangements for people with terminal illness. Mrs Jones got the necessary form, completed it, and left it with the receptionist at the GP's surgery, who said she would get the GP to countersign it and forward it to the Benefits Agency. Having heard nothing, Mrs Jones telephoned the Benefits Agency two weeks later. They had not received the form, and further enquiries revealed that it had been filed at the surgery. Eventually, the money came through. Mr Jones was becoming too weak to stand unaided.

Phase 2

One Saturday evening Mr Jones got out of bed by himself to use the commode, and fell. The nurses had advised Mrs Jones that, if he were to fall, she should call the ambulance service for help in lifting him. So Mrs Jones called the ambulance service, expecting that they would help her to get him back into bed. Instead, they examined him, and took him off in the ambulance to the local accident and emergency department, ten miles away. Mr Jones was not able to cope – physically, intellectually or emotionally – with this situation on his own, and some time later his wife was called to the hospital. Fortunately a neighbour was able to give her a lift and stay with her at the hospital.

Phase 3

After more tests that night, Mr Jones was admitted to hospital and Mrs Jones went home. Mr Jones's bed was in a general medical ward housing mainly younger patients. A urinary infection was suspected and a drip set up to reduce his dehydration.

When relatives visited the following day (Sunday), they found that he had been left alone at the end of the ward furthest from the toilets, without a call bell, bottle or commode, and was therefore unable to cope with going to the toilet. The humiliation of wetting the bed was horrible.

Phase 4

On the Monday morning, the hospital started Mr Jones on a course of antibiotics for the suspected urinary infection (which had not yet been confirmed). The reason for prescribing an antibiotic was not given to the relatives, or to the GP who visited later that day.

By the end of Monday, Mr Jones had been fitted with an extremely uncomfortable continence aid, and was deeply distressed and unhappy. He told his wife he was lying there 'trying to die'. All the parties to his treatment – relatives, nurses, and the GP – had questioned why he was in hospital. The hospital social workers were contacted to arrange care for him on his return home.

Phase 5

Two days later, care had been arranged. The ambulance service had been contacted, and on Wednesday he was taken home. On arrival at home, the ambulance staff helped him walk up the two flights of stairs to his bedroom – a task that took more than half an hour. That evening the first carers arrived from the private care service that had been called in by the social services department. No one had been informed by the hospital that Mr Jones had a urinary infection, so the antibiotics were stopped.

Phase 6

By the following weekend, Mr Jones was very ill. He had slept for an entire day following the exhausting task of walking up two flights of stairs. He was incontinent and in severe pain from the ineffective continence aids that were being used. His daughter had to arrange a case conference with the GP and nurses to get these arrangements changed. Mr Jones's mind was wandering, and he had become incapable of co-operating in his care. For the only time in his whole illness, he was rude to his carers.

A week of extreme stress for Mr Jones, his wife and his daughter ensued, during which they had to do the following:

■ adjust to twice daily visits from carers and explain the situation to every new carer who arrived
■ deal with the fact that the professionals often arrived while lunch (the main meal of the day) was being cooked or about to be served
■ explain to a number of different nurses what the circumstances and difficulties were and persuade them to do something about it
■ deal with the fact that very few of the visitors realised that Mr and Mrs Jones had poor hearing and were therefore often unable to understand what the visitors were saying, even when this was pointed out to them
■ chase around the area finding pharmacists who could supply appropriate continence aids, as well as collecting prescriptions, aids and adaptations
■ learn the working arrangements of Crossroads care attendants, twilight nurses, nightcare nurses, MacMillan nurses, hearing aid suppliers, collectors of contaminated refuse, community dentists and the private company supplying care assistants.

There had still been no assessment or review visit from the social services department. It took more than two weeks to resolve the problems triggered by the decision to remove Mr Jones to hospital. However, no long-term harm appeared to have been done and a new and more stable situation then emerged.

Our perspective on these events can never be the same as that of the Jones family, so there are no right answers. Our notes were as follows.

Phase 1
Psychological safety: good – Mr Jones at home, with Mrs Jones in charge and providing security.
Physical safety: becoming problematic because Mr Jones is now too weak to stand unaided
Accessibility/responsiveness of services: GP seems to have been accessible and responsive, organising nursing support; social services department was accessible, but not very responsive; no help given in contacting the Benefits Agency.

Phase 2
Psychological safety: lost.
Physical safety: temporarily improved.
Accessibility/responsiveness of services: ambulance service responded quickly; no help offered to Mrs Jones to get to hospital.

Phase 3
Psychological safety: completely absent – Mr Jones in despair, having been placed in a situation where he has lost all autonomy; Mrs Jones not able to be present to co-ordinate action and family very upset.
Physical safety: satisfactory.
Accessibility/responsiveness of services: no evidence of an assessment having been made of Mr Jones's needs.

Phase 4
Psychological safety: totally destroyed.
Physical safety: treatment plan changed without apparent consultation or information given to GP or family; drugs prescribed without explanation; continence aid causing great discomfort (applied for convenience of staff?).
Accessibility/responsiveness of services: hospital very slow in deciding on discharge and in beginning to make arrangements for Mr Jones to return home.

Phase 5
Psychological safety: improving.

Physical safety: making Mr Jones walk up two flights of stairs exhausted him; still unclear whether antibiotic was needed.
Accessibility/responsiveness of services: carers arrived promptly.

Phase 6
Psychological safety: for Mr Jones, poor at the beginning of this phase, but then gradually improving; Mrs Jones now under great stress, because co-ordination of care is almost entirely in her hands.
Physical safety: poor at the beginning of this phase, but improving, especially after the painful continence aid was changed.
Accessibility/responsiveness of services: professionals slow to deal with problem of continence aid; plenty of services available, but responsibility left with carers to call them in and co-ordinate them; professionals unable to recognise and respond to Mr and Mrs Jones's poor hearing.

Now let's turn to the other three issues identified by the Jones family as problematic:

■ who was empowered to make what decisions
■ the effectiveness of the communication between all those involved
■ the effectiveness of the integration of the various services involved.

ACTIVITY 9.6

Identify for each of phases 2–6 of the case study, the key decisions made – apparently without consultation with Mr Jones or his family – that had adverse consequences for psychological and physical safety. In each case, what alternative decision might the Jones family have preferred, had they been consulted?

Once again, there are no right answers, but here are our suggestions.

Phase 2
Ambulance staff decided to take Mr Jones to the hospital's accident and emergency department. (Could they have put him back in bed?)

Phase 3
The accident and emergency department decided to admit Mr Jones to hospital. (Could they have sent him home, or could he have been admitted to a more suitable ward, with access to a call bell?)

Phase 4
The hospital decided to prescribe an antibiotic for the suspected urinary infection and to provide continence aid. (Was either necessary?)

Phase 5
Ambulance staff decided to help Mr Jones to walk upstairs. (Should he have been carried?)

Phase 6
The social services department did not arrange an assessment or review visit (perhaps this was the result of the lack of a decision). (Should they have arranged a co-ordinated care package?)

Mr Jones's story is not untypical. However competent all the individual care staff, this did not prevent a severe illness and a very stressful episode. The Jones family identified the two major – and related – inadequacies in the services provided to Mr Jones as failures in communication and a lack of integration between services. The individual professionals took actions that appeared sensible to them at the time, but which did not take into account Mr Jones's overall state of health and well-being. Each handed Mr Jones on to another person, without being aware of the consequences of their actions.

It is perhaps in managing the communication between your service and other services that relate to it – and thus contributing to the integration of services – that you, as a manager, can make the greatest contribution to the development of better outcomes for patients and service users. The individual professionals who work in health and social care are, almost inevitably, reactive: it is your job to be proactive. Mr and Mrs Jones's story would almost certainly have been very different if a multi-agency care plan had been in place from the outset.

David Hands (1999) presents a useful analysis of the need for integration between services because of the potential for boundary difficulties to arise. He describes this with reference to the health service, but it is not too difficult to see that his points have equal relevance to social care. There is a need for integration between:

- component parts of the total system (the separate organisational entities that are responsible for prevention, primary care, secondary care, tertiary care, continuing care and rehabilitation)
- different stages in the treatment of a specific condition (from initial tentative diagnosis through investigation, testing, final diagnosis, assessment, treatment and aftercare)
- different parts of the same provider organisation (for example, the various parts of a hospital, such as clinical, diagnostic, outpatient, ward and hotel services)
- different health professions and different specialities within the same profession (for example, doctors, nurses and the professions allied to medicine)
- separate provider organisations of the same or a similar kind (for example, general practices, hospitals or specialist service providers in different locations)

- health services and related services (for example, social services, housing, transport, environmental health, voluntary organisations and the Benefits Agency)
- commissioners and providers of services
- managers and clinicians
- different treatment and care regimes for different diseases or conditions for the same patient
- patients, their families, their homes and their social context.

ACTIVITY 9.7

For the main service for which you are responsible, identify one other service that lies on its boundary. It might be another service within the same organisation or part of a different organisation. It might be part of the health service, social services or the voluntary sector.

1 Describe briefly how you work with it.
2 Are there differences between its methods of working and yours that help or hinder you?
3 Describe briefly any areas of conflict between these two services.
4 How effective is the communication between you that directly affects patients or service users?
5 How could you work together more effectively to improve outcomes for patients or service users?

Partnership development

An organisation works more effectively when it has mutually beneficial partnerships, built on trust, sharing of knowledge, and integration with its partners.

(European Foundation for Quality Management, 1999)

Improving integration

Gorman (1998) has identified a number of principles that can assist partnership working, and thus help to provide more integrated services for patients and service users.

- Reciprocity is at the heart of all partnerships. A partnership will fail unless there is something in it for both partners. The benefits do not have to be symmetrical, although that helps.
- Successful partnerships often have someone who plays the role of convenor. This individual has respect across the agencies involved in the partnership and understands the issues as they affect the individual partners. He or she acts almost as the physical embodiment of the partnership.
- A partnership has to work at all levels. The nuts and bolts of multi-agency agreements are often thrashed out by teams of middle managers. These agreements will come unstuck if they are not in tune with the thinking of senior management or if they cannot or will not be implemented by front-line managers and staff.

- Successful multi-agency partnerships actively engage with the differences between the partners, just as multidisciplinary teams bring together values and mindsets that can be in conflict with each other. Partnership working is about managing the differences and getting the best from them. Bring the differences out into the open and work with them honestly.
- Wherever possible, adapt existing structures to suit the needs of partnership working.
- Focus on specific projects and tasks. This helps to clarify the issues, and brings key questions, benefits and problems to the surface so that they can be addressed.
- Focus on outcomes. Partnership working is only valuable if it leads to better outcomes for patients and service users.
- Be clear about your own concerns and priorities. Be prepared to listen to and understand the concerns and priorities of others. Look for points of agreement and build bridges based on them. Be prepared to negotiate and, where necessary, to compromise.

We began this chapter by considering the importance of being clear about the purposes of the services for which you are responsible and identifying and measuring their intended outcomes. We then explored the various levels at which you can enable service users to participate in the design and delivery of your services – informing them, consulting them, engaging in partnership with them, or delegating control to them.

We concluded by focusing on the importance of managing the boundaries between your services and others. As a manager in health or social care, it is likely that you will be increasingly required to work collaboratively with other services to seek more effective outcomes for patients, service users and carers. A good understanding of the part that your service plays within the whole process of care is important. This will help you to spot opportunities for service development and improvement, to take a service user perspective and to manage more effectively.

REFERENCES

Berry, L., Zeithaml, V. and Parasuraman, A. (1985) *A Practical Approach to Quality*, Joiner Associates Inc.

Department of Health (1995) *A Policy Framework for Commissioning Cancer Services: A Report by the Expert Advisory Group on Cancer to the Chief Medical Officers of England and Wales*, Department of Health.

Department of Health (1999) *The National Service Framework for Mental Health*, Department of Health (http://www.doh.gov.uk/nsf/mhexecsum. htm).

Department of Health and Department of the Environment, Transport and the Regions (1999), 'Better care, higher standards', Joint Circular, December, Service First Unit, Cabinet Office, London.

European Foundation for Quality Management (1999) *The EFQM Excellence Model*, EFQM.

Gillis, C. R. *et al.* (1996) 'Survival outcome of care by specialist surgeons in breast cancer: A study of 3786 patients in the west of Scotland', *British Medical Journal*, 312: 145–8.

Gorman, P. (1998) *Managing Multidisciplinary Teams in the NHS*, Kogan Page.

Hands, D. (1999) 'Integrated care', in M. Lugon and J. Secker-Walker (eds) *Clinical Governance*, pp. 33–48, The Royal Society of Medicine Press.

Living Options in Practice (1992) *Achieving User Participation: Planning Services for People with Severe Physical and Sensory Disabilities* (Project Paper No. 3), King's Fund Centre.

Riley, C. and Riley, J. (1998) 'Outcome indicators: Friends or enemies?', *Managing Community Care*, 6(6): 246–53.

QUALITY IN SERVICES

Though 'quality' is an elusive concept, you will be well aware of the pressure there is on managers in health and social care to improve it. Knowing who your customers are, understanding what they would like from you and using your resources appropriately to meet their requirements are essential ingredients in providing quality services.

It is important to consider what 'quality' means. We begin by looking at various definitions of quality to help you identify what quality means for your area of health and social care services. This is the first step towards recognising where you are delivering good quality and diagnosing any quality problems you may have.

A great deal of attention has been given to quality in recent years. But why is quality important? In particular, why is it important in health and social care? We examine why quality is important both to those who use your services and to your staff. Quality has many dimensions and it is important to identify all those that affect your services and your customers' perceptions of them.

WHAT DOES 'QUALITY' MEAN?

So what does this elusive word 'quality' mean? If you buy jewellery from a Bond Street jeweller in London, you might think that this gives some guarantee of quality – but what about the jeweller who sells work in your local craft market? He or she might use gold and precious stones too – so can this be work of a high quality? And how about the differences between taking a cruise on the *Queen Elizabeth II* and cruising around Poole Harbour on Joe's pleasure boat? Can we expect quality from Joe?

There are always at least two points of view – the customer's and the provider's. One key to defining quality in health and social care is to look at differences in points of view between those who use services and those who provide them. Any definition of a quality service must incorporate the perceptions of both service users and service providers.

Quality means different things to different people. For example, your parents might offer you a top quality jacket, perhaps made of the best traditional materials. However, you know that you would never wear it because it is not a style that you would choose or one that you would want to be seen wearing. It does not fit in with the image you are trying to create. Is that a quality item of clothing? The answer is 'yes' for them but 'no' for you.

In health and social care, people see quality (or lack of quality) both in the way in which they are treated while they are using a service and in the outcomes they derive from it. If a mother with young children is moved into more appropriate housing, she will have an opinion about how she was consulted and supported during the process, as well as an opinion about the new housing and how this has changed her living conditions.

Defining quality

Quality was recognised as an important issue in developing successful services and businesses in the early 1980s and the influence of writers at that time is still important. The list below contains several definitions of quality, some of which are still widely used.

Quality is . . .

- fitness for purpose (Juran, 1986)
- conformance to requirements (Crosby, 1984)
- the totality of features and characteristics of a product or service that bear on its ability to satisfy stated or implied needs (International Standards Organisation, 1986)
- the degree of conformance of all the relevant features and characteristics of the product (or service) to all aspects of a customer's need, limited by the price and delivery he or she will accept (Groocock, 1986).

These definitions have many similarities. They all indicate that quality is about meeting the customer's requirements – whether they are stated or implied. If quality is about meeting customers' or service users' requirements, it is important to discover what these requirements are. If you provide services with extras that service users don't want, you will not be adding quality. So how do those who provide the services they think are needed match their ideas with those of service users who often know what they want and need? If you provide what you think are high-quality services because they are provided by well qualified and caring professionals who know what is best, will the service users agree with the professionals and think that they are receiving a high-quality service? Not necessarily! Let us consider which of the definitions we offered earlier are most useful for health and care services.

Fitness for purpose

This is a useful definition when considering what sort of support to deliver or which drugs or equipment to use. If an item fits the purpose for which it is intended, it is a quality product. On the other hand, if an item embodies the latest features or technology but is not suitable for the task in hand, it is, in this context, of poor quality. For example, if an older person needs help with shopping and cleaning, that is the support that he or she requires of a quality service. Providing a place in a residential home would not meet his or her needs, however much better the accommodation and services might seem to the provider.

Conformance to requirements

Crosby's definition means that the requirements must be specified. Such a specification is frequently described as a 'standard' and the specification should give a clear indication of what must be done if the standard is to be met. It should be easy to assess whether a standard has or has not been achieved. Standards are increasingly used in this way in health and social care services, and organisations are often required to conform to standards that are set nationally.

The totality of features and characteristics of a product or service that bear on its ability to satisfy stated or implied needs

Many requirements of those who use health and social care services are implied rather than stated. We can fairly easily predict that patients and service users simply want to improve their health or social well-being as quickly and as painlessly as possible. But they might not always know exactly what services will meet their needs. They might even expect or want services that are inappropriate or potentially harmful. To meet this definition fully, you need to tease out from patients and service users what their implied expectations are. This can be difficult and time-consuming, but the effort is often worthwhile in improving co-operation and mutual understanding.

The degree of conformance of all the relevant features and characteristics of the product or service to all aspects of a customer's need, limited by the price and delivery he or she will accept

You might have preferred Groocock's definition because this is the only one that considers the relationship between meeting customers'

John Oakland (1989) often asks students whether his watch is a quality watch. It has, he says, been insulted all over the world. Typical responses are 'No, it's cheap', 'No, the face is scratched', 'How reliable is it?' and 'I wouldn't wear it'. Rarely is he told that the quality of the watch depends on what the wearer requires from it. Oakland claims he does not need a piece of jewellery to give an impression of wealth. What he requires is a timepiece that also gives him the date in digital form. In his view, he has a quality watch.

requirements and cost. Cost is usually a constraint in the provision of health and social care services. A quality service cannot usually meets all service users' wishes at any cost. Some residents in care homes or patients in hospital may, for example, want their own room with a private telephone and a television. However, managers would probably take the view that the value that customers put on this extra service would not justify the cost. One solution might be to make these extra facilities available but make a charge for them.

The quality chain

You may have a number of customers with very different requirements. Your management role may not involve delivering services directly to patients or service users, but may be in a service that supports a number of activities, for example, a finance or information or personnel service. The concept of a 'chain' of quality is useful in considering the implications of these complex relationships. Quality is an issue in every aspect of a service so, when there are a number of different stages, and links between these stages, there is often the potential for things to go wrong. The *quality chain* uses the idea that the quality of each element and each link is crucial in determining the quality of the whole chain.

People within organisations are often customers of each other's services. For example, you are a customer of your finance department when you receive financial services but, when you provide information to the finance department, it is your customer. Often services are delivered by a sequence of different people – the receptionist may receive and record the arrival of a service user, someone else may interview them to clarify their requirements, someone else may carry out tests and someone else may give them information about what will happen next. This *process* is often referred to as a quality chain. Each person or service in the organisation is both a customer of the preceding person or service and a supplier to the following person or service (Figure 10.1). The quality delivered to the ultimate patient or service user will be a result of services meeting requirements all along the chain. For a quality service to be delivered, requirements have to be met both inside the organisation – between internal suppliers and their customers – and across the organisation's boundary – between internal and external suppliers. Increasingly, people from different health and social care organisations are contributing to a quality chain to deliver more integrated services.

The quality chain may be broken at any point by a person or a piece of equipment not meeting the requirements of the customer, internal or external. In most cases this failure eventually finds its way to the patient or service user, reducing the quality of service provided. In addition, such failure both adds unnecessary costs to the whole activity and has a negative effect on staff morale. Have you experienced the

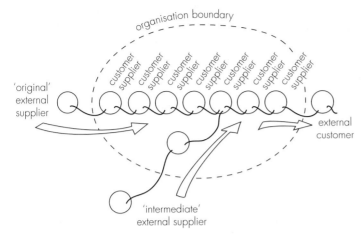

Figure 10.1 The quality chain

frustration of not being able to do your job as effectively as you would wish because of a failure earlier in the quality chain?

So quality is about meeting the needs of all customers, internal and external. Even if your position in the chain in a long way from the final customer, you should think both about your immediate internal customer and about the effect of what you do on the final customer – the patient, service user or carer.

> Quality is needed at every link, otherwise the chain will be broken, and the failure will usually find its way sooner or later to the interface between the organisation and the patient. It is those who work at that interface who experience the problems of records or X-rays not being available, or transport not arriving, or the lack of clean laundry or shabby furniture which adversely affects the service given to the patients, but the failure has occurred some time previously at some other point in the chain.
>
> (Morris, 1989)

Perspectives on quality

To builders constructing an extension to a house, quality might mean principally the standard of workmanship they can put into it and the speed with which they can finish it. The time taken to complete the job would also be important to the householder, but on top of that would be the amount of disruption caused. To the householder, the courtesy of the builders would be a major factor, as would how far the householder felt properly consulted on decisions like where to put the window and what materials to use. The perspectives of providers and customers are different.

In an organisation that gives proper attention to quality, staff will

An example comes from a study of hotel conference services. The hotel staff judged the quality of the coffee breaks they provided for delegates in terms of the flavour of the brew, while the delegates mentioned factors like the speed of delivery, the timing of the coffee break, the space available for conversation and the proximity to toilet facilities.

have working definitions of quality similar to those of their customers. If staff have definitions that are very different from those of their customers, or do not properly understand customers' requirements, customers are likely to be dissatisfied.

Consider the different perspectives that might be held by users of services, providers of services, commissioners of services and the general public. Here are some of their concerns about quality (Table 10.1).

Table 10.1 Different perspectives on quality

Interested parties	Concerns about quality
Service users	Access to services Quality of experience Waiting time Caring and supportive environment
Providers	Professional excellence Concern for patients and service users Efficiency
Commissioners	Number of patients and service users who receive services, related to demand Number of complaints Cost per episode or treatment Concern for patients and service users Information about quality
General public	Fairness Value for money

Patients, service users and carers will be concerned about the outcomes of their treatment and care, about the way they are treated by staff, and about the nature and comfort of their environment. All these will differ for different groups of service users with different expectations and cultural backgrounds.

For providers, there should not necessarily be a conflict between professional excellence and customer requirements. Each profession has a responsibility to ensure that part of what is valued by senior members of the profession is a commitment to meeting all the requirements of the customer. However, providers are not necessarily a homogeneous group and different professional groups may have different points of view. For example, a physician may wish to treat a patient with a new drug because he or she believes that it will offer the quickest solution or be the one with least side effects, and therefore be the 'best' for the patient. However, if this treatment takes longer than conventional treatments, it may prevent the contracted target number being reached by the provider organisation.

Commissioners are likely to share patients' and service users' concerns about access to services and the effectiveness of treatment.

Figure 10.2 Quality means different things to different people

They will be particularly interested in the number of patients treated and the cost per treatment. They will also require a considerable amount of information about quality standards in provider organisations.

Although many members of the public have used health or social care services, they may also have broader concerns, in particular about fairness, access and value for money.

ACTIVITY 10.1

1   Which groups of people influence quality in your area of activity?
2   In what ways do these groups differ in their perceptions of what constitutes a quality service?
3   How could these differences be reconciled?

Though your room for manoeuvre may be limited, part of your job as a manager is to reconcile different perceptions of quality. Ways of thinking that might help towards reconciliation include:

- 'putting the patient or service user first' as a way of setting priorities and cutting through competing requirements
- remembering that health and social care organisations are designed to cope with populations, but it is individuals who are patients and service users
- facilitating good communication between the different parties by being open about any differences
- not exaggerating the differences – even the pressure to cut costs can be mitigated if providers and commissioners agree that quality is important.

Meeting all the requirements of customers, stated or implied, while keeping costs to a minimum, is often far from easy. It is well worth investing the effort in reconciling requirements because:

- it will give you a better idea of what you are aiming at
- you will be better able to monitor and demonstrate the performance of your service
- if all your staff are on the same wavelength, your team's energy can be directed towards providing the service, rather than resolving differences.

Managers play an important role in ensuring that service users' expectations and perspectives about quality in service delivery are respected, even if they cannot always be met.

WHY IS QUALITY IMPORTANT?

In one sense, attention to quality must be worthwhile if people are concerned about it. We would go further, however, and suggest that attention to quality is important for three main reasons:

- it is important to service users
- it is important to your staff
- it helps you reduce costs.

Importance to service users

Service users not only benefit directly if their requirements are better met, but also indirectly if they feel confident that, next time they visit you, they will also be treated well.

Service users and their relatives are often worried, anxious, stressed, frightened and vulnerable. Such feelings are exacerbated by long waits, insufficient information, insensitivity to their needs and poor facilities. All that can be done to lessen these feelings and improve the quality of their experiences will be well received. When you are well, you can cope with a long wait in the supermarket, showers not working in the sports centre and a patronising bank manager – all aspects of poor quality in other service organisations. When you are in need of treatment or care, however, you are not so resilient to or tolerant of bad service and your appreciation for the good service you have received is all the greater.

Importance to staff

The majority of staff who work in health and social care have a real desire and commitment to care for people in need, often sacrificing opportunities for more money or more convenient working hours. If a service is not organised properly, staff are likely to find it more difficult to provide the level of care that they wish to and become frustrated and demotivated.

A well designed quality improvement programme, empowering staff to decide what can be done and then supporting them in their efforts to improve quality, is one way out of this spiral. The benefits to you and your staff are likely to include:

- increased job satisfaction
- less frustration
- greater self-worth as your department's reputation grows in the community
- better feedback from patients or service users.

Importance for reducing costs

It is not difficult to persuade people that improving quality will be better for both service users and staff. But it is often less easy to persuade them that improving quality can also save money.

Consider a company making microwave ovens which has, on average, 5 per cent of its products defective in some way. If it does not improve the quality of its basic processes, it will have to employ teams of checkers to pick out the ovens that are defective. It will then need to rework the defective products, incurring still more costs. Ovens may be returned by dissatisfied customers, incurring both transport and repair or replacement costs. Perhaps most importantly, the company will acquire a poor reputation and fewer people will buy its ovens. All this is a recipe for going out of business.

The cost of reducing the frequency of such problems will be small by comparison. Moreover, if quality had been built in when the plant was first designed, the extra cost of providing better quality would have been lower still and the company would have had a competitive edge both on quality and on cost.

The costs of poor quality in service industries may be more difficult to estimate, but they are nevertheless still evident, as shown in the following quotations.

> Service companies waste anywhere from 30–35% of their operating costs by not doing things right.
>
> (Hutton, 1988)

> In 1988 it was estimated that up to 25% of [National Westminster Bank's] operating costs were absorbed in the difference between the costs actually incurred in accomplishing a task, and the costs that would be incurred if a 'right first time' approach were to be successfully adopted.
>   The iceberg effect of failure costs demonstrates that above the water line are the obvious costs of failure – rework, rechecking, query handling, complaint handling, and waived fees. Below the line, and representing a far greater problem, including lost repeat business, lost customers, staff overtime, machine downtime, and bad employee morale.
>
> (Department of Trade and Industry, 1990)

In health and social care services too, studies have estimated the costs of not doing things right:

> Good quality may not always save money, but poor quality always costs and usually wastes money.
>
> (Carruthers and Holland, 1991)

At Doncaster Royal Infirmary such costs were estimated at 28 per cent of the revenue budget. At Cheltenham General Hospital, the costs of not doing things right amounted to £4 million – over 20 per cent of total costs. These costs could never be brought down to zero, but the scope for large savings and increases in the quality of care is considerable.

DO YOU HAVE A QUALITY PROBLEM?

In each of the situations in Table 10.2, there are implications for patients, for staff and for costs arising from poor quality.

It may be that these examples do not map precisely on to your service, but it should not be too difficult to see that flaws in service always carry implications further along the quality chain, particularly in terms of the time needed to sort out problems after the event. Quality, then, is not just about making things better for service users and other customers: it is also about cutting out unnecessary costs.

Table 10.2 Quality problems

Description	Implications for service users	Implications for staff	Cost implications
Health records missing or out of date	Frustration at having to repeat history Wrong treatment offered	Histories need taking again Internal inquiries	Extra time spent searching or taking histories Extra consultations Expensive/complex remedial treatments
Insufficient car-parking facilities	Patients late for appointments	Staff late for appointments Low morale	Staff (or patients) kept waiting Capital equipment not used to fullest capacity
Discharge delayed because drugs to take home are not available	Longer stay	Unnecessary work for all staff	Repeated appointments Higher accommodation costs Slower throughput
Porters not available to move patients to operating theatre	Delays in operations Sicker patients Patients in for longer	Delays in operations Inter-staff tensions	Expensive staff and plant underused More costly treatments for patients' worsened conditions
Patients kept waiting over an hour for prebooked appointments	Stress and frustration Car parks full	Ambulances held up Staff on the defensive	Higher accommodation costs Extra staff time on explaining and mollifying Need for larger waiting rooms and car parks

ACTIVITY 10.2

Estimate:
1   What percentage of time is spent by you and your staff in sorting out problems? (Consider all problems, including those caused by people outside your department.)
2   What percentage of these problems are new ones?
3   How many major quality problems can you identify in your own area of activity?

This Activity should suggest to you that there is the potential for reducing costs by better attention to quality in your department. Typical responses by managers outside health and social care services are up to 98 per cent for item 1 and 4 to 5 per cent for item 2. How did you compare? Is there a fundamental message here? If there is, it will help to pinpoint the major quality problems affecting your area of activity. From your encounter with the notion of quality chains, you will probably already be able to identify which of these problems are:

■ your own responsibility
■ upstream of your responsibilities
■ downstream of your responsibilities.

Having established where there are problems that you are aware of, it is also important to check that you have considered all aspects of quality in your area of work. So we now turn to the different 'dimensions' of quality.

DIMENSIONS OF QUALITY

Quality has many components. It is not sufficient to satisfy some requirements but not others. The aim should be to meet *all* the requirements of customers, stated or implied. Robert Maxwell of the King Edward's Hospital Fund for London proposed six dimensions of quality in health care that have been used widely by health authorities. Table 10.3 presents these in a slightly adapted form so that they are equally applicable to quality in social care.

Table 10.3 Dimensions of quality in care services

Dimensions	For example . . .
Access to services	Are services convenient geographically? Are waiting times for services, the physical design of buildings, the availability of transport and car parking acceptable?
Equity	Are services provided to all potential service users, whatever their cultural, racial or social backgrounds?
Relevance to need	Do services reflect the needs of the population served? Are there any gaps in meeting needs?
Social acceptability	Is the way services are provided acceptable to the people they are intended to serve?
Efficiency	Are services delivered as efficiently as possible within the resources available? Are services cost-effective and appropriately staffed?
Effectiveness	Do services achieve the intended benefits and outcomes in terms of the health and social care of the people served?

(Source: adapted from Maxwell (1984) 'Quality assessment in health' *British Medical Journal*, 13: 31–4, with permission from the BMJ Publishing Group)

These dimensions have proved very useful for evaluating services. They also offer managers a checklist for setting standards for a service.

However, for day-to-day management, it might also be useful to have a set of factors that relate more closely to the requirements of individuals. For example, although each service user would like to be treated 'efficiently', he or she might have a number of more personal concerns. The Department of Health (1989) listed seven dimensions of quality that need to be satisfied for an individual patient. Slightly adapted so that they are relevant for managers in any health or social care setting, they are:

■ appropriateness of treatment and care
■ achievement of optimum clinical or social care outcomes
■ all clinical procedures and professional actions should minimise complications and other preventable events
■ an attitude that treats service users with dignity and as individuals
■ an environment conducive to the safety, reassurance and comfort of service users
■ speed of response to service users' needs and minimum inconvenience to them (and their relatives and friends)
■ involvement of service users in their own care.

The next Activity invites you to consider how these two sets of dimensions of quality map on to your services and your customers.

ACTIVITY 10.3

Make a note of the dimensions of quality from Maxwell's list or the Department of Health's list that are most relevant to your main customers. Add any additional dimensions that are not on either list.

From this Activity you should be able to judge which classification is most useful to you, or whether you need to devise a special set of dimensions of quality for the services for which you are responsible.

The relationship between perceptions and expectations

Finally, three further pointers on quality in services may be useful to you in establishing exactly what quality means for your area. These derive from research by Berry *et al.* (1985), who carried out in-depth interviews of customers for a wide range of services.

Customers judge quality by comparing their perceptions of what they receive to their expectations of what they should receive. This point is important to understanding and controlling service quality because both expectations and perceptions are experiential states of mind rather than necessarily being real. A customer who waits, knowing it will be 30 minutes before he or she is served, may be happier than one who waits only half as long but does not know how long the wait will be.

(Haywood-Farmer, 1988)

■ *Consumers' perceptions of service quality result from a comparison of their expectations with their actual experience of the service.* The quality of a service is not just determined by the customer's reaction to it. It also depends on the customer's expectations. For example, an airline offering inter-city travel in the United States was experiencing problems with a flight scheduled to leave at 8 a.m. and arrive at 8.40 a.m.: it frequently arrived late. However, when they changed the schedule to say that it would arrive at 9 a.m., the plane was never late and passengers' perceptions of quality were much improved!

■ *Quality perceptions are derived from the service process as well as from the service outcome.* Service users remember the process as well as the outcome. This is, of course, well recognised by staff in health and social care. One example is that of maternity services. Coming home with a healthy baby, while of prime importance, is certainly not the only matter of concern for the baby's parents. What kind of a time they had and how they were treated will be remembered for the rest of their lives.

■ *Service quality is of two types, normal and exceptional.* First, there is the level of quality at which the normal service is delivered. Second, there is the level of the quality at which exceptions and problems are handled. If, for example, you were to compare the quality of service provided in different department stores, your analysis would not be complete without finding out how each store handled customers wishing to return goods.

This chapter has concentrated on definitions of 'quality' and why quality is so important for service users, staff and budgets. A key element in most definitions of 'quality' is the relationship between providers' and customers' requirements and expectations. This relationship is no simple matter in health and social care services, in which expectations and requirements among the many parties in the system may be very different from each other. None the less, we have analysed some of the key dimensions of quality that health and social care services should meet, and offered you opportunities to match them against your own workplace experiences. You should now be able to begin to identify whether there are quality problems in your service and what they are. In the next chapter, we consider how to set quality standards and ensure that they are achieved.

REFERENCES

Berry, L., Zeithaml, V. and Parasuraman, A. (1985) *A Practical Approach to Quality*, Joiner Associates Inc.

Carruthers, I. and Holland, P. (1991) 'Quality assurance – choice for the individual', *International Journal of Health Care Quality Assurance*, 4(2): 9–17.

Crosby, P. B. (1984) *Quality Without Tears*, McGraw-Hill.

Department of Health (1989) *Working for Patients* (CM555), HMSO.

Department of Trade and Industry (1990) *The Case for Costing Quality*, HMSO.

Groocock, J. M. (1986) *The Chain of Quality*, John Wiley & Sons.

Haywood-Farmer, J. (1988) 'A conceptual model of service quality', *International Journal of Operations and Production Management*, 8(6): 19–29.

Hutton, M. (1988) *Total Quality Management: The Crosby Approach*, Crosby Associates UK.

International Standards Organisation (1986) *Quality Vocabulary: Part 1, International Terms*, ISO.

Juran, J. M. (1986) 'The quality trilogy', *Quality Progress*, 19(8): 19–24.

Maxwell, R. (1984) 'Quality assessment in health', *British Medical Journal*, 13: 31–4.

Morris, B. (1989) 'Total quality management', *International Journal of Health Care Quality Assurance*, 2(3): 4–6.

Oakland, J. (1989) *Total Quality Management*, Heinemann.

CHAPTER 11

WORKING WITH STANDARDS

Quality is not achieved simply by trying a bit harder. You can be confident that you are achieving – and continuing to achieve – high-quality results only by setting up a system that will enable you to monitor them. This involves identifying what quality means for your area of work and then setting standards related to the outcomes required. Without clear and achievable quality standards, staff cannot have sufficient clarity about what is required, and have no way of knowing whether they have achieved what is required of them.

The process of setting standards, monitoring to measure results against them and taking action if they are not fully achieved is similar to setting personal objectives, monitoring whether they are being achieved and taking appropriate action if they are not. As with objectives, standards need to be clear and unambiguous if you are to monitor quality effectively. However, there is an additional issue: expectations of quality change. Once a quality standard is achieved, there is often an expectation that this will be used as the basis for improvement. Quality is not something that can be achieved and then maintained at the same level for ever. Most quality standards need to improve steadily, even if slowly, to match the rising expectations of service users. In this session we discuss the role of standards, how they can be set, and how they relate to the outcomes required of a service.

Because it is important that a standard should be measurable, there is a temptation to emphasise aspects of a service that can readily be measured. But much work in health and social care is difficult to measure in ways that seem meaningful. For example, it is easy to measure how many people have been visited in their homes, but it is much less easy to measure whether a visit resulted in an appropriate outcome. There may be a tendency to direct activities towards achieving standards that are easy to measure and to neglect areas of work for which standards do not yet exist. Similarly, when standards are set and measured nationally, there may be an over-emphasis on particular areas of work. None the less, managers are increasingly expected to understand how to work with standards and to be able to use them in effective and meaningful ways in their areas of work.

WHAT IS A STANDARD?

When you set a standard for an activity you are:

- explicitly stating a view of your customers' requirements
- communicating to staff that these requirements are important
- establishing that this is the target to be achieved at the present time.

A useful way of visualising the role of standards in quality management is shown in Figure 11.1. The standard is the chock that prevents the quality of service ball from rolling back down the hill. The position that has been achieved is the standard at the moment and is the position to be maintained. For example, you may have a standard that service users will be seen within 30 minutes of their appointment time. The chock is currently at 30 minutes, but to achieve real excellence it needs to be moved nearer the top of the hill, by resetting the standard to a shorter waiting time. There is, however, likely to be a cost implication of deciding to raise a standard. Resourcing levels and ways of working often have to change in order to achieve higher standards.

However, once you have achieved the current standard, you will usually be expected to push the ball further up the hill and to place the chock at a higher level. This process continues until you reach the top of the hill and customers' requirements are fully met. But even when you reach the top of the hill you will find another hill – there will always be further scope for improvement. Customers' requirements are likely to change, and research and evidence-based practice will affect the standards you set. The process is never-ending and is one of continual improvement.

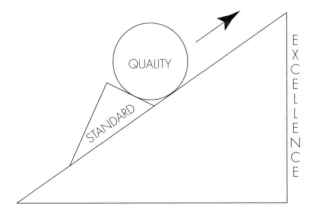

Figure 11.1 Quality 'ball on the hill'
(Source: Koch, 1991)

ACTIVITY 11.1

A health authority defined a standard as 'an agreed level of performance negotiated within available resources'.

Is this comprehensive enough? Or are there other requirements for an effective standard? Make a note of the qualities you think an effective standard should have.

Compare your notes with the following suggestions. Standards should be:

Measurable and capable of being monitored

If they are not, you will not know to what extent they are being met. Measurement does not have to be numerical, but it does involve assessing something that can be seen to have been achieved or not. You need to consider how easily a standard can be monitored – the last thing health and social care services need is more paperwork!

Realistic and attainable with available resources

It is no good having standards that cannot be achieved with the resources available to you. This would only lower motivation and morale. If the standard you can achieve at the moment is not what your customers require, you may need to make improvements in stages. You could develop a standard that goes some way to meeting customers' needs, while informing commissioners and service users that this is just an interim standard that you are making efforts to improve. The example quoted earlier is a case in point. No one would pretend that a wait of 30 minutes is ideal, but it was set because it could be achieved and it may be possible to improve on it later.

Real and important indicators of quality

There is always a temptation to set standards that are easy to monitor but are not necessarily central to service users' experiences. Numbers of people seen is an example – neither high nor low counts necessarily express the quality of the experience.

Expressed clearly and unambiguously

There should not be confusion about whether or not standards have been achieved.

Consistent with service aims and values

Your department and organisation must be able to demonstrate that they have a strategy to achieve their stated aims.

Set in conjunction with the people who will be asked to achieve them

If they are not, staff may be alienated by the standards rather than motivated by them. A key question in setting standards is who should participate in their development. If your team are to be committed to achieving a higher standard, it is often helpful to involve them in setting the standard and in planning how the new level can be achieved.

Frameworks of standards

It is important to be explicit about how standard setting fits in with your department's overall policy on quality management. You need to think about all the stages in a service user's experience and examine the quality problems that occur at each stage. Otherwise you may find that you are developing excellent standards in one area but ignoring other areas that are equally important to service users.

Setting standards in health and social care is not solely your prerogative and that of your staff. Increasingly, national standards are being introduced through National Service Frameworks, Performance Assessment Frameworks and (in England) by the recommendations of the National Institute for Clinical Effectiveness. Comparisons between the performance of different organisations against national standards are important both in relation to 'best value', which requires local government to review services to ensure that they are providing value for money, and in relation to inspections by, for example, the Social Services Inspectorate, the Audit Commission and the Commission for Health Improvement. In setting standards you need to pay attention to the national policy context, research into the effectiveness of alternative treatments and care interventions, the results of inspections, and the policies and strategies of your own organisation.

Standards in many areas of professional work have traditionally been set and monitored by professional bodies and have often not been expressed in such measurable terms as we are proposing. Some health

Standards are not set to overrule or ignore good professional work and judgement but to acknowledge that performance in any area of care and service can vary both with individual members of staff over time, and between them.

(Koch, 1991)

and social care professionals are not convinced that standards are appropriate in their work. They argue that it is impossible to specify what a professional should do in all situations, that it is necessary to exercise professional judgement and that the aim of professional training and qualification is to prepare professionals to make appropriate judgements.

Others argue that standards based on professional consensus about good practice are useful, even if there will occasionally be circumstances that require different actions. Standards do not replace professional judgement, but set targets that can be understood by everyone involved – including both professionals and others who contribute to achieving the standards, and service users who are expecting a service of the quality indicated by the standards. The test of the usefulness of a standard is whether it is helpful in monitoring and improving the quality of service provided.

When standards are set by Government agencies or commissioners, and are linked to inspection or funding, the role of managers is to organise their area of service delivery to ensure that the standards are achieved. This is often not easy because most health and social care services are essentially responsive – they are offered to those who need them when they need them. To some extent, the volume of demand can be predicted, but there are times when demand outstrips the ability of services to respond, as in flu epidemics or in very cold weather when those who can normally live safely in their own homes may need extra care. If standards are set in the expectation that demand will be steady, it is often not possible to achieve them fully when the level of demand increases suddenly. In such circumstances standards might be seen as indicators of a problem, as 'tools' to help managers to keep track of the extent to which the service is under pressure rather than as 'rules' that must be followed to avoid some sort of punishment.

Another problem is that there may be a tendency to direct work solely towards the achievement of a standard, rather than to focus on delivery of a service that meets the needs of the service user. In some cases, the emphasis on achieving standards can even lead to a temptation to subvert standards, for example, by not putting people on waiting lists so that the lists appear shorter.

However, especially when standards are agreed with the involvement of those who will work to achieve them, they can be very helpful in improving the quality of services. National standards provide a framework of expectations as the basis for developing services that offer equally high quality to service users wherever they live. The use of standards in health and social care is increasing and the ways in which standards are used can be expected to develop and change.

DEVELOPING A STANDARD

In many areas of health and social care, there are not yet standards for teams to work towards and managers are often asked to develop appropriate standards. The aim should be to develop realistic standards that will encourage people towards their achievement. The approach you take will depend on your understanding of the abilities, commitment and motivation of the people in your team.

ACTIVITY 11.2

Choose one aspect of the service(s) for which you are responsible that is in need of improvement and for which no standard is set currently. Who should participate in setting the standard? List all those you would include.

Patients, service users and carers are sure to come near the top of your list. It will doubtless include the professional, administrative and technical staff involved in your area of activity, as well as other managers and commissioners. You might also include members of staff who have had experience of developing standards in other areas. To what extent each of these groups is involved is an issue for you to decide, but it is important that none of them feels excluded from the process.

ACTIVITY 11.3

Imagine that you are managing a department responsible for providing physiotherapy services. The department's job includes:

■ defining criteria for service provision
■ receiving and recording referrals
■ making appointments
■ recording patients' attendances
■ assessing patients' needs for therapy
■ planning the treatment for each patient
■ making sure that equipment appropriate to patients' needs is available
■ delivering therapy treatments
■ supervising therapy treatments
■ recording the outcome of each therapy session in a patient's notes.

What information would be available to you if you were setting standards for performance in this area of work? What methods could you use to gain more information?

There may be standards that have been set nationally, for example, standards for waiting times. There may be standards that have been developed by those commissioning the physiotherapy services or by the hospital to which this department belongs, either in this area of work or in similar areas. Previous managers or staff in this area of work may have already done some work that provides a starting point for setting standards.

A number of approaches are available if you need more information:

- You could carry out a time study for frequently repeated routine tasks such as assessing patients and recording attendances, in order to establish target times that staff are confident can be achieved. However, it is also important that the standards identify the different components of what should be achieved within the target time, for example, assessing a patient within a particular period of time, completing the form used for recording the assessment accurately and passing the information to the appropriate person.
- You may find it useful to carry out sample surveys of the most frequently performed functions. For example, you might check the availability of equipment and whether it is functioning properly. Some equipment may be shared with wards and not kept in the physiotherapy department, making the task of ensuring its availability for clinic sessions more difficult.
- You might look at past performance to establish, for example, how many patients have been seen each week in the past three months. This might be useful as a basis for establishing how many patients can be treated each week, but it may not reveal how many patients need to return for further treatment and thus have to be counted two or more times. The standard should reflect aspects of good practice that are meaningful to staff in your area.

In using any of these methods, you will have to involve the staff concerned if they are to feel committed to the standards of performance that are eventually defined.

Whatever standards are being set, for whatever purpose, two key considerations always apply:

- *It is no use setting a standard unless there is a way of measuring performance.* It can be argued that, merely by setting a standard, performance can be improved even if there is no way of measuring it. However, people will realise fairly quickly that there is no monitoring, and other standards, which can be monitored, may be thrown into disrepute.

■ *The best standard is one that enables the person doing the job to see fairly easily when performance is satisfactory.* It is helpful for staff to be able to use standards to monitor their own performance. Consider, for example, drivers collecting people from their homes to bring them to a day centre. There is scope here for setting a standard that allows drivers to be flexible while still meeting a time target. They might need a target that allows them to adjust their schedule to accommodate any local difficulties that develop with individuals as they are collected.

It is important to set standards that are achievable and that help the process of service delivery rather than presenting obstacles. If standards do not enable staff to be flexible in responding to the needs of individual service users, both staff and service users will find the standard a hindrance rather than a benefit. If a standard takes a lot of work to monitor and seems to address a trivial aspect of service delivery, staff will find it tedious and irrelevant. It is also important to recognise that standards are set to address performance under fairly stable conditions and there may be times when it is impossible to achieve them.

ACTIVITY 11.4

Choose one of the key processes of your department or section. Devise one appropriate standard against which to measure the successful outcome of part of this process.

Now test this standard against the following criteria and tick each one that it meets:

	Yes	*No*
Is it measurable?	❏	❏
Is it attainable?	❏	❏
Does it address quality (not just numbers)?	❏	❏
Is it clear and unambiguous?	❏	❏
Is it consistent with service aims and values?	❏	❏

If your standard does not meet all of these criteria, try to amend it so that it does.

It is often useful to subdivide a standard into a number of component parts when an activity is complex. Smaller components can make monitoring the achievement of the standard easier. In the following example a standard developed for social workers (Smyth *et al.*, 1999) is subdivided into five elements.

Standard: The social worker works in partnership with individuals and, where necessary, carers to assess needs and to agree and plan a response to meet needs.

Element 1: The social worker seeks consent to carry out an assessment of need with service users and involves carers and others where appropriate.
Element 2: The social worker, in partnership with service users and where necessary and appropriate carers, carries out an assessment of need, taking risk factors into consideration.
Element 3: The social worker and service users agree priorities and ways of working together to meet identified needs and risks.
Element 4: The social worker and service users identify and confirm support and resources to implement the action plan.
Element 5: The social worker co-ordinates and records the agreed action plan.

Each element is then subdivided into performance criteria that clearly and specifically describe the work to be undertaken. For example, here are the performance criteria for Element 1.

■ The role and responsibilities of the social worker and the purpose of assessment are explained to service users.
■ The consent of service users is obtained to consult with others to carry out an assessment and to take any immediate action necessary within an agreed time-scale.
■ Any immediate action necessary is carried out and any services are agreed as temporary until endorsement by a full assessment.
■ Reasons for and use of assessment information given by others are clearly explained.
■ Service users are empowered to exercise their rights to give feedback . . . on the quality of services and to make complaints.
■ Service users are advised of advocacy services available within the area.

This approach provides a great deal of detail about how the standard should be achieved.

Another technique is to proceed in steps. This is useful when a new standard is introduced into an area of work and it is expected that staff will speed up as they become used to the new way of working. Consider, for example, a standard to complete care plans for all patients who have been in hospital for more than 24 hours. If it is not practicable to achieve this immediately, interim targets might be set as in Table 11.1.

Table 11.1 Proceeding in steps

Months to	Percentage completed
December	70
March	85
June	95
September	100

This gives staff time to change their practices – and perhaps additional resources to be provided – to achieve the target fully.

Basing standards on dimensions of quality

In order to ensure that standards are real and important measures of quality, it is often helpful to base them on dimensions of quality. One way of doing this is to use the dimensions proposed by Maxwell (1984) – access, equity, relevance to need, social acceptability, efficiency and effectiveness. To set the standard, you need to consider quality issues relating to ensuring that the service is accessible to everyone, meets specific needs in a way that is socially acceptable and is delivered in a way that is both efficient and effective.

Another framework for dimensions of quality is the NHS Performance Assessment Framework, in which the dimensions are health improvement, fair access, effective delivery of appropriate health care, efficiency, patient/carer experience and health outcomes of NHS care. Table 11.2 shows how this framework has been used to set standards for the provision of a cervical cytology screening programme.

STRUCTURE, PROCESS, OUTCOME

Some standards are easy to measure – such as the waiting time we discussed earlier, or that an ambulance should respond to an emergency within 14 minutes in an urban area and 19 minutes in a rural area. It is relatively easy to identify such standards and to monitor whether they have been achieved. But what about setting standards for services that might be delivered over a longer period or that are more complex? Services in which it is harder to set numerical standards might include the care of older people or of people with learning difficulties. These areas require more sophisticated standards that reflect some of the complexities of the service, rather than simple counts of outcomes.

Issues like these led Avedis Donabedian (1980) to distinguish three critical components for written and measurable standards of care:

Table 11.2 Quality standards for the provision of a cervical cytology screening programme

Areas	Aspects of performance	Standard	Criteria
Health improvement	Overall health of populations, reflecting social and environmental factors and individual behaviour as well as care provided by NHS and other agencies	Health authority should only offer screening to women for whom it has been agreed that it is appropriate	Women between 20 and 65 should be offered screening every three years unless there are sound medical reasons not to do so Women who have had full hysterectomies or are already undergoing treatment should be excluded If last smear positive, women over 65 should be offered screening until they have had three negative smears
Fair access	Fairness of provision of services in relation to need on various dimensions: ■ geographical ■ socio-economic ■ demographic (age, ethnicity, sex) ■ care groups (e.g. people with learning difficulties)	Health authority should ensure that all women have access to cervical cytology screening programme (if appropriate) at least once every three years and that this access should be made as easy as possible	There should be a register of all women in the health authority's area All appropriate women should be invited to attend for screening at least every three years Screening should be offered by all GPs and health centres Women should be able to make their own appointments Letters sent to women should be informative
		All appropriate women should be offered screening regardless of their race, creed, social class and geographic location	Access to screening services should be available in all locations in district Screening should be offered to all women residents Reminder letters should be sent to all women in district Health visitors should follow up all women who either fail to attend an appointment or fail to make one
Effective delivery of appropriate health care	Extent to which services are: ■ clinically effective (interventions or care packages are evidence-based) ■ appropriate to need	Health authority should minimise number of women who die of cervical cancer	Mortality rate from cervical cancer should be lower in population of women accepting screening than in population not accepting screening

continued . . . .

Table 11.2 continued

Areas	Aspects of performance	Standard	Criteria
	■ timely ■ in line with agreed standards ■ provided according to best practice ■ delivered by appropriately trained and educated staff		All appropriate women should be screened every three years Health authority should attain nationally and/or locally agreed targets for percentage coverage of women eligible for screening
Efficiency	Extent to which NHS provides efficient services, including: ■ cost per unit of care/outcome ■ productivity of capital estate ■ labour productivity	Service should ensure that smears are taken, processed and reported on without undue delay and at lowest cost possible, while ensuring that service remains effective and acceptable	All recall letters should be sent within three years of date last smear was taken All smears taken should be sent to appropriate laboratory within three working days All results should be reported to woman (if appropriate), place smear was taken (e.g. GP's surgery or clinic) and central register controlling programme
Patient/carer experience	Patient/carer perceptions of delivery of services, including: ■ responsiveness to individual needs and preferences ■ skill, care and continuity of service provision ■ patient involvement, relevant information and choice ■ waiting and accessibility ■ physical environment ■ courtesy of administrative arrangements	Screening service should be acceptable at all stages to women resident in district	Letter sent inviting women to attend should be sensitively expressed Rooms where smears taken should ensure women are given privacy Letters sent informing women of results should be sensitively expressed and women with positive results should be informed in person rather than by letter
Health outcomes of NHS care	NHS success in using its resources to: ■ reduce levels of risk factors ■ reduce levels of disease, impairment and complications of treatment ■ improve quality of life for patients and carers ■ reduce premature deaths		

(Source: adapted from Department of Health, 1998)

- *Structure* – the physical and organisational framework within which care is given. This includes the staff, facilities and equipment available, the environment within which the care is delivered and the documentation of procedures and policies.
- *Process* – the actual procedures and practices implemented by staff in the design, delivery and evaluation of care.
- *Outcome* – the effect of that care on the service user plus the costs of providing that care.

An example of the use of these headings is given in the following description of an adult mental health service.

Structure, process and outcome in mental health

Structure refers to aspects of the physical environment (e.g. quality of decor and furnishings, accessibility of unit to clients) and to certain characteristics of the social environment (e.g. staffing ratios, skill mix). These are all relatively static factors or fixtures which generally do not change much during an episode of client contact.

Process is concerned with events during a treatment episode. Typical process factors include the nature and speed of response to referrals, allocation of cases, decisions about treatment or therapy, therapist time per client, and case-note recording.

Outcome refers to the results of the team's intervention. It can be considered in terms of the extent to which the client has been helped or her/his problem resolved, and is a direct measure of the clinical effectiveness of treatment or therapy. Other outcomes might relate to the degree of client satisfaction with the service or the extent to which the need for other specialised or costly services (e.g. acute psychiatric admissions) has been reduced.

(Burbach and Quarry, 1991)

All three areas of structure, process and outcome are important to any health or social care service, though possibly with differing emphases, depending on the nature of the service. In the case of services for people with learning disabilities, some researchers – such as King *et al.* (1971) – say that the process area may be the most important. In relation to health care in general, Koch (1991) says that, 'Outcome is more difficult to define than structure and process standards and is arguably the most important of the three.'

For an example of how the headings of structure, process and outcome can be used in practice, have a look at Table 11.3, which is a standard for an occupational therapy service.

Table 11.3 Standards for the occupational therapy service of Fife Health Board

Standard statement The occupational therapist will ensure that any child who attends Robert Hennyson School and lives at home will have an annual home visit to enhance a continuity of approach between school staff and parents and up-to-date knowledge and provision of specialist equipment.

Structure	Process	Outcome
Occupational therapist will have access to the child's record of needs	Occupational therapist will discuss child's needs and abilities with parents in areas of seating, bathing, toileting, feeding, positioning, and others as indicated by earlier assessment	Every child living at home and attending Robert Hennyson School will be visited in home by occupational therapist at least once a year
Occupational therapist will have access to other members of school staff to discuss child's current needs and functioning	Occupational therapist will offer advice and guidance to parents in above areas, and reinforce their role in using particular techniques or equipment	Parents will understand practice and principles of occupational therapy and equipment used with child, and reinforce approach used in school in home setting
Occupational therapist will discuss child with physiotherapy and community occupational therapy staff to assess need for joint home visit	Occupational therapist will discuss with family the range of statutory and non-statutory services available to them	Parents with children attending Robert Hennyson School will have access to specialist occupational therapy advice regarding home environment
Occupational therapist will ensure that time outside normal school hours is made available to carry out home visits	Occupational therapist will assess suitability of house for child and family and, where present environment is unsuitable, make recommendations as to adaptations required, or support rehousing application	Therapist will be able to meet parents outside school setting to ensure greater understanding of home situation, and parents will have opportunity to discuss child's functioning at home in that setting

continued . . . .

Table 11.3 continued

Structure	Process	Outcome
Occupational therapist will contact parents to arrange mutually convenient time to carry out visit	Occupational therapist will review with parents any equipment in the home, its use by them and its appropriateness in meeting current needs of parents and child	Written evidence will be available as to appropriateness of home environment and recommendations for any action to improve this
Occupational therapist will have transport suitable for visit	Occupational therapist will record home visits in keeping with Fife Health Board's occupational therapy policy and forward this to team members	Team members working with child will receive annual update on child's functioning in home environment, with particular emphasis on activities of daily living and use of special equipment
Occupational therapist will have records of his/her previous contacts with child in keeping with local occupational therapy policy	Occupational therapist will record home visit in monthly returns	Occupational therapy register will identify frequency of home visits with child
	Occupational therapist will contact social work department's occupational therapist regarding any additional requirements for equipment	

(Source: based on Kitson, 1986)

ACTIVITY 11.5

Consider how you might apply Donabedian's classification to your work area, using the headings 'structure', 'process' and 'outcome'. Choose an aspect of your service for which there is no existing standard. Many people find that it is helpful to think first about what outcome is to be achieved, then to consider what processes would achieve that outcome and finally to consider what structures are required to carry out the processes.

Once you are confident that you can draft a standard, you will be in a good position to review and revise standards for your area of work. Perhaps standard setting should be an agenda item for a meeting with your staff. Developing standards may seem like a daunting task. But many examples of good practice exist – whether in the form of standards from other parts of your organisation, from other organisations or from professional bodies. Adapting these may provide a helpful starting point.

MONITORING STANDARDS

Developing service standards is a time-consuming process, but it can focus attention on problem areas and suggest improvements that can be quickly implemented. However, the main benefits come from sustained monitoring of performance against standards to establish the extent to which they are being met. If the service is not meeting its standards, there is work to be done to find out why and to rectify the problems. If performance is better than expected, it is still important to investigate the reasons for this in order to discover ways of continuing to improve. Hugh Koch summarised this process neatly as shown in Figure 11.2.

Monitoring means 'continuous or regularly repeated observations of important parts of the service structure, process, output or outcome'.

(Morgan and Everett, 1991)

In designing a monitoring procedure there are many decisions to be made:

■ what to monitor
■ why you want to monitor it

Figure 11.2 Monitoring standards
(Source: Koch, 1991)

- how often you should monitor it
- the level of detail required
- who will collect the information and how
- how reliable the information will be
- if the information could be fed into a computer for analysis
- who should receive the information
- how the information will be used.

Monitoring can take many forms, for example, counting how many people are on a waiting list or in a waiting room, measuring service users' satisfaction with carefully designed questionnaires, or noting how long it takes a patient to recover after an operation. Deciding what to monitor and how to do it is a key task. Sensitivity may be needed to avoid monitoring being intrusive to staff or service users. Involving staff in making choices will be important in gaining their commitment to recording accurate measurements.

The methods chosen for monitoring depend to some extent on how the standards have been drawn up. Though many different factors might be measured and compared, there are essentially two main approaches:

- Count the percentage of occasions when the standard is achieved (for example, the percentage of service users who were seen within 30 minutes of their appointment time).
- Record whether the standard has been achieved, partially achieved or not achieved in the period being considered. This is especially useful where standards are set using the structure–process–outcome model. Table 11.4 shows a form from an occupational therapy service, on which a record of results can be made as well as notes of further actions to be taken.

ACTIVITY 11.6

Look back at your notes for the previous Activity. How could you monitor these standards for structure, process and outcomes?

Your answer might have included planning who should keep records of what and how frequently. You might have considered whether records should be paper-based or computer-based and how the information should be stored and used.

Monitoring is essentially about ensuring that information on whether standards are being achieved is collected regularly and in sufficient detail. In order to improve and develop service provision, the results of monitoring must lead to action.

Table 11.4 Monitoring form for an occupational therapy service

Statements of quality assurance	Achieved	Partially achieved	Not achieved	Further action to be taken
Provision of an area of privacy for treatment				
Provision of a quiet and acceptable area for patient treatment				
Provision of adequate up-to-date equipment for patient treatment				
Regular maintenance programme that keeps equipment in safe working order				
Correct staffing levels for: – inpatient treatment – outpatient treatment – day patient treatment – community patient treatment				
Fully-staffed service in line with current establishment				

(Source: Koch, 1991)

Audit

Audit is another form of monitoring that can be a vital part of maintaining and improving the quality of a service. The term 'audit' is widely used in health care and includes clinical, medical and nursing audits. Its scope can be illustrated with two quotations, beginning with a definition of an audit:

> the systematic, critical analysis of the quality of medical care including the procedures used for diagnosis and treatment, the use of resources and the resulting outcome for the patient.
> (Davison, 1990)

> Audit should allow the objective peer review of patterns of care, sensitive to the expectations of patients and other clinical disciplines and based on scientific evidence of good medical practice.
> (Shaw, 1991)

Because the term has associations with investigation and appraisal, an audit needs to be carried out in a supportive atmosphere to allow open and honest discussion of the results. Though audit can contribute much to the management of quality, it tends to be a closely focused activity, examining one particular aspect of a service rather than the service as a whole.

The basic philosophy of quality management is getting the process and the outcomes right first time. In complex services, where many different types of staff and many different areas of work contribute to the delivery of a service, it is particularly difficult to ensure that all the stages in the process and the links between them are of an equally high quality. A well managed quality chain goes some way towards ensuring high-quality outcomes, but the outcomes for any individual service user will be viewed from a personal perspective.

Setting standards and monitoring performance against them provide a process through which quality can be managed. It is important that the standards be realistic and meaningful and that they represent aspects of the service that are worth measuring. It is helpful if the staff who are to contribute to achieving the standards are involved in setting them at a level that they agree is attainable. Once you have standards in place, performance can be measured against them. This provides the basis for taking managerial action if the standards are not being consistently achieved, and for improving the standards in due course.

REFERENCES

Burbach, F. R. and Quarry, A. (1991) 'Quality and outcome in a community mental health team', *International Journal of Health Care Quality Assurance*, 4(2): 18–26.

Davison, A. (1990) 'Action on audit', *International Journal of Health Care Quality Assurance*, 3(6): 14–16.

Department of Health (1998) *A First Class Service: Quality in the New NHS*, Department of Health.

Donabedian, A. (1980) *Definition of Quality and Approaches to its Assessment*, Health Administration Press.

King, R., Raynes, N. and Tisard, J. (1971) *Patterns of Residential Care*, Routledge and Kegan Paul.

Kitson, A. (1986) 'Rest assured', *Nursing Times*, 27 August, pp. 28–31.

Koch, H. (1991) *Total Quality Management*, Longmans.

Maxwell, R. (1984) 'Quality assessment in health', *British Medical Journal*, 13: 31–4.

Morgan, J. and Everett, T. (1991) 'Introducing quality management in the NHS', *International Journal of Health Care Quality Assurance*, 3(5): 23.

Shaw, C. (1991) 'Specifications for hospital medical audit', *Health Services Management*, June, pp. 124–5.

Smyth, C., Simmons, I. and Cunningham, G. (1999) *Quality Assurance in Social Work – A Standards and Audit Approach for Agencies and Practitioners*, National Institute for Social Work.

MANAGEMENT CONTROL

This chapter begins by considering some of the benefits of effective management control. It then introduces the 'control loop' – the idea that control is a cyclical process of setting standards, measuring performance, comparing performance with the standards and taking corrective action if necessary. We then look at some of the issues in measuring and comparing, and at the different ways in which control can be exercised. We conclude by focusing on how corrective action can be taken to ensure that standards and objectives are achieved.

The chapter does not set out to give you rules to work by. Its aim is to give you some ideas that you are invited to think about in the context of your own job. By the end of the chapter, you should have developed some ideas of your own as to how control fits into your managerial tasks. You should also have developed some ideas about how you can help your staff in the control they have to exercise, and what control your manager or supervisor is (or should be!) exercising over your activities and those of your department or section.

WHY CONTROL?

If you accept that part of a manager's role is to control the flow of work, you may feel that there is no need to ask this question. However, there are more benefits from control than you might at first recognise. Some of the most significant are:

- Without effective control, much of the effort that has gone into planning will be wasted, since you will not know whether your objectives have been achieved.
- Effective control helps you to obtain the best results from the available money, people, equipment and time.
- With effective control, a work group – a team, a department or a whole organisation – can be steered consistently towards its objectives.

- The standard-setting and monitoring elements of control enable systematic action to be taken to keep on target, thus reducing argument and conflict.
- Effective control can give your team a feeling of confidence, cohesiveness and purpose.
- Effective control, through measuring and comparing, provides a basis for forecasting, estimating and planning.
- Effective control of people's work helps you to assess them for promotion, transfer or training.
- With an effective control system, staff can assess their own performance and adjust their approach, leading to greater commitment and more job satisfaction.

ACTIVITY 12.1

Describe briefly a situation from your experience in which each of the statements below applied.

1   Effective control saved the day. (Was there a strong 'controller' in the lead?)
2   Absence of control resulted in damage to the organisation's interests. (What would you have done, had you been responsible?)
3   Absence of control did not cause problems. (Then ask yourself whether there was truly an absence of control.)

'Control' is an emotive word that sparks a hostile and resistant response from many people. Some find the notion of managers attempting to exercise control over staff offensive. Some writers have insisted that only inanimate items like resources, expenditure and events can be 'controlled' and that people must be 'managed'. The distinction between management and control is a fine one and you must make up your own mind about the difference.

Another reason why hostile responses might arise is that the word 'control' can be used with a variety of different meanings, some of which have overtones of coercion and exploitation. The managerial sense of the word, as used in this book, is much more akin to the control that a driver exerts over a car, keeping things on the planned course to make sure of a safe arrival at the intended destination. One of the contributions that systems thinking has made to management thinking is by providing a model of the control process. This is known as the *control loop*.

THE CONTROL LOOP

Let's take the driving analogy a little further. A minibus driver picking up people from their homes to take them to a day centre takes care that each passenger is seated comfortably and safely in the minibus. While the passengers are chatting and looking out of the windows, the driver is controlling the journey. To do this, the driver:

- continuously monitors the instruments that provide information about the minibus (its speed, its fuel consumption and reserves, the temperature of the engine, and so on) and continuously monitors the progress that the minibus is making from the final pick-up to the day centre
- compares this information with the usual progress along the normal route, to check that everything is going according to plan (for example, that the minibus is still on track to arrive at the planned time and has adequate reserves of fuel left to reach its planned destination)
- takes corrective action if things are not going according to plan (this might include very minor interventions, such as stopping to allow another vehicle to pull out, more significant changes, such as taking a different route to avoid roadworks, or even implementing a contingency plan and diverting to a new destination if circumstances require it).

These three steps – *monitoring* what is happening, *comparing* what is happening with the plan, and *taking corrective action* where necessary – are the essence of management control.

The same three steps can be seen in health and social care. For example, if an older man who lives alone has an accident that reduces his ability to take care of himself, he may need temporary help from care services. A care plan will be prepared, the situation will be monitored as he recovers, and the level of care will be reduced and eventually discontinued when he is fully recovered.

Another example is the management of a patient in intensive care. A range of instruments provides information about the patient's condition. The medical staff monitor these instruments continuously and compare the patient's condition with what should be happening. If the data from the instruments are not following the course that they should, the staff might have to take corrective action – perhaps by administering a drug to bring the blood pressure or pulse rate within acceptable limits, or perhaps by some more drastic intervention. These processes of monitoring, comparing and taking corrective action if necessary will continue until the patient is out of danger. When, in due course, the patient leaves intensive care, the same processes of control continue, though perhaps less obtrusively. The patient is no longer wired to the monitoring instruments because it is no longer necessary to have continuous information, but the staff carry on monitoring the patient's progress by gathering information in other ways (ward rounds, observation, examinations, scans, and so on) and they compare this information with what they would expect for that particular patient. If the patient's progress is not going according to plan, they might need to take further corrective action but, if the patient is on course for recovery, they need do no more than continue to monitor his or her progress.

These three steps underlie all forms of managerial control, though in 'normal' management, such as running a section or department, the steps may be less obvious and clear-cut. Nevertheless they are there, and can be represented by the control loop shown in Figure 12.1.

The control loop implies that you must start with a plan that specifies goals (where you are going) and objectives (detailed statements of measurable standards to be attained). Your next task is to *measure* what is actually happening. You then *compare* this with what is supposed to be happening – the level and direction of performance specified in the plan. If all is well, you need only to continue monitoring. If things are not going according to plan, you need to take *corrective action* to bring the performance back on course.

ACTIVITY 12.2

List four reasons why the separate steps indicated in the control loop might appear less obvious and clear-cut in 'normal' managerial work than they do in driving a vehicle or managing the care of a patient or service user.

Figure 12.1 The control loop

There are many reasons why 'normal' management control is more complex. Very few managers have a plan that is as detailed and specific as the plan a driver has for a journey. Even where the destination or goal is fairly clearly defined, the standards to be attained and maintained cannot always be specified exactly. And even if some standards can be specified fairly precisely, it is rarely possible to measure what is actually happening in the workplace with anything like the same accuracy – as quickly – as is possible in a vehicle procedure or in many medical procedures. For example, there is often a significant delay between an event happening and the availability of data about it. Nor are the data always reliable. Moreover, a driver is controlling only one car, whereas most managers are controlling several different activities at the same time, each of which may be at a different stage of development. And a driver does not usually have to break off in the middle of the journey and turn his or her attention to something completely different such as the absence of a member of staff, a disciplinary problem or a casual interruption.

Nevertheless, the separate steps in the process of managerial control – setting standards, measuring, comparing and taking action to correct performance – are important. Many managers find the concept of the control loop extremely useful. It is a way of helping to make sense of the apparent muddle of managerial work. It helps managers to recognise the essential role of planning and objective setting. It also emphasises the fundamental importance of gathering accurate and timely information about what is going on, so that appropriate corrective action can be taken before emergency action is needed.

A systems view of control

Another equally helpful way of viewing management control is closely related to the control loop but extends some of the ideas in it. It is based on systems thinking. At the heart of systems thinking is a *process* with *inputs* and *outputs* (Figure 12.2).

You can think of most working activities in this way. It is the task of the manager to control an activity to ensure that the inputs and the process result in the desired outputs.

It could be argued that the outputs (or outcomes) are the most important. The process is ineffective and the inputs are wasted if the outputs are not right. So the manager's first task is to ensure that the outputs are right. But it is impossible to know whether the outputs are right unless they have been specified in detail beforehand. The manager's first job

Figure 12.2 The systems process

Figure 12.3 A feedback loop

is therefore to specify the standards that the outputs must meet. These standards might be specified in terms of quantity, quality, cost, time, or other measurable characteristics. (You will recognise that this is another way of saying that the objectives must be specified in advance. You will also recognise that, up to now, this is exactly the same first step as in the control loop.)

However, systems thinking adds a new idea – that an activity cannot be controlled unless there is a *feedback* loop carrying a flow of accurate and timely information about the outputs that are actually being achieved (Figure 12.3).

The manager's second task, based on the systems way of thinking about control, is to ensure that arrangements are made for obtaining accurate and timely information about the outputs. The control loop glosses over this all-important step. It implies that managers will be able to measure performance themselves or will have ready access to a flow of information. Adequate information is not always easy to obtain.

The third task is to ensure that the information flowing along the feedback loop is used to determine whether it is necessary to take action. This is the same process as that described in the control loop. Information about what has been achieved is compared (by the *comparator*) with the standards. If significant discrepancies are detected, an *actuator* calls for corrective action (Figure 12.4).

The control loop does not make it entirely clear how or where corrective action can be taken. The systems loop, however, shows that managers have three separate areas in which they can apply corrective action.

ACTIVITY 12.3

Look carefully at the systems loop in Figure 12.4 and identify the three separate areas in which managers can, if they think it necessary, take corrective action.

Figure 12.4 The systems loop

The most obvious area for taking corrective action is in the *inputs*. The inputs will vary greatly with the kind of work that is being carried out. They may include people, skills, equipment, accommodation, raw materials, time, finance and information. If there is a difference between the planned standards and the standards actually being achieved, managers must decide whether changes in any of these inputs might ensure that objectives could be met. For example, an additional team member might be necessary to ensure that the work is achieved within the desired time-scale.

Alternatively, managers might consider changing the *process*. This is the way in which the work is carried out. Many factors determine how work is done, for example, custom, precedent, rules and regulations, professional training and statutory requirements. Some of these can be influenced by the manager, while others might be more difficult to change in the short term. Nevertheless, corrective action might require the process to be modified.

Finally, as we saw earlier when considering the control loop, corrective action might, in some cases, require that the original plan be modified and the standards might need to be revised.

MEASURING AND COMPARING

Standards provide a basis for measurement and comparison. As we said in the last chapter, if you set standards but do not measure performance to compare it with the standards, you lose most of the benefits of defining the standards. It is the processes of measuring, comparing with expectations and then taking action to bring performance more closely in line with expectations that enable quality to be managed.

Measuring the measurable

At whatever level measurement and comparison take place, you can only measure the measurable, yet this rather obvious point does need to be considered quite carefully. It does not mean that you should avoid setting standards if there is no existing method of monitoring them but that, where there is a worthwhile standard, it is worth making an effort to find a means of measuring whether you are achieving it. However, you must be sure that your measure is a true indication of performance against your standard.

For example, put yourself in the position of the domestic services manager of a hospital. You want to measure and monitor your department's performance on cleaning work and compare it with that of the private-sector contractor that cleans a neighbouring hospital. You discover that your teams take twice as long to undertake the cleaning as do the private-sector people. You set an objective that, within one year, you will match the private-sector contractor. Six months later you have achieved your target and are very pleased.

Then someone points out that, instead of carrying out all the cleaning tasks as they did previously, your teams now do only the major ones: wiping floors and cleaning wards, corridors, sluice areas and toilets. They haven't polished the floors for six weeks, they no longer wipe down shelves and skirting boards in the wards, and they pay scant attention to clearing rubbish discarded during outpatient clinics. You believe that the private-sector cleaners have not been doing these tasks either, but you cannot be sure. You then realise that it might have been better to measure, compare and control the types of job rather than the working hours.

There will be instances when it is not possible to identify a reasonable and straightforward approach to measuring performance, even when the ultimate objective is desirable and definable. In these cases, one of the following approaches may be adopted.

Objectives in sequence

Identify a number of sequential steps necessary to achieve the objective. For example, if you have a long-term objective to ensure that all the staff working in your office have appropriate training plans, you might set an initial objective of carrying out appraisals within a short time-scale. You could set training plans for each person once their development needs have been identified.

Objectives in parallel

You might subdivide the overall objective into a number of separate objectives so that each staff group can have its own objective and control progress towards it for themselves. You would then need to ensure co-ordination between the groups so that you are satisfied that your approach results in them all working towards your overall objective.

No clear objective to start with

You might tell the people concerned that you don't yet know exactly what steps will have to be taken and so have no obvious objectives that can be used to measure progress. Make your overall intention clear and start working in that direction. While the work proceeds, look for controls that can be used (inviting staff to suggest ways of monitoring can be useful).

ACTIVITY 12.4

In each of the following situations, identify how you would set objectives and standards and monitor progress. You should consider, for example:

■ how much information you might have at the beginning
■ the extent to which conditions might change
■ the accuracy of your information
■ the flexibility with which the tasks can be carried out
■ how much feedback you would need.

1   You are the co-ordinator of a community project to upgrade a large old house to a half-way home for five people with learning dis-abilities, using a team of about 30 relatively unskilled volunteers. (Can you follow the progress of the project if you supervise all 30 volunteers yourself? Can you forecast the project's progress? How will you maintain morale? Do you know what materials will be needed?)
2   You are the hospital works officer – without authority over other managers – advising five separate departments on the plan for moving two miles down the road into a new building. (You might have problems with staff reluctant to move, managers reluctant to listen, security of records, continuity of work, etc.)
3   You are using three temporary clerks for one week in the medical records office to assist your three experienced staff to 'pull' clinic notes for busy outpatient sessions.

We thought that, if you were the co-ordinator in case 1, the volunteer workers might not take too kindly to being controlled, so you would have to approach this carefully. You are unlikely to be able to use rigid direction and close control – if you do, the chances are that the volunteers will go home. It might be best to set objectives for completing major sections of the work (for example, plumbing, electrical, timber fixings) and to use section leaders to control the work of their own teams. Do you know of examples at work where a sensitive team of people needs to be managed (controlled) in a similar way?

If you were the hospital works officer in case 2, we felt that it would be important to consider how you could influence your colleagues and set objectives that would help all of them to move with the least disruption. If you could persuade everyone to agree overall objectives and time-scales, you might influence them to stick to the plan by having regular progress reports and by holding meetings at which you consider together how to deal with any issues that are delaying progress.

In case 3, you might decide to delegate control to your three experienced staff. They could agree together what objectives and time-scales they need to achieve in order to be prepared for each outpatient clinic. Perhaps each could manage one of the temporary staff to ensure that they meet their objectives.

Management by exception

Management by exception is one way of getting more returns for less effort. It involves setting up controls in such a way that you concern yourself only with those results that are significantly different from the plans you have made. Results that are within acceptable limits – that give no cause for concern – are ignored. Only those results that fall outside acceptable limits are reported so that action can be taken if necessary.

This may seem obvious. If it is so obvious, why do so many control and information systems provide enormous volumes of data, leaving the manager to wade through them and find out whether anything requires attention? To a considerable extent, management by exception relies on having staff who are competent and on whose judgements you can rely when they tell you that everything is going according to plan. It also relies on the data presented to you being up to date and sufficiently accurate. There are, therefore, potential dangers in using management by exception and in defining, for example, what level of performance is outside acceptable limits.

Some examples of exception reports are:

The paper for next week's meeting will not be ready by five o'clock today as requested.

The chest X-rays of 1,492 patients are complete; there are four that we are not entirely happy about.

Salary awards of 6 per cent are to be made generally. Could we talk about two members of staff who should perhaps be treated as special cases?

We are 10 per cent below target on reducing the waiting list for speciality X, but all other waiting lists are within the limits agreed.

'Dear Sir, I am writing because I have been waiting for a hip replacement for far too long.'

Although the schedule of appointments generally kept to time, 10 per cent of service users waited more than 30 minutes.

ACTIVITY 12.5

Think of an instance in your work where exchanges of information would be simplified if the principle of management by exception were applied. This might be an area of work on which regular reports are made that often seem to be a waste of time because they rarely contain information that requires action to be taken. If management by exception was applied, would it:

	Yes	No
■ make your job less interesting?	❐	❐
■ clarify the picture?	❐	❐
■ allow more effective action to be taken?	❐	❐
■ save time and effort?	❐	❐
■ allow you to get to the point more quickly and with greater accuracy?	❐	❐

Identify one aspect of your management work in which you would like to adopt the principle of management by exception.

TAKING CONTROL AS A MANAGER

There are a number of ways in which a manager can take control of an area of work. In some organisations there are systems and procedures that set out what should be done.

Procedures and systems

You may have come across a 'manual of procedures' at work. *Procedures* are the way in which your organisation requires certain activities to be carried out; they are often specified in great detail. For example, an organisation may have procedures for:

■ completing the late arrivals book
■ making a weekly record of absentees and informing the personnel officer
■ paying expenses to people who attend for job interviews; here you may find a number of different procedures, for example:
  – where the sum is £30 or less
  – where the sum is more than £30 but less than £100
  – where the sum is more than £100
  – where the interviewee is currently employed by the organisation at another location
  – where the interviewee is not currently employed by the organisation.

Figure 12.5 illustrates a typical procedure. It deals with the method of recording and approving incoming invoices in a finance department. You do not need to understand what is being explained in the procedure, but it is important to appreciate the significance of the amount of detail and the careful specification of what is to be done. (The procedure refers to 'attachments', since it is usual to include examples of relevant forms with procedures, but they have been omitted here as they do not help to explain the principles.)

Note how effective this procedure is as a control. The correct method (the standard) is defined. If anything goes wrong, the activities performed can be checked against the standard and any differences can be recognised. You should be able to relate the various aspects of the control loop to the use of this example of a procedure.

Systems are collections of procedures. It is to the system that we ascribe a purpose or an objective; the procedures are the means of operating the system. Let's look at an example.

You are running the storeroom in a general practice and realise that you need a stock control system. You specify the objective of the system – to balance the quantities in the store with the forecast demand for goods based on historical data. The inputs to the system are data on stock used and new stock purchased. The system processes the information by adding, deleting and adjusting the information about each item. These are then output in the form of stock lists, low stock warnings and, perhaps, purchase orders.

PURCHASING ACCOUNTING PROCEDURES	Section: 5.1.1
Incoming invoices	Date: 23.2.99

Step	Procedure narrative

DAILY PROCEDURES

Finance department

1   Receive invoices from suppliers and date stamp as received.
2   Prepare invoice payment authorisation form (IPA), two copies (attachment A), entering:
- the name of the department of origin (the department that requisitioned the expenditure)
- the supplier's name
- the invoice number and date
- the invoice value in words and figures.
3   Check IPA form for accurate completion.
4   Enter in invoice register (attachment B):
- IPA number
- date of receipt
- supplier's name
- amount of invoice
- invoice number and date
- name of department of origin and date IPA was sent.
5   Hold a copy of IPA on open file until invoice is returned.
6   Send invoice with IPA to originating department.

Department of origin

7   Check invoice for:
- receipt of goods or services
- price, extensions and additions.
8   Authorise invoice by completing IPA showing net payment to be made, after deductions for advances, retentions or other withholdings. Sign IPA.
9   Return IPA and invoice to finance department.

Finance department

10   Enter in invoice register the date returned and note any amendments made.
11   Enter invoice in purchase day book showing:
- invoice date
- IPA number
- supplier's name
- invoice amount gross
- allocation to appropriate column.
12   Sort IPAs by supplier in alphabetical sequence.
13   From purchase day book, post invoice amounts to individual creditors' accounts.

MONTHLY PROCEDURES

14   Total columns in purchase day book and agree cross costs.
15   Post totals of individual columns of purchase day book to the debit of the appropriate accounts in the nominal ledger and the total to the creditor's control account in the nominal ledger. Journalise exchange differences arising in the creditors' ledger.
16   Agree creditor's control account in the nominal ledger to the creditor's control amount in the creditors' ledger and the total of the list of balances of the individual creditors' accounts.

Figure 12.5 Example of a procedure

In this example, the procedures might be:

- booking in goods received
- issuing goods to GPs' surgeries and clinics
- calculating the value of goods to the practice as a whole
- calculating the value of goods to individual surgeries and clinics
- counting each stock item
- gaining approval to purchase new stock
- approving incoming invoices.

Each of these procedures is a control device. Each defines what is to be done and the procedures thus set the standards for the system. Performance against these standards can be monitored and, if the procedures have not been adhered to (that is, the standards have not been met), either the future performance or the existing standards might be adjusted.

ACTIVITY 12.6

Are activities in your area of work done in an appropriately systematic way without going overboard on regulation? For example, are there systems and procedures for dealing with problems that arise regularly?

You might have identified areas of work in which it would be helpful to have a more systematic approach. In particular, if there are activities that are carried out frequently but inconsistently, it might be helpful to develop a written procedure that everyone could use. This is particularly helpful when staff are new to an area of work, because it helps them to perform effectively without immediate supervision. If you felt that there was room for improvement, you might discuss your ideas with your manager.

People factors

Up to now we have considered management control as the process by which managers ensure that everything stays on course or that necessary corrective action is taken. This would be a relatively easy task if the process to be controlled were entirely mechanical, but it is made infinitely more complex by the need to take account of people.

Control as a management process consists largely of encouraging people to do certain things and not to do others. How you encourage them is a measure of your managerial skills in motivating people. There are a number of factors to bear in mind:

- Individuals work in organisations to satisfy their own needs and their needs vary greatly.
- Individuals are influenced by rewards, satisfactions and punishments – in most cases more strongly by the attractiveness of rewards and satisfactions than by the fear of punishments.
- The effectiveness of rewards or punishments diminishes rapidly as the time between performance and feedback increases and the link between them becomes less obvious.
- Standards that people see as being too easy or too difficult to attain have little effect on their performance.
- Targets must be seen as desirable and achievable, and should not bear unreasonably heavily on some people and more lightly on others.
- Participation by the individual in setting a standard will increase his or her determination to achieve it.

It is most important when setting standards to obtain people's agreement to targets (either directly or through their representatives). This is often difficult and time-consuming, but it is such a key factor in managing that it must be done with determination, understanding and sensitivity.

Timing of control

Control can take place at three different times:

- *before* the activity – feedforward control
- *during* the activity – concurrent control
- *after* the activity – feedback control.

Feedforward control

Feedforward control is used to try to anticipate problems or deviations from plans before they occur. Setting budgets is an example, in that it involves establishing levels of expenditure across time, which are then monitored by means of regular budget statements that show actual expenditure against the plan.

'Dummy runs' are also a form of feedforward control. For example, if a new computerised data-processing system is being implemented to replace a manual system, there might be a dummy run when both systems run so that the manual system is still available if the new system fails or is inadequate in some way. This allows potentially expensive and time-consuming faults to be ironed out before the new system is fully operational.

Another example of feedforward control is setting up pilot projects. A pilot project provides the opportunity to apply an idea on a small scale and assess its impact before changing the direction of the entire organisation and then perhaps coming to the conclusion that the idea is unworkable in practice. A pilot project is often used to try out a change on a small scale when major changes would be opposed. It provides an opportunity for the supporters to demonstrate their case and the opponents to be persuaded.

Concurrent control

This is sometimes referred to as 'steering' control because any corrective action that is necessary can be taken almost immediately. An example of concurrent control is in the production of sterile packs in a hospital's central sterile supplies department. The operator of the sterilising unit has a visual control over the standard to be achieved because there is a strip on each pack that changes colour to indicate that the contents of the pack are sterile and fit for despatch to an operating theatre or clinic. The advantage of concurrent control lies in the speed at which the feedback is available.

Feedback control

All control systems provide some form of feedback, but often a considerable time after an activity has been completed. There may then be no opportunity for the outcome of the activity to be changed or modified. However, the feedback provides managers with an opportunity to influence the outcome of similar future activities. An example is an organisation's monthly or four-weekly cycle of budget reports. The financial results in certain areas of activity during the period just ended may have deviated from those planned and little can be done to correct them. But an investigation of the cause of the deviations will allow corrective action to be taken in an attempt to ensure that future periods are not affected.

Surveys of patients and service users are another example of feedback control. They can provide valuable feedback on the quality of care, and can be used in making decisions when you review services.

Types of control

Control can be exercised in different ways:

- an informal approach versus a formal approach
- a qualitative approach versus a quantitative approach.

Informal versus formal control

In exercising control, it is important to make an appropriate choice between an informal and a formal approach. A formal approach might involve a sequence of steps that include defining a standard, monitoring performance and taking management action. An informal approach may not be discerned as control, but merely the application of common sense and experience. That does not make the informal approach any less powerful; used in the right way with the right people, it can be very effective. Consider the two statements below. The first is formal and systematic, the second informal. Both could result in effective control.

General manager to commissioning officer:
The budget for commissioning the new orthopaedic ward is shown on this computer tabulation as £100,000. We've got £10,000 for beds, £10,000 for linen, £20,000 for lockers and sundry furniture, £7,000 for soft furnishings (window curtains, bed curtains and tracking), £10,000 for utility room equipment and the balance for orthopaedic equipment. As the orders are placed according to the agreed time-scale, the costs will be allocated against the project. I will receive an updated report from the Finance Department. Please keep an accurate record of items delivered to the new ward and report to me in writing no later than five days prior to our regular Steering Group meeting.

Commissioning officer to assistant:
I'd like you to keep an eye on the delivery of furniture and equipment for the new ward. Please give me a ring each Monday afternoon and let me know how things are going.

If you choose to use an informal method, you must know the abilities of the person you are dealing with and pitch your approach accordingly.

Qualitative versus quantitative control

This distinction concerns the nature of the information and its monitoring. In the qualitative approach, the targets are defined as statements of quality rather than in numerical terms. For example:

Unless the assistant cook can improve the co-ordination of residents' meals, I'll have to transfer him to vegetable preparation duties.

> All maintenance staff required to work away from their base will be provided with changing facilities in keeping with their status.
>
> The paint colours for the office extension should be matched as nearly as possible to the existing scheme.

The quantitative approach puts the targets in terms of numbers. For example:

> Unless the assistant cook can ensure that the cooked food is ready for loading on to the lunch trolleys for despatch by 12 noon, I'll have to transfer him to vegetable preparation duties.
>
> Facilities for maintenance staff working away from their base will be as follows:
>
> | | |
> |---|---|
> | Changing room facilities | 1 square metre per person |
> | Lockers | 1 per person |
> | Showers | 1 per 3 people |
> | Toilets | 1 per 10 people. |
>
> The paint colours for wall surfaces in the office extension should be matched to British Standard 1575.

Which type of control should be used?

Our aim in defining the various types of control is to make you aware of the differences. We have not proposed any clear guidelines as to where each type of control should be used. We have, however, suggested some types of problem and some types of people to which each approach may be appropriate.

In exercising any form of control, a large element of judgement is required on the part of the manager. Regardless of the form of control imposed on you from above, you must decide whether the same or a different control technique will be most effective in managing your area of work. This is a difficult but crucial aspect of exercising control. Important considerations are 'How will this action be construed by the people who are to be controlled?' and 'Will it be effective and achieve my objectives?'

ACTIVITY 12.7

Consider the relevance of some of the points made in this section to your own work.

1   Identify from your experience a situation in which each of the following has occurred.
    ■   A target has been set without agreement, and has caused resentment and discouraged effort.
    ■   A target has been set after consultation, and has motivated people towards achievements.
    ■   A target has been set, and fear of failure has driven people to achieve it.

2   Identity a situation in which you have used each of the following or it has been used on you.
    ■   Feedforward control.
    ■   Concurrent control.
    ■   Feedback control.

3   Identify one example of each of the following types of control that you have used or that has been used on you. (You may be able to identify an example that fits more than one category.)
    ■   Informal.
    ■   Formal.
    ■   Qualitative.
    ■   Quantitative.

4   Do any of these examples show a different approach used on the controller (i.e. down the line of command as far as the controller) from that used by the controller for the same task?

TAKING CORRECTIVE ACTION

In this section we consider some of the ways in which corrective action can be taken – the last element of the control loop.

Resetting standards

We have seen how the control loop allows you either to adjust the activities that are aimed at achieving the standard or to adjust the standard itself. There are several circumstances in which resetting the standard may be justified:

■   when it is clear that external factors have made the standard unrealistic

- when the standard is recognised to be no longer meaningful
- when the people trying to achieve the standard do not have the skills or abilities to succeed
- when the leadership has been inadequate and the standard cannot therefore be achieved in the time available.

It will not always be clear which of these reasons is the most significant in any particular case. Nevertheless, it is important to consider why the standard needs to be reset so that you can select and plan an appropriate course of action.

When you feel that the standard should be reset, you need to consider whether you will cause more problems by changing it than by holding firm. For example, by changing the standard would you:

- undermine acceptance of both the old and the new standards?
- encourage people to ignore any future standards you set?
- remove an incentive to get as close to the standard as possible, even if it cannot quite be achieved?
- make those who have really exerted themselves feel it was a waste of effort?
- unduly affect other aspects of your department's work or that of other people?
- be setting a new standard that is no more realistic than the previous one?

You could, no doubt, add to this list. The important point is that you need to think through the effect of changing a standard of performance. When trying to decide whether to modify a standard, start by asking yourself, 'Would it be unreasonable to keep things as they are, even though a change is desirable?'

We have already said several times that there is little value in setting standards unless you monitor against them. Similarly, there is little value in setting standards unless you are willing to take action to ensure that the standards are met. Your choices might include incentives, motivators, persuasion, cajoling, bribing, training and coaching but, ultimately, you must be prepared to enforce discipline.

Where methods of working are laid down, objectives set or standards defined, there will be instances where:

- people work deliberately against them
- the standards are known but ignored
- the targets have not been understood adequately.

In the first two of these situations, disciplinary action may be needed to ensure that the targets are not undermined or ignored. In the last, the problem may be poor communication or lack of training.

Levels of control

Another choice that you have to make in setting up effective controls is about who should control what. Consider the treatment room in a large general practice (Table 12.1). There will be a number of different levels of control operating.

You will probably be able to identify performance measurements, comparisons and actions from your own experience to add to this example. There may, for example, be a group of staff in your department or section that has its own informal measures and standards. There may be another level of management with direct influence over the work of your area. There may be a supervisor who has identified worthwhile monitoring measures that you could also use.

Table 12.1 Levels of control in treatment room of a general practice

Staff member	Performance measurement	Comparison with standard	Action
Nurse	Am I seeing an appropriate number of patients in each session?	Is the number changing over time?	Discuss referral patterns and training needs.
Senior nurse	How many patients are seen each week? Are all nurses seeing an appropriate number of patients in each session?	Time keeping; idle time; time spent with individual patients (average and range).	Reorganise duty rosters and/or appointment systems.
Senior receptionist	Is treatment room reception working well? Is paperwork completed by the end of each day and is it accurate?	What are acceptable delays and lapses?	Review organisation and procedures.
Practice manager	What are the costs? What income is generated?	Can efficiency be improved?	Reduce costs or increase income.
GP	Is work being delegated appropriately? Are nurses adequately trained?	How might delegation be improved?	Review referral procedures.
Primary care group manager	Is the practice employing adequate numbers of nursing staff?	Local and national figures.	Encourage good practice; review staff budget.

ACTIVITY 12.8

Identify an example of each of the following from your own experience.

- Control has been exercised solely within the group by the responsible manager.
- Individuals have successfully exercised control over their own activities.
- Individuals' control over their own activities has not been successful.

In each of these cases, consider how control could have been put in place differently and more effectively.

For control to be effective, it must be appropriate to the situation and to the staff, as well as being designed to enable measurement of performance against the appropriate standards. If control is delegated to teams and individuals, they may need training so that they understand how to manage the control process. One of the benefits of training staff to understand control is that they can then work with you more effectively to set standards that they believe are worthwhile and achievable.

We have described the process of management control by depicting it as a control loop. Look again at Figure 12.1. Each element in the control loop is an important part of your managerial role and requires considerable skill and judgement. The way in which you exercise control as a manager is at least partly a matter of personal style, although your organisation may expect you to adopt a particular approach. You may feel that imposing control over your staff is unnecessary. This may be appropriate if your staff are willing and able to control their own work to ensure that standards are met. However, meeting standards is increasingly important, and controlling activities to ensure that standards and targets are met is one of the main responsibilities of a manager.

MANAGING PROCESSES

Examining how your service is delivered in order to identify opportunities for improvement can be quite challenging. If you are to make effective improvements, you need to be clear about the areas over which you have authority and to decide which staff to involve in defining, planning and implementing change. You also need to recognise the boundary issues to be dealt with – to identify any parts of your service area that link with or overlap with other organisational or professional areas. While you are thinking about these matters, it is important to be aware of how patients or service users view any change, to ensure that you are making improvements that will benefit them. This chapter offers some signposts and tools to help you in this complex process.

Our focus is on the 'pathway' that patients and service users follow through the range of services that they encounter in health and social care. This may involve several boundaries between services and professions. If you work in a large and complex organisation, such as a hospital or a social services or social work department, you may have limited scope to influence many elements of the pathway. However, in a smaller organisation – perhaps an advisory service or a small voluntary organisation, you may be able to influence the whole range of service delivery more directly.

Whatever your situation, you may be called on to participate in reviews of the effectiveness of service delivery, to contribute ideas for improvement, and to implement and monitor improvements or changes that have been agreed. This will require you to focus on values, purposes and results. You will need to make use of feedback from patients, service users and carers, use your 'people management' skills to help your team to contribute ideas and adjust to change, and use your skills in setting standards, handling information and feedback, planning and monitoring.

DEFINING AND MAPPING PROCESSES

It might be helpful at this stage to clarify a few of the terms used in talking about service delivery processes. *The New Oxford English Dictionary* suggests the following definitions of a process:

> a continuous series of actions, events or changes . . . especially a continuous and regular action or succession of actions occurring or performed in a definite manner; a systematic series of actions or operations directed to some end.

A process consists of a number of *activities* that are organised into an appropriate sequence and co-ordinated to achieve a specific purpose. We could describe a process as a number of activities that transform inputs into outputs: inputs (materials, skills, etc.) are transformed into outputs by the application of the process.

A *service* is made up of a number of processes that work together to deliver the service. The word *system* is used to describe all the services, processes, activities (and people) involved in the delivery of a particular aspect of health or social care. The contact that an individual patient or service user has with particular processes and services as they move through the system can be described as a *pathway*.

These concepts can be examined from different perspectives. For example, a system may look very different to a patient or service user from the way it looks to you as the manager of a particular service. Let's consider the sort of experience a patient or service user might have. His or her first encounter with a health or social care service is likely to include a number of discussions and possibly some tests. These activities may be followed by a decision about providing some help or treatment that should lead to a successful outcome. In 'systems thinking' terms, this can be described as a *transformation process* (Figure 13.1).

Figure 13.1 shows inputs being transformed into an output by a process. However, this diagram does not give us any information about the nature of the process or processes that contribute to the transformation. The inputs may not all necessarily happen at the same time or only once. Nor may the outputs necessarily all happen at the same time. Figure 13.2 is a more helpful diagram that illustrates how a process may involve a series of inputs being made at different times, with a number of different activities contributing to the achievement of the output or outputs.

Figure 13.1 A transformation process

Figure 13.2 Flow of transformation processes

Process flow

The sequence of inputs, activities and outputs can be described as the *process flow*, implying that there is a smooth progression from one activity to the next until the output is achieved. This way of thinking helps to identify where improvements to processes can be made. Once the flow of a process is understood as a sequence of inputs and activities with links between them, it is possible to identify where there are bottlenecks or blockages in the flow of the process. By examining each input in relation to each activity, you can be more precise about the resources that are needed to provide each input and when they are required to carry out each activity.

The following case study illustrates how this way of thinking can be applied to improve a service area. It describes the work of a steering group that is seeking to improve the pathway (or trail) patients follow through elective surgery.

ACTIVITY 13.1

As you read the case study, focus on each activity and the inputs that contributed to it. Remember that inputs can include staff as well as materials and equipment. Make a note of the sequence of activities and the inputs that contribute to each.

The Steering Group has generated a series of process flow diagrams for the various stages of the 'patient trail' – which begins with an outpatient department referral and consultation, and ends (it is hoped) with the cured patient's discharge. Members of the Steering Group have also been speaking with staff, at all levels, involved in theatre work.

One of the diagrams shows the segment of the trail which takes the patient through the operating theatre. Let us assume that you are the third patient on the morning list for theatre 4 on Wednesday, and that the operation concerns a hernia repair; this should take around 45 minutes 'at the table'. The list for this theatre session will have been drawn up some days ago, but will only have been finalised on Tuesday afternoon or evening. For many different reasons patients 'drop out' from and are added onto the list up to the last moment. When the second patient's operation is drawing to a close – say, with about ten minutes to go – the theatre sister fills out a 'patient request ticket'. She takes this to the holding area and either gives it to a porter or puts it on a board for the next available porter to collect. The porter then walks to the ward to collect you, and brings you down to the theatre suite with your ward nurse as escort. All patients must be escorted by a porter and a qualified nurse. When you get to the theatre holding area the ward nurse transfers you to an operating department assistant and they check your details to make sure that you are indeed expected. You are then transferred onto a special theatre trolley and wheeled into the anaesthetic preparation room outside the operating theatre. This is where you wait until the previous operation is over and the theatre has been made ready for you.

If something goes wrong with the previous operation, you could be here for some time. If the nurse on the ward has given you any pre-medication, you should be relaxed and free from anxiety. Here also you meet again your anaesthetist, who visited you on the ward yesterday or this morning to check that you were fit to anaesthetise. When the theatre and surgeon are ready, the anaesthetist will induce anaesthesia, give you a breathing tube, and wheel you into the theatre where the team will lift you onto the table.

The surgeon is now ready to start your hernia operation. A typical surgical team includes the surgeon, anaesthetist, a senior registrar, a scrub nurse (who looks after the instruments), an operating department assistant (who supports the anaesthetist) and one or more theatre nurses to assist too. When the surgeon has finished, the anaesthetist reverses your anaesthesia and removes your now redundant breathing tube. Seeing that all is going well, one of the nurses or the operating department assistant wheels you into the recovery area where the anaesthetist leaves you, if all is still well, to return to the theatre and to attend to the next patient. You are now in the temporary care of the recovery nurses, who phone your ward when you are fit to travel back with a porter and your escort nurse.

(Buchanan and Wilson, 1996)

Table 13.1 is the chart we made to show inputs to each of the activities. This chart is one way of mapping a process flow. It is not necessary to use a table as we have here – many people find that it is more immediate for them to draw a flow diagram freehand and note the inputs at each stage in a different colour.

Table 13.1 The patient's pathway

Inputs	Activities
1 Theatre sister Request ticket	Give patient request ticket to porter or put on notice board
	↓
2 Porter and ward nurse (escort) Bed or trolley	Collect patient from ward Deliver to theatre on bed or trolley
	↓

3   Operating department assistant
    (ODA) and ward nurse
Patient notes
Trolley
	Check patient details
	Move patient on to theatre trolley
	    (if on bed)

	↓
4 Anaesthetist Equipment	Induce anaesthesia
	↓
5 Anaesthetist and ODA Equipment	Wheel patient into theatre Lift onto operating table
	↓

6   Surgical team (including surgeon,
    senior registrar, anaesthetist,
    scrub nurse, ODA, theatre
    nurses)
Operating theatre
	Surgeon performs operation, assisted
	    by senior registrar

	↓
7 Anaesthetist Nurse or ODA Trolley	Reverse anaesthesia Wheel patient to recovery area
	↓
8 Recovery nurses Operation record forms	Recovery nurse waits for patient to recover enough to go back to ward Operation record form completed
	↓
9 Nurse and porter	Wheel patient back to ward

This particular example looks only at the part of the patient's pathway immediately surrounding the actual operation. It excludes the visit to the GP, preliminary diagnosis, referral to the outpatient clinic, attendance at the clinic, pre-admission preparation, admission to the hospital, post-operative nursing, going home and care at home. Each of these processes could be mapped in a similar way.

PROCESS MAPPING

The first stage in process mapping is to select the process that you intend to map and to make a checklist of the activities that are included in that process. Selecting a part of your service to examine in this way presents quite a challenge. Your service may be only a small part of the patient's or service user's pathway. It may, however, make an important contribution to his or her overall comfort and satisfaction. For example, financial assessment and billing for a service may be done separately from assessment of need and provision of the service, but these can contribute significantly to a service user's anxiety. It is important to identify the process as it is viewed by service users so that its component parts can be considered in terms of their impact on them.

The next step is to think about the output or outcome of the process. Thinking in terms of what the customer receives is helpful in identifying the outputs of any process, whether your customers are patients or service users or staff in other departments of your organisation. It is therefore important to consider exactly who the customers are for the process you are intending to map.

Once the outputs and customers have been identified, you are in a position to consider what your customers need, want and expect of your output. This is important in reminding you of the quality that the process must achieve.

Next, you need to identify all the people who carry out the activities that make up the process you want to map. In our operating theatre example, a considerable number of people were identified, but probably fewer than you would have been able to identify if you were a manager in that area and were familiar with all the activities. It is important to include the staff from support services that contribute to the process as well as those who carry out the more obvious tasks. For example, medical records staff would have been involved at various stages of the operating theatre example.

Once you have assembled this information, you are in a position to define the process in the form of a clear statement that names the process and identifies the output(s) it is intended to achieve. You are then ready to prepare a map of the process.

Here is a summary of the main features of process mapping as it is carried out at Leicester Royal Infirmary (1998):

Select a process

1   Make a list of the activities included in the process.
2   State the output or outcome of the process (the product or service that is created by the process and is handed over to the customer).
3   List the customers for your output (the person or persons who use your output: customers may be internal or external; they may use your output as an input to their work processes).
4   List your customers' requirements of your output (what your customers need, want and expect of your output).
5   List the process participants (the people who carry out the steps of the process – as opposed to those who are responsible for the process).

Define the process

Map the process

Working systematically in this way will help you to be clear about how far you want to go in looking at parts of the patient's or service user's pathway over which you have no control. You may decide that it is important to look at the parts of the pathway that affect patients or service users immediately before and after they encounter your service.

ACTIVITY 13.2

You may like to try process mapping to help to make improvements in your own area of work.

1   Select a process from your working environment that you think could be improved.
2   Make a list of all the activities that contribute to the process.
3   Identify the output of the process.
4   Identify the people who use this output.
5   Make a list of what these people want or need or expect from your output.
6   List the people who contribute to carrying out activities in this process.
7   Write a definition of the process. This should include the purpose, the inputs, the transformation and the output(s).
8   Map the process, showing the inputs and activities, as in the example of an operating theatre. Base the map on the patient's or service user's pathway through the process. Identify:

- the people involved
- any travel or transport required
- any professional or service boundaries crossed
- sources of feedback and information
- points at which decisions have to be made
- points at which delays occur
- any specialist equipment required
- other factors that are important in your process.

9 Consider the importance of this process to your organisation and who would be the major stakeholders in any proposed changes. (For example, a care management or childcare assessment process cannot be changed unilaterally by any one team, although the way it is applied in a particular team may be capable of improvement without reference to other teams.)

If there is a possibility of making some changes in your service, you will need to involve your staff, relevant partners and other stakeholders in this exercise – improving processes is easier when those affected by them have been involved in identifying the problems and designing the solutions.

Once you are confident that the process map includes all the relevant information, the next step is to analyse it to find opportunities for improvement.

Identifying weaknesses in the process

The process map is the starting point for improving the process. You are likely to have a number of sources of information that will help you identify the strengths and weaknesses in your process. For example, you will know, from supervision and appraisal sessions with your staff, which elements of the process they find most problematic. Feedback from patients or service users may indicate where they experience difficulties with the way in which the service is run and where the outcomes of their contact with your service have not been satisfactory. Feedback from your management control will have made you aware of problems to be overcome, and you will know where standards – either local or national – are proving difficult to attain. Conversations with colleagues responsible for services at the boundaries of your process may be able to highlight difficulties your service causes them.

If you do not have some of this information, consider whether the information you collect and your record keeping are adequate for your management needs. It is usual to keep appraisal and supervision records confidential, but information about common concerns and training needs can be drawn from them. If you do not have feedback from your patients or service users, you may need to conduct a survey or arrange a meeting with a group of them to find out their views. You may need to improve your records of the extent to which standards are being achieved. You may also recognise that you have insufficient opportunities to exchange views with others who contribute to the process that you have mapped.

In the operating theatre example, the Steering Group identified several problems by talking to staff and patients. Many of these involved delays of one sort or another arising from the ways in which the activities were carried out:

- the way in which the theatre list is put together (a mix of different types of procedure, the learning needs of junior surgeons, etc.) may cause difficulties in predicting operation times and in keeping to schedule
- some of the professionals may see only their part in the process and not the 'big picture' as perceived by patients or other staff
- the surgeon is late
- the anaesthetist waits for the surgeon before initiating anaesthesia
- extra demands on porters at peak times
- the previous operation takes more or less time than anticipated.

The consequences of such delays can include cancelled operations, and thus anxiety, discomfort and inconvenience for patients and their families. They can also mean that staff are unable to keep to shift times, so that they have to work longer hours than intended. There is wasted time and the potential for muddle in the links between some activities. It is not clear who is overseeing the pathway of the patient in this example or who would take action to minimise the risk and discomfort to the patient if there is a delay in any activity that contributes to the overall process.

The process map can be used to define the current situation in terms of its strengths and weaknesses, and to identify opportunities for improvement. Four useful types of analysis can be applied to identify weaknesses in the process – value-added, handover, elapsed time and process cost analyses.

Value-added analysis

An important criterion in evaluating a process is to identify whether value is added at each stage for the patient or service user. Each part of the process can be assessed to see whether or not it represents a gain. For example, a long waiting time between referral and seeing a social worker, or between procedures in an outpatient clinic represents no gain for the service user. Time spent wandering around a hospital looking for the X-ray department also represents no gain. Activities carried out efficiently, for example, taking a blood sample or supplying home care speedily when it is needed, represent added value. Procedures carried out inefficiently, perhaps because of faulty equipment, reduce the amount of value added.

Handover analysis

This involves examining how each activity is completed and the next initiated. Once again, the experience of the patient or service user on the pathway through the whole process is the basis of the analysis. Any handover involves time and effort in passing a patient or service user from one person or one part of the process to another. Each handover is an opportunity for delay, confusion, and loss or distortion of useful information. As a patient or service user, it can also include the frustration of telling your story to yet another member of staff!

Elapsed time analysis

This refers to the time elapsing between and during different parts of the process. You can identify the usual lengths of time involved and note the reason for each. It is useful to pay particular attention to the time taken by activities that are not essential parts of the process. For example, it takes longer for a patient to walk through hospital corridors to widely dispersed sites – X-ray, pathology, and so on – than to move from one to the other within an outpatient suite, and it takes time for a mobile service to reach a service user. Sending information online is quicker than sending it by post. Again, the experience of the patient or service user in following the pathway through the process is the starting point for this analysis.

Process cost analysis

How much are inefficiencies in the process costing you? In seeking to improve processes, it is important to be clear about the nature of the intended benefits – are they about increasing quality or reducing costs or both? Experienced process redesigners tell us that process improvements for cost reduction alone are harder to implement because people are often less committed to making this kind of change. You also need to be aware that reducing costs in one area may only shunt them to another: if this happens to be another department or organisation, it can create friction. Some process improvements may require capital investment in new equipment or moving equipment and staff to be nearer the user. You may not have the power to implement such changes at the moment, but you can argue the case for modest process improvements now, and present a case for the benefits and potential savings of more radical change as a later option.

Each of these analyses may have suggested potential improvements.

Identifying potential areas for improvement

If you have found that some of the activities offer no – or very little – added value to the patient or service user, you could consider why they are carried out at all. Sometimes activities have been retained simply because no one has questioned whether they are still necessary. New technologies and materials can reduce the need for preparatory activities or for activities to take place in specially designed accommodation.

If staff are trained to develop a broader range of skills, it may be possible for one member of staff to carry out several activities in order to avoid handing the patient or service user from one person to another. The location of activities is also important: how easy is it for a patient or service user to move from one area of activities to another? If there are significant distances between activities that are frequently sequential in a pathway, it may be possible to reduce these distances. Historical reasons may have led to the locations of particular services and staff, and managers may not think of challenging this unless the implications for service users are considered.

The time taken between activities is important in contributing to the length of a process, and there are often opportunities to reduce this time by handing over from one activity to another in a different way. The handover part of a process often includes handing over information, records or notes as well as people. If time is to be saved, all of the necessary information must be handed over promptly so that the next activity can take place on time and effectively.

Saving time usually results in a reduction in costs. It may seem cost-efficient to make service users wait for professionals whose time is valuable, but people who are waiting cost resources in space, furniture, support staff, heating, lighting, and the provision of refreshments and toilets. Many of these costs could be reduced if waiting areas are needed for only one or two people at a time. Also, if people are left waiting for services, their condition can deteriorate. Once a patient or service user has been assessed as needing a service, it is likely that the service will be most cost-effective if it is supplied immediately.

If your process pathway crosses boundaries between your area of responsibility and others, you are likely to have to negotiate your ideas for process improvements with those who manage these other activities. This may involve more senior managers than yourself or managers from another organisation. You may need to clarify who takes responsibility for the overall care of patients or service users as they progress through the different activities along the pathway. You will also need to consider whether changes in your process may cause disruption to other activities or processes and, if so, how you could minimise such disruption and gain co-operation in making changes.

ACTIVITY 13.3

Using the information you have about the strengths and weaknesses of the process you have been examining – from appraisal or supervision, patient and service user surveys, monitoring, and so on:

1 Apply added value, handover, elapsed time and process cost analyses to your process map.
2 List the main problems emerging from your process map and analysis.

As in the previous Activity, if you are working with colleagues on a potential process improvement you will need to carry out the analysis of the process map in collaboration with them.

You should now have identified some opportunities to improve your service for the benefit of patients or service users. You should also have some relevant information to present to colleagues and decision makers to support your proposals. You may have identified improvements to quality that would also represent cost savings for your organisation. Once you have clear ideas about potential improvements, you need to present a clear argument for implementing them. It is often helpful to present proposals of this kind either as a written report or as an oral presentation, backed up with visual aids that support your argument. Once others are convinced that improvements can be made, the next step is to design the process improvement.

DESIGNING PROCESS IMPROVEMENTS

The design stage of process improvement may include:

■ stimulating and using the creative and innovative talents of your staff, colleagues and other stakeholders, whether in making incremental or 'breakthrough' improvements
■ discovering and using new process designs, operating philosophies and enabling technologies
■ using surveys of patients and service users and other forms of feedback to determine their perceptions of existing services and their needs and expectations of services in the future
■ designing and developing both improved and new services to meet the needs and expectations of patients and service users.

For example, here are some of the proposals that were generated by consultations with staff in the operating theatre example:

The *senior nurse manager* in the surgical directorate has seen some recent publications on business process re-engineering. She sees a review of the theatres as a major opportunity to introduce new working practices. Re-engineering, she notes, can involve multiskilling, process teams, flatter organisation hierarchies, 'case managers', and more employee 'empowerment'.

The *business manager* in the directorate is sympathetic to this view, but feels that it is the administrative staff who assemble patient documentation, who arrange appointments and who draw up the theatre lists, who are isolated and not effectively involved in the patient trail. The hospital's computerised Theatreman system captures a lot of information about the patient flow, including operation times, outcomes and delays. This information, however, is not used systematically to monitor what is happening and to trigger improvements.

The *theatre sisters and operating department assistants* claim that the theatre lists would run to time more often if they did the scheduling themselves – once the surgeons had determined each patient's priority.

The *consultants*, however, who can claim the highest status and expertise in this context, argue that the problem lies simply with the lack of adequate numbers of ward staff and porters, and with the way these staff are used and controlled. The problem could be solved, in their view, with more nurses, more porters, more effectively managed. The data in the Theatreman computer, they feel, is inaccurate and unreliable, as information is recorded by operating department assistants and nurses under pressure, and keyed up by clerical staff who sometimes need to rely on 'informed judgement' when coding the information. They would like to see some straightforward remedial action taken immediately, to help them, to help their staff, and to help patients. A major organisational review would take time, and is not really necessary.

(Buchanan and Wilson, 1996)

What lessons can we learn from the reactions of each of these groups of people?

- Consultation with the patients in this situation is difficult because they are anaesthetised during most of the significant time. However, their views on how they experience the time they are awake – and the consequences of actions taken while they are asleep – would be informative.
- People sometimes think in terms of 'episodes' rather than in terms of 'processes' – they see problems from the perspective of their own part of the process, without perceiving the overall picture.
- Some people have higher status than others and can enforce their points of view, making it difficult for others' views to be heard.
- Major organisational review and change may be required to improve the process.

- Major change carries significant implications for costs and for disruption of services.
- Sometimes major change is not required.
- People do not necessarily agree about what the problem is.
- Problems arising from poor management of the implementation of change can lead to the usefulness of existing activities being undermined.
- There can be differences of opinion about who should be included in the 'process team'.
- New ideas take time to be accepted sufficiently to be incorporated in the creative thinking of a team.
- Some solutions can require major financial investment (for example, new information systems) which the immediate members of the process team do not have the resources or the authority to implement.
- Not everyone welcomes innovations.

ACTIVITY 13.4

Return to the process from your own work area that you examined and consider how you and the other people involved can set about designing improvements to it. Make two lists – one identifying things you need to do to redesign the process, and the other identifying things you must avoid doing as you redesign the process.

You may find it useful to refer to our lists below, which draw largely on the case study material. Your list may need to include other things specific to your working environment.

Dos and don'ts in service design and redesign

DO

Decide who the 'process team' includes and make sure they are all involved.

Check language and understanding.

Check that existing procedures are being used properly and effectively.

Think of appropriate ways to consult patients and service users that suit the situation.

Try to achieve a consensus about what the problem or problems are.

Look for technological opportunities.

Listen carefully to all points of view.

Give equal weight to all points of view.

Encourage people to think 'process' rather than 'episode' and to see their place in the overall picture.

Consider how the parts of the process fit together and communicate with each other.

Encourage creative thinking – for example, by brainstorming.

Keep your eye on the purposes and values of the service.

Make use of any outcome information.

Create opportunities for discussion and 'sparking' of ideas.

Be prepared to review the service standards to be met.

Be clear about your own powers and responsibilities.

Be prepared to think flexibly about responsibilities and skills.

Be prepared to incorporate new national standards.

Be prepared to incorporate research and good practice from elsewhere.

Consult stakeholders.

Think small before thinking big.

Check whether there are relevant National Service Frameworks.

DON'T

Force the pace.

Assume that everyone has the same understanding of the words and concepts in use.

Leave important players out of the process team.

Move to solutions before the problem is clear and has been analysed.

Forget key stakeholders.

Allow fixed patterns of thought ('this is how we do it here') to prevent creative thinking.

Underestimate the time and energy this activity may take.

The establishment of the NHS Learning Network is an attempt to disseminate good practice across the NHS. The Service Delivery Practice Database contains examples of service improvements, such as booked admissions and waiting list initiatives that have delivered benefits to patients. The idea is to encourage replication and sharing of good practice and innovative solutions to service problems more widely across the NHS. Copying ideas is to be encouraged!

The ways in which processes are carried out make a very important contribution to the quality of services. This chapter has taken you through the technique of process mapping and analysing process maps in order to identify opportunities for improvement in your own area of work. We concluded by considering some of the issues involved in the redesign of a process.

REFERENCES

Buchanan, D. and Wilson R. (1996) 'Next patient please – the operating theatres problem at Leicester General Hospital NHS Trust', in J. Storey (ed.) *Blackwell Cases in Human Resource and Change Management*, pp. 190–205, Blackwell.

Leicester Royal Infirmary (1998) *Patient Process Redesign Toolkit*, Leicester Royal Infirmary NHS Trust.

CHAPTER 14

PLANNING AND MANAGING PROJECTS

It is one thing to analyse your service delivery processes to identify and design improvements, and quite another to implement them successfully. Implementing change involves bringing all your management knowledge and skills to bear in planning the resources required in order to complete the project within the required time-scale.

A project is something that needs to be done in addition to – and occasionally instead of – the normal day-to-day tasks of managing. It is usually a one-off non-repeated activity that is intended to achieve specified objectives and quality requirements within a time limit. Maylor (1996) defines the characteristics of a project in the following terms:

■ It has a clear beginning and end.
■ The whole activity is directed at achieving the defined output or outcome.
■ It has a set of constraints that limit and define what can be achieved.
■ Its output can be measured in terms of performance against agreed indicators.

A project, almost by definition, involves change. Planning for change involves you, as a manager, working with the impact of the change on all the people involved – patients, service users, staff, carers, service providers with whom you work in partnership and other stakeholders.

And planning is itself a process. That might seem so self-evident as to be hardly worth stating. But planning is often such a messy, iterative and confusing business that the underlying process may be completely obscured. This chapter focuses on that underlying process in order to help you plan in a systematic way. Planning is rather like preparing for a journey. You need to work out the best way of getting from where you are now to where you want to be.

PLANNING A PROJECT

Jean is the manager of a day centre for adults with learning disabilities. We are going to illustrate the planning process in the context of a project to implement an improvement in her service. At each stage, we describe what she did and invite you to consider how these stages would be similar or different in planning a service improvement in your work setting.

Jean works for a large voluntary organisation providing services for adults with learning disabilities. It has recently received a critical inspection report on its day services, is concerned about the impact of the National Service Framework for Mental Health and is anxious not to lose its contracts with local authorities. A planned major improvement is to extend the 'shared action planning' process to all its service users, and a steering group of managers from each of its day centres has recently agreed a timetable for this. Jean now has the task of implementing this in her centre.

Jean's centre has space for meetings and activities for about 40 people with learning disabilities, ranging from people with physical as well as learning disabilities to people who lead fairly independent lives. Some of them have mental health problems in addition to their learning disability, and some have epilepsy. About half of them live in group homes or hostels, and the rest live at home with their parents or other relatives. The local population includes people from different ethnic minorities, and this is reflected among the 40 service users and the 15 members of staff.

Shared action planning enables the organisation to deploy the skills of its staff to achieve its mission, which is:

To ensure that people with learning disabilities are able to express their wants, needs and concerns, that plans will be made and action taken with them and with their carers to meet those wants, needs and concerns, while due regard is paid to any risks of harm involved, and steps taken to support and protect from harm with the minimum reduction in life chances and choices.

Jean's service has the following features:

- Each service user has a key worker.
- The role of the key worker is to ensure that the service user has an opportunity to express his or her wishes and needs, and to try to make available the life chances he or she hopes for.
- Assessments of need are carried out and updated annually.

- The key worker acts as a focal point for communication, liaising with the people who influence the service user's life – including parents and other relatives, adult education tutors, employers, therapists and health and social services staff.
- The key worker sets up review meetings with relevant parties on a regular basis to ensure that shared action plans are implemented.
- The key worker – together with the service user – keeps records of assessments, review meetings, key events and incidents, and actions taken to implement shared action plans.

At present, only the service users who live in group homes and hostels have a shared action plan. The aim now is for all the service users to have one. This means that the process will have to be introduced to 20 more people and their families, and some staff who have not previously acted as key workers will need to take on this role. There will be more meetings between staff, service users and others, and more records to be kept.

To give herself some time to think about the implications of this change, Jean arranged for one of her deputies to cover for her for a day. She considered shutting herself in her office, but realised that she would have so many interruptions that she would achieve little or nothing, so she found herself a quiet place at home. Her aim for the day was to give enough thought to the major issues to be able to prepare an agenda for a special meeting of her senior team, who would be vital to the successful implementation of the project. She wanted them to think about the issues, and to play a prominent role in planning what needed to be done and in preparing staff, service users and families for the changes to come.

In order to clarify what she needed to do to steer the process, Jean asked herself the following questions, based on what are often described as the seven phases of the planning process:

- Phase 1 – What are we trying to do?
- Phase 2 – What is the best way of doing it?
- Phase 3 – What are we going to have to do?
- Phase 4 – In what order should we do things?
- Phase 5 – What resources are we going to need?
- Phase 6 – Let's review the plan: is it going to work?
- Phase 7 – Who is going to do what – and when?

She scanned quickly through the seven phases, making brief notes about each. She realised that she would have to return to all the phases in more detail later, but this first look gave her a sense of what had to be done. Here are her notes.

Phase 1: What are we trying to do?

This is not problematic – shared action planning has been done before and is familiar to staff and service users in the centre. There is no need to develop a new statement of purpose. However, it might be helpful to revisit both the purpose of the centre and the purpose of shared action planning as part of making sure that all staff, service users and families understand what is involved and are prepared for the change.

Phase 2: What is the best way of doing it?

Shared action planning has proved to be an effective means of delivering the centre's purpose, and it will not be necessary to spend much time reconsidering its appropriateness. It can be implemented only if all parties have a good understanding of what it involves and are prepared to play their roles in it. Making sure that everyone is clear about these things is going to be vitally important. Drawing up a plan for clarifying everyone's roles, delegating tasks and putting together a communication strategy need to be items on the agenda for the meeting with senior staff.

Phase 3: What are we going to have to do?

This will be an important item on the agenda. The senior staff's knowledge of their roles and the aspects of the work of the centre for which they are responsible is going to be vital in assessing the current position and making sure that they anticipate what has to be done and what problems may arise. They need to take 'ownership' of the implementation process by setting agreed objectives.

Jean came up with a long list of things to do grouped under four headings.

Tasks involving everyone

- Gain the co-operation of staff and service users in extending shared action planning.
- Review the workings of the existing scheme to ensure that valuable experience is built on and not lost (this may also be a good way of allowing people to say 'goodbye' to the things that they will lose by the change).
- Understand the anxieties engendered by change and take steps to reduce these where possible.
- Set up a familiarisation strategy so that everyone involved understands what shared action planning is and the demands it will make on them, whether they are staff, service users, families or partner agencies. It is about co-ordination of all the parties who impact on the life of a person with a learning disability.
- Anticipate some of the likely changes that will be initiated by service users through the new opportunities they have to express their views about their lives, including the impact on their families.
- Anticipate any risk factors that may emerge.

■ Think about the needs of service users and families for whom English is not their first language.

Tasks involving staff

■ Discuss anticipated changes in staff roles and working practices with the trades union.
■ Appraise the new skill requirements of staff and set up any training required.
■ Revise staff rotas to take account of changes in working practices.

Tasks I have to do (or delegate)

■ Monitor both the implementation of the change and the effectiveness of shared action planning for all clients.
■ Plan the timetable for extending shared action planning.
■ Develop a reporting strategy to inform the local authorities with which the centre has contracts of plans, progress and anticipated problems.
■ Make sure that my own needs for developing new skills are met.

Resources

■ Identify the resource implications of introducing new record-keeping systems, changing roles for staff and additional review meetings.
■ Calculate the costs of implementation.

Now that Jean has identified the main things that need to be done, let's pause for a moment to explore how you can apply the first three phases of planning to a project in your own workplace.

ACTIVITY 14.1

Think of an improvement that you would like to make in your area of work. Review the first three phases of planning for your project and make notes about what will need to be done under the headings:

■ Phase 1 – What are we trying to do?
■ Phase 2 – What is the best way of doing it?
■ Phase 3 – What are we going to have to do?

(You may wish to keep a project file of your notes on this and subsequent activities in this chapter.)

Now we return to Jean's notes.

Phase 4: In what order should we do things?

At the meeting with senior staff, we'll need to draw a chart showing the sequence of the main activities that will need to take place. We'll also have to consider whether a phased process of introduction would be appropriate. Timing of training for staff and service users will be a key issue and phasing in the new arrangements would avoid having to do all the training at once.

Phase 5: What resources are we going to need?

This will be another item for the senior staff meeting. In addition to freeing up staff time for training and to do new tasks, some new equipment will be needed (including filing cabinets for storing the additional records) and space for more frequent meetings. We'll need to review how space is currently being used in the centre and plan for any necessary changes.

ACTIVITY 14.2

Make brief notes on phases 4 and 5 of your project:

- Phase 4 – In what order should we do things?
- Phase 5 – What resources are we going to need?

The next step for Jean was to review whether the ideas she had so far would be likely to work in her setting. Here are her notes on the remaining phases of the planning process.

Phase 6: Let's review the plan: is it going to work?

There will be many opportunities for senior staff to review the project as we work together. The shared action planning process includes provision for monitoring progress with individual service users. An overview of progress should be a regular item on our agenda to ensure that key targets are being met and to adjust the plans if it is necessary to make changes.

Phase 7: Who is going to do what – and when?

Delegation is going to be crucial. Appropriate people will need to have delegated authority for each of the activities on the schedule chart. Each person will have to have clear objectives and targets, including dates for the delivery of their parts of the plan. Each person will need to be given the time to undertake their tasks and will also need to have – or have the opportunity for developing – the necessary skills.

By the time Jean had completed her review of the seven phases of planning, she had created the agenda for the first meeting of the senior staff. She now realised that they would need to set up a series of meetings to deal with all the planning issues and to monitor progress.

ACTIVITY 14.3

Complete your project plan by considering phases 6 and 7:

■ Phase 6 – Let's review the plan: is it going to work?
■ Phase 7 – Who is going to do what – and when?

How easy will it be to make changes?

Stocking (1985) identified a number of factors that assist the rapid diffusion of innovation in a health service, many of which are equally relevant in social care:

■ The existence of identifiable enthusiasts – those who invented or discovered the idea, who are keen to disseminate it, who have reasonable status in their profession or occupational group, and who are prepared to invest considerable time and energy in promoting it – people who will 'champion' the project.
■ The innovation should not be in conflict with current national policies, organisational policies or established climates of opinion among professionals and other groups.
■ It needs to have local appeal to those who have the power to promote change.
■ It has to meet the perceived needs of patients, service users and staff, must 'add value', must not require major role or attitude changes, and should be simple to organise.
■ It should be adaptable to suit local circumstances.
■ Little financial or other resources should be required, unless such requirements can be hidden or increased resources can be made available.

Here are Jean's notes about how closely her plan fits with Stocking's criteria:

The existence of identifiable enthusiasts

I certainly see myself as a 'product champion'. Two of my deputies, several of the other staff and many of the service users are very positive. The cook is particularly keen, as she likes catering for the individual preferences of service users. Some of the parents of service users living in hostels have found shared action planning helpful and campaigned for it to be introduced for all service users.

The innovation should not be in conflict with current policies or established climates of opinion

Shared action planning fits well with national and local policies. Most of the centre's staff have become familiar with it during the five years since it was first introduced, although some find it cumbersome and time-consuming. Some staff are new to it.

It needs to have local appeal to those who have the power to promote change

There might be some difficulty here. Some opinion-formers in the local Mencap group are in favour of shared action planning, but others have campaigned against changes that they see as putting their sons or daughters at risk.

It has to meet perceived needs and add value

Shared action planning is designed to meet the needs of service users, and to enable them to enlarge their horizons. But it can appear threatening to those who think that people with learning disabilities should be protected from the responsibilities and difficulties of life.

It must not require major role or attitude changes

Becoming a key worker is part of the professional ambition of some staff, but for more senior staff it may represent loss of the status they had previously. It requires staff to use their skills wisely, to listen to service users and to recognise that professionals do not always know best.

It should be simple to organise

Shared action planning can lead to substantial reorganisation of activities to accommodate the needs and wants of service users.

It should be adaptable to suit local circumstances

Provided that the principles of good communication, key working and co-ordination are maintained, shared action planning is very appropriate to our local circumstances.

Little finance or other resource is required

This depends on how the key worker role is developed. If it is linked to grades and pay, some staff may expect promotion and pay rises, and some may feel that they are losing out. There may also be costs incurred by the service users in taking up new activities.

Jean found this analysis of the centre's situation helpful in identifying the areas on which she and her team wou'' need to concentrate. Judged by Stocking's criteria, they were going t   particular attention to:

- worries of parents and families, espe·   perceived risks to service users
- issues about staff roles and grading
- the impact of changes in working practices on everyone involved.

ACTIVITY 14.4

Make notes on how the process improvement you were planning in Activities 5–7 match Stocking's criteria.

Which areas will need special attention when you are implementing your plan?

MANAGING PEOPLE AND CHANGE

Jean is responsible for the use of a building and the physical resources within it, but she knows that the effective implementation of a process such as shared action planning is dependent on the willingness and ability of those who take part in it to make it a success. Their contributions are far more important than the physical resources.

A number of factors influence how people respond to change, and you need to put yourself in the shoes of each of the participants to understand what the change means to them. Some questions to consider are:

1   Who will be active and who will be passive in the process of implementing the project – who are likely to be proactive initiators, passive objects, or victims of the proposed change?
2   For whom will the proposed change lead to a change of identity?
3   What meanings do the *status quo* and the proposed change have for each of them?
4   Who will experience a change in status or image of themselves as a result of the proposed change?
5   How may the proposed change affect their motivation?
6   What will they win or lose?

You will almost certainly find it helpful to discuss the proposed changes with each group of people – or even each individual. This will be a major task, but may well save a lot of time later.

KEEPING ON TRACK

In this section we focus in rather more detail on two of the phases of planning a project that we described – sequencing activities (phase 4) and scheduling activities (phase 7) – for which a number of techniques are available that you may find useful.

Sequencing activities

Phase 4 of the planning process concentrates on sequencing activities – arranging them in the order in which they need to be done. It is important to identify activities that cannot start until others have been completed. These activities will determine the overall sequence in which you carry out your project because you have no option but to do them in that order. Other activities may be less critical. It may be possible to undertake some of them in parallel: you can do them at the same time. It may be possible for some activities to take place at any time: you can decide when is a suitable point to fit them in.

Two techniques for sequencing activities and representing them in diagrammatic form are *logic diagrams* and *Gantt charts*.

'The art of implementation is to establish priorities and sequences of action carefully.'

(Sir Roy Griffiths, speaking at the 1989 IHSM Conference 'Management in the 1990s')

Logic diagrams

One way of sorting out the relationships between a sequence of actions is to use a logic diagram. The name sounds rather daunting, but this is quite a simple technique that can readily be done on the back of an envelope.

A logic diagram is a network of lines that shows the logical sequence of activities and, in particular, which activities must be completed before others can start. For example, in the diagram in Figure 14.1, activity H must be completed before activity I can start. Activity H can be taking place at the same time as activity F, but both must be completed before activity I can start.

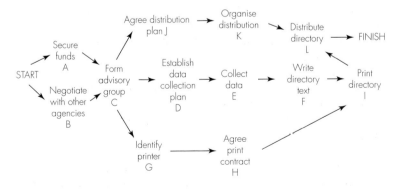

Figure 14.1 Logic diagram for the production of a directory

ACTIVITY 14.5

Sketch a logic diagram for the sequence of activities that you will need to carry out in the project that you have been thinking about.

Logic diagrams are only concerned with showing the sequence of activities. They make no attempt to show the length of time that an activity will take: the lengths of the lines in the diagram do not represent the durations of the activities. To give a more detailed picture of the project – including the time required for each activity – it is helpful to draw a Gantt chart.

Gantt charts

The Gantt chart (named after the man credited with inventing it) is one of the most commonly used techniques for planning a sequence of activities and showing how long each will take. Each activity is drawn as a bar against a time-scale. The length of each bar represents the expected duration of that activity.

A Gantt chart presents the project plan in a visual form that can readily be understood by everyone involved. It can be used at any stage in the planning process, from initial outline planning to the detailed planning of individual tasks. Figure 14.2 is Jean's Gantt chart, showing how she will extend shared action planning.

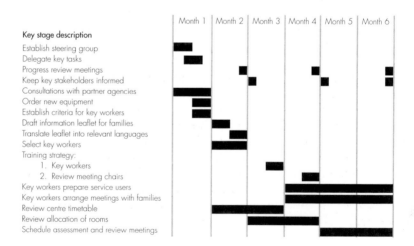

Figure 14.2 Gantt chart for extending shared action planning

You can see from Figure 14.2 that:

- A Gantt chart shows the sequence and durations of activities and thus reveals any options for changing the sequence.
- It shows those activities that can be carried out concurrently.
- Bars need not be continuous.

This technique can be used for planning complex projects as well as simple ones. However, for bigger projects, each bar on the master chart might have to be drawn as a more detailed separate Gantt chart. In Jean's example, the bars dealing with selection, training and the tasks of key workers would have to be planned in more detail, although the overall duration of the activities involved would still need to be completed at the times shown in Figure 14.2.

ACTIVITY 14.6

This is an opportunity to turn the logic diagram that you drafted into a Gantt chart. List all the activities needed to implement your project in sequence in the column on the left. Decide the likely overall duration of the project and head the rest of the columns as days, weeks or months. Draw in the bars to indicate the length of time each activity will take.

A Gantt chart can help you to think about whether you can complete a project on time. You may have started with the first activity and just worked down the list, putting in the time you thought each would take. If so, you will be lucky if the chart shows that you will meet your deadline for completing the project. If you have a deadline, you could start with the final activity and work your way back. If this reveals that you are not able to complete the project on time (or that you should have started it a few months ago!), you can consider how to adjust the plan.

You have a number of choices. It may be possible to carry out several activities in parallel, instead of one after another. You may be able to reduce the scale of the project to eliminate some of the activities. You could increase the resources available (usually the number of people carrying out activities). This might be appropriate if the outcome is important and is needed by a particular deadline. Another option is to negotiate an extension to the deadline to enable all the activities to be completed without increasing resources.

Scheduling activities

Phase 7 of the planning process – deciding who is going to do what, and when – is the final stage before implementation. Up to this point, the plan has been largely hypothetical – working out what you are trying to do, and how you will do it if the necessary resources are available. It is all conditional. But when the conditions have been fulfilled, and the plan has been approved and is about to be put into practice, a further step is needed. You need to specify how the plan will be converted into action. This means being clear about who is to do what and by when, so that all those who will be implementing the project know precisely what is required of them. This also ensures that you, as the manager responsible for it, can co-ordinate and control the often complex range of activities and resources that are needed to implement it.

The specification prepared in this phase goes under various names. It is often referred to as an 'action plan'. Another way of describing this phase is to refer to it as 'scheduling'. The schedules are the part of a plan that sets out the details of who will carry out which parts of the work, and when they are to do it.

Two useful approaches to scheduling activities are *key events planning* and *milestone planning*.

Key events planning

One of the simplest ways of representing a plan in an easily understood way is to list the key events and the date (sometimes even the time) when each event is planned to occur. By 'event', we mean an action or activity that is planned to occur at a particular time. It is different from a 'process', which takes place over a period of time. So 'order publicity material' and 'complete review of publicity material' are events planned for a particular time and could appear on a key events plan, but 'prepare publicity material' is a process rather than an event because the activity would take place over a period of time. 'Key events' are the most important events in the plan; the lesser events cluster around them.

There are two main uses for key events planning:

■ to specify the overall framework of a project so that other people can prepare their detailed plans to fit in with the key events
■ to identify the target dates in a large project plan that must be met by the people involved in only one part of that plan.

Let's consider an example. A local charity has raised a substantial amount of money to build a hospice. The building is nearing completion and will be opened by a VIP. The commissioning officer is planning the opening ceremony in close consultation with the protocol officer (the VIP's representative) and has drawn up the key events plan shown in Table 14.1.

Table 14.1 A key events plan for the opening of a hospice

Date	Key events	Other events
2 July	Planning meeting	Receive project status reports Issue detailed plans for each department
6 July	Outline plan of ceremony to VIP	Distribute ceremony plan internally Receive departmental updates Receive building, plant and equipment status report
16 July	Visit of VIP's protocol officer	Receive draft of publicity material Agree press arrangements Confirm catering plans Agree guest list
24 July	Receive comments from protocol officer	Distribute comments Order publicity material Confirm press arrangements Check status of whole project
27 July	Handover of building	Check that equipment installation complete Test equipment
30 July	Planning meeting	Review handover Receive final lists of problems from departments
2 August	Rehearsal	
6 August	Final planning meeting	Review publicity material Review status of any problems
13 August	VIP visit	

This is not a comprehensive list of everything that must take place to achieve a successful opening ceremony. Its purpose is to highlight the dates on which key events are planned to occur and by which the activities contributing to those events must be complete. It enables the people responsible for the different aspects of the ceremony (publicity, catering, finishing the hospice, etc.) to adjust their own plans to fit in with the dates of the key events and to identify any possible problems in meeting them.

By the addition of an extra column to Table 14.1, it would be possible to indicate who was responsible for ensuring that each event occurs as scheduled. Each of these people could then produce more detailed schedules of who was going to do what and by when.

Table 14.2 Part of a milestone plan

Milestone	Main activities	Other activities
30 June	Building complete Services 90% complete	Computer installation commenced
31 July	Services complete Planning starts for moving medical records	Budgets completed Staff informed of individual tasks

Milestone planning

Milestone planning is very similar to key events planning. The difference is that, whereas a key events schedule lists the main events irrespective of the time intervals between them, a milestone schedule lists a series of dates at fixed intervals (the milestones). It shows the stage that each of the main activities is expected to have reached by those dates.

Milestone planning is often used to monitor and control events to ensure that they remain on course. The manager calls for progress reports to be submitted at the fixed dates, so that he or she can check whether everything is going according to plan. The technique is illustrated in Table 14.2.

PROBLEMS WITH PLANNING

The seven phases of planning a project that we have described are an idealised and rational sequence. Planning starts at phase 1 and moves smoothly forward. If managerial life were as simple as that, planning would be merely a matter of moving steadily through the phases to the point when implementation begins. Thereafter, the manager would cease planning and start controlling – ensuring that everything was going according to plan.

But life is often not as simple as this. Countless complexities may conspire to make the planning process more like a game of snakes and ladders than the neat linear process that we have depicted. Nevertheless, even a game of snakes and ladders has an underlying logic: the aim is to progress in a particular direction, despite the hazards and despite having to visit old ground time and again. Similarly, planning has an underlying logic, with the aim of progressing in a particular direction. But in the hazards of real life, there is a risk of losing that sense of direction. Our aim in spelling out the phases has been to give you a 'map' to help you keep on track throughout the planning process.

All sorts of things make planning a good deal more complex – and less rational. Let's look at two common problems: you can find yourself going round in circles, and your objectives may be vague. We then conclude the chapter by looking at a solution – making contingency plans.

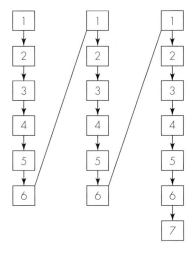

Figure 14.3 Multistage approach

Going round in circles

You may have to go back over the same ground several times, refining and modifying as you go. One way of describing this inevitable revisiting of old ground is to refer to it as *multistage planning* (Figure 14.3), implying that you go through the whole process once, and then again, and then again, until your plan is sufficiently refined to be put into action.

Multistage planning is likely to be a necessary part of implementing a project within your own service or department. It is likely to be even more necessary when developing major plans at the corporate level. Here is how one planner working in the health service described the process.

First stage
This would be the production of a plan in general terms, outlining the overall aims and objectives, a rough estimate of the costs and the time required. This would be an outline plan that would be in sufficient detail to show that there would be a reasonable likelihood that it could be carried out.

Second stage
A plan would then be produced which would still be fairly broad, based on rough estimates. All the people involved in the project would contribute to the plan and identify the activities required of them to achieve it. A number of options would be developed, listing the alternative ways and means of meeting the aims and objectives. These would be considered by the participants and a preferred option should emerge once everyone has

ascertained the feasibility of achieving their respective contributions. A consolidated plan would be produced.

Third stage

If the second stage plan seemed feasible, a final plan would be produced. This would be more detailed than the previous plans and would provide an action plan for implementation.

In this illustration, the terms 'first stage', 'second stage' and 'third stage' are used to emphasise that planning is a multistage process rather than a single pass as implied in the 'rational' seven-phase approach. These terms are not generally used, but the principle of multistage planning is widely practised.

An alternative way of viewing this multistage process is to regard it as being *cyclical*. Each cycle takes you through all the seven phases (Figure 14.4). At the very least, you will need to go round the loop two or three times as you refine your plan. The first time round you will probably do little more than identify and resolve some of the major problems, finishing up with the broad outline of a plan. The second time round (if all is going well) you will be able to add more detail and begin to make decisions. The third time round (if you are lucky) you might finish up with something that could be put into effect with a reasonable chance of success. It is little wonder that you often feel that you are going round in circles when you are planning – you *are* going round in circles, but you are gathering more information and refining the details as you do so.

In real life, you are rarely likely to be able to maintain forward progress round the circle for very long. You will often need to drop back a couple of phases, just as in snakes and ladders, before you can make further progress. So the process is better described as *iterative* rather than cyclical, acknowledging the fact that your forward progress may be interrupted by having to return and adjust something that you

Figure 14.4 Cyclical approach

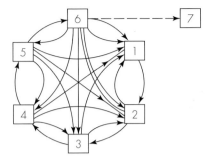

Figure 14.5 Iterative approach

have just settled. The idea of planning as an iterative process is illustrated in Figure 14.5, which demonstrates why planning can seem such a confused and confusing process.

However you look at it, planning is rarely a straightforward process. It is usually necessary to go over the same ground several times, refining the plan and adding more detail as the route becomes clearer.

Vague objectives

How often, when you are planning, have you sat down and carefully worked out precisely what you are trying to achieve? Unless you know what you are supposed to be achieving, it is very difficult to plan to achieve it.

It may be difficult to describe clear and precise objectives because the situation or task is unclear. Sometimes, however, we are our own worst enemies and we describe objectives in vague terms even though we have all the ingredients we need for precision. One way of avoiding this problem is to check that your objectives are SMART (specific, measurable, agreed, realistic and time-bounded).

The objective 'Go on holiday in the summer' is definitely not SMART (but it may be a goal). The objective 'Take a walking holiday for two in the Black Forest in the middle two weeks of June at a cost not exceeding £600' is very SMART and you can see the difference at a glance.

When you apply the SMART test to your objectives, you may find they are not sufficiently precise. The action that is then needed may be as simple as adding in more detail (which was available but you had forgotten to include it). Alternatively, you may realise that more work is needed before you can improve the wording of an objective (which may take you into the iterative approach illustrated in Figure 14.5).

Contingency plans

We have focused on some of the factors that make planning hazardous. We all know that events have a remarkably perverse way of evolving in unexpected directions. It is not surprising, therefore, that plans often appear to 'go wrong'. In fact, they don't go wrong. They just don't quite fit the reality that finally emerges, and they need to be adjusted if they are to remain operable. It is often possible to make the necessary adjustments so that the plan is still workable, and it is one of the tasks of managers to keep plans continuously under review and to adjust them as circumstances demand. Flexibility is therefore one of the most important characteristics of any plan – and of any planner.

But circumstances can sometimes change quickly and dramatically so that the original plan is no longer operable. Suppose a key member of staff were to leave Jean's team just as her project is to be implemented? She would need a contingency plan. Perhaps she could train another member of staff to cover the same tasks. Perhaps someone could be seconded to Jean's team from elsewhere in the organisation or from another organisation. Perhaps the plan could be rescheduled or partially implemented.

Throughout the planning process, you should keep on asking, 'What if this goes wrong? What if that goes wrong?' If the answer is that it doesn't matter, a contingency plan may not be necessary. But if it does matter, a contingency plan is essential. You should be constantly on the look-out for contingencies that could have significant consequences, and prepare contingency plans to deal with them if they do occur.

Planning is not a simple process. Even when planning quite a modest project, it is often necessary to go round in circles, revisiting old ground repeatedly and adjusting as you go. However, it is helpful to use a structured approach – to keep the seven phases of planning in mind to ensure that you include all the important elements. You need to maintain some order within the chaos in order to make progress towards improving services.

REFERENCES

Maylor, H. (1996) *Project Management*, Pitman Publishing.
Stocking, B. (1985) *Initiative and Inertia: Case Studies in the NHS*, Nuffield Provincial Hospital Trust.

SERVICE PLANNING, ACCOUNTABILITY AND RISK

Planning publicly funded health and social care services in most countries is a function of Government. Government policy has a profound influence on the proportion of national income spent on health and social care, and on the ways in which services are provided and priorities are set. This influence extends to health and social care organisations that are not directly funded by Government because of the ways in which the processes of commissioning services operate. Managers who are planning service provision must therefore take account of Government policy whether they are planning for:

- a large national organisation such as the NHS
- a local council, as in the case of social care
- an independent service provider in the voluntary or private sectors
- a provider of an integrated service that no longer sits squarely in any one of these sectors.

We begin this chapter by examining the process of business planning, which enables organisations to translate Government policy, the resources available to them, and the needs and aspirations of local people into plans focused on making the best use of resources to achieve their objectives. Your organisation's business plan provides the background against which you have to manage your service or department.

We then consider what accountability means to you as a manager in health or social care services.

We conclude by examining the responsibilities that you have for the safety of your staff and service users, and how you can assess and manage risk in your service or department.

PLANNING HEALTH AND SOCIAL CARE SERVICES

Health and social care services in all countries in the United Kingdom are strongly influenced by changes in Government policy because they are funded as public services. It may be tempting to think that changes at Government level are unlikely to have much effect on your service. You may think that running a children's home or a hospital ward or assessing and providing for service users' needs is essentially the same process – with the same management challenges – whatever Government is in power.

However, if there is a change in the level of resources provided by Government or in national or local Government policy, there may be a need to make major changes in how health and social care services are delivered. New policies can include changes of priorities in funding, different attitudes to collaboration or competition, and different values relating to the purposes of public services. These in turn can produce changes in emphasis, new opportunities and new organisational structures that may provide you with opportunities for improvement, change and innovation.

Consider, for example, the requirements of 'best value' (Department of the Environment, Transport and the Regions, 1998). This is an approach that national Government requires local authorities to follow to demonstrate that they are spending public money effectively. Local authorities are responsible, through their social services or social work departments, for commissioning social care provision from independent organisations, as well as providing their own services. They are required to undertake regular and fundamental performance reviews to ensure that continuous improvements are made to all services, not just to those where there are serious shortcomings.

The main outcome of a best value review is a set of performance targets that incorporate national guidance on best practice. These should include strategic objectives, cost efficiency, effectiveness, quality and fair access. There is also a requirement to draw up an action plan to demonstrate how the targets are to be achieved. Each local authority has to explain why the targets have been set as they have and why it has chosen a particular route to achieve them. Best value reviews:

- *challenge* why and how a service is being provided
- *compare* the performance of a service with the performance of similar services offered by other providers across a range of relevant indicators, taking into account the views of both service users and potential suppliers
- *consult* with local taxpayers, service users and the business community in setting new performance targets
- embrace fair *competition* as a means of securing efficient and effective services.

Reviews of this nature, with an emphasis on increasing and improving partnership working between health and social care organisations, can lead to quite different approaches to service delivery.

Planning guidance

Government policy directives provide the main building blocks for planning in publicly funded health and social care. In England, for example, health authorities are required, in collaboration with all relevant agencies, to produce health improvement plans. Local authorities must produce children's services plans that take an overview of services rather than focusing on provision by individual organisations. This approach to planning is based on the concept of integrated care pathways, thus promoting the development of services that are integrated across organisational boundaries. The requirement for services to work across traditional boundaries to provide more integrated responses to the needs of service users is seen as a national priority because failure to make appropriate links between services decreases public confidence and increases costs.

As a front-line manager, you are not likely to be responsible for the preparation of a plan that involves other organisations and service providers. You may, however, be asked to contribute information to such a plan, and to develop your own service to meet the objectives of integrated service plans in your locality. If you are a manager in an independent organisation, you need to keep your eye on developments that may affect your position as a service provider, and you may be asked to contribute to the planning process.

Business planning

Organisations in health and social care have to plan their own activities within the overall plans that have been developed for services in a geographic area. Each organisation develops a *business plan* to ensure that it can continue to make a valuable contribution to service provision by using the resources available effectively to meet appropriate performance standards.

Business plans are inevitably complex to develop because of the number of separate health and social care organisations that need to be involved in providing services and because organisations have to demonstrate that they offer good value, in terms of both value for money and standards of performance. Comparisons are increasingly made between services provided in different areas of the country, with the aim of bringing all services up to an equivalent standard. This approach emphasises continuous development of service provision, and managers at all levels can expect to be involved in measuring performance against standards and in planning for improved performance.

Business planning can be described in terms of three main features – it should be continuous, user-driven and outward-looking.

■ Business planning is unlike planning a task or a project because it has no clear end-point. There are always aims and objectives in a business plan, but they are regularly updated and replaced. Thus business planning is a *continuous* process.

■ Business planning is *user-driven* because every organisation, if it is to remain successful, has to meet the needs and expectations of patients and service users and the objectives set by commissioners. Four types of stakeholder have an interest in your services – beneficiaries, participants, payers and specifiers. Failure to be sensitive to the needs of any of these can lead to failure to meet performance targets. If an organisation is unable to meet its targets, its future may be in jeopardy, particularly if there are other local organisations that are more successful.

■ The focus of attention in business planning is partly on the organisation itself, but it must also be *outward-looking* – it must take account of external factors that could influence its future. For example, there may be imminent changes in national service frameworks or new standards may be introduced. Business planning needs to take account of comparisons with other organisations that are doing better and what any potential competitors are doing.

Since business planning is a continuous process, which implies that a business plan is constantly changing, is it worth writing it down? The answer is 'Yes'. Organisations need a written business plan because the information it contains needs to be shared both within the organisation and with stakeholders and the public. All the interested parties need to know:

■ What are we trying to do?
■ What is the best way of doing it?
■ What resources are we going to need?

Although continuous change is to be expected, some elements of a business plan will be more enduring than others. For example, organisations rarely change their overall purpose or core activities. Most organisations plan to build on what they already do successfully.

There are no absolute rules about what should be included, but a business plan will usually:

■ Make clear the purpose of the organisation.
■ Describe the organisation's vision of the future.
■ Set out broad aims and more specific objectives that will move the organisation towards its vision of the future.
■ Describe the services being offered and to whom they are offered.
■ Describe any intended changes in services.

- Set short-term targets for activity levels and outcomes.
- Set targets for income and expenditure.
- Describe how the organisation intends to keep in touch with the needs and expectations of patients or service users to ensure that its services are responsive.
- Describe quality standards and how they will be met.
- Describe the implications of the plan for staff, including how their development needs will be met.

Business plans are often written with different levels of detail for different audiences. For example, most health and social care organisations produce a business plan that covers these issues in sufficient detail to enable members of the public to be involved in consultation about them. Staff need more detail about some aspects of the business plan in order to make detailed plans for their own areas of work.

ACTIVITY 15.1

Use this list to reflect on whether you have a clear understanding of the plan for the service for which you are responsible. Put a tick against each item that you feel that you could explain to your staff and your service users.

The purpose of your service	❏
The vision of the future for your service	❏
Your service's broad aims and specific objectives	❏
The service offered and to whom it is offered	❏
Any intended changes in the service	❏
Short-term targets for activity levels and outcomes	❏
Targets for income and expenditure	❏
How you keep in touch with the needs and expectations of service users	❏
The quality standards and how they are met	❏
The implications of the plan for your staff and how their development needs will be met	❏

If your organisation has a business plan, obtain a copy and study it. This should help you understand how you can contribute both to working towards achieving its objectives and to developing future business plans. If any aspects of the plan are unclear to you, you may wish to discuss these with your manager or other colleagues. If your organisation does not have a formal business plan, discuss with your manager whether it would be helpful to develop one. In the absence of a plan, it is difficult for staff at any level to set objectives that contribute to the aims of the organisation and thus to work towards a common purpose.

In addition to the characteristics of the business planning process that we described earlier (it is continuous, user-driven and outward-looking), you may have noted that a business plan includes:

- components that can be described as strategic (for example, vision and aims) and those that are operational (for example, targets for income and expenditure)
- a range of different time-frames, from the long term (vision) to the short term (objectives and targets).

Your task is to identify how your service is going to contribute to improvements in the health and well-being of your local population, in the context of national and local policy. Business planning should enable managers at all levels in an organisation to contribute to the planning process and to take responsibility for organising activities that are directed towards achieving the purpose, aims and objectives of the organisation.

ACCOUNTABILITY

If you are *accountable* for something, you are the one who has to explain or is held to account if something goes wrong (or right!). It implies that you have *responsibility* – that you have to undertake duties and make decisions. Organisations give *authority* to job holders so that they can carry out their responsibilities and be accountable for the outcomes. Organisations also design structures that define who is responsible for each area of work and to whom each manager is accountable. These hierarchies are called *lines of accountability*.

Accountability and responsibility thus go together. As a manager, you may be asked to account for the areas of work for which you are responsible. Your organisation is accountable for the quality of the services it provides and the resources it uses in providing them. Accountability is more than responsibility, in that it also brings an expectation that the responsible person or body will be able to provide evidence of the way in which the responsibility has been carried out. It includes being able to demonstrate that management control has been exercised over the use of resources to maintain quality standards. The reality in most workplaces is that, while senior managers are accountable for the overall quality of the service, first-line managers carry the responsibility for ensuring that the services directly available to patients or service users are the best possible within the resources available.

Accountability in health and social care organisations

Health and social care are public services, and must therefore be accountable to the public. They deal with vulnerable and ill people, and carry important responsibilities in relation to the mental and physical health and the protection of individuals and communities. Governments are aware of the importance of these responsibilities, and have set up structures and processes to ensure 'good governance' – that responsibility lies with people who can be held to account for the quality and fair delivery of health and social care. Health authorities, primary care groups and trusts, general practices, hospital and community trusts, independent sector management committees and trustees, and local authorities all have specific responsibilities for which they are accountable.

National performance assessment frameworks have been created for health and social care services, and commissioners of services are required to report on their own performance and that of organisations that provide services. National targets are set for particular initiatives – for example, the Quality Protects initiative to improve children's services in England. There are national institutions that focus on identifying and disseminating good practice, such as the National Institute for Clinical Excellence, and the Improvement and Development Agency for Local Government. There are also institutions that focus on reinforcing good practice, such as the Social Services Inspectorate, the Audit Commission and the Commission for Health Improvement, which carry out reviews and inspections of the performance of health and social care organisations. There is provision within the structures of the Department of Health for the audit of clinical, financial and performance standards, and the Government has powers to intervene if organisations are seriously underperforming. Registration and inspection authorities regulate the work of all service providers, whether statutory or independent, and have the power to close down services that do not meet the required standards. Codes of conduct – for example, for members of local councils and trustees – spell out the standards of behaviour expected of people occupying these offices.

Clinical governance

The notion of 'governance' has become important as a means of focusing on organisational accountability in health and social care. The four main components of clinical governance for health service trusts were spelled out in *A First Class Service* (Department of Health, 1998). They are:

■ clear lines of responsibility and accountability for the overall quality of services, including clinical care

- a comprehensive programme of quality improvement activities
- clear policies directed towards managing risks
- procedures for all professional groups to identify and remedy poor performance.

The first of these includes:

- the trust's chief executive carrying ultimate responsibility for assuring the quality of the services provided
- a designated senior clinician being responsible for ensuring that there are systems for clinical governance and for monitoring their effectiveness
- formal arrangements for trust boards to discharge their responsibilities for clinical quality, for example, through a clinical governance committee
- reports to trust boards on the quality of clinical care being given the same importance as financial reports
- an annual report on clinical governance.

There is a similar expectation that quality in social care will be regularly reviewed and improved, but the systems are different because of differences in the structure of provision. Each local authority's responsibility for social care is regulated by inspection and by being required to demonstrate 'best value' (which, as we have seen, includes measuring public services against similar services provided by the voluntary or private sectors).

Although there is some variation in detail from country to country, similar expectations of quality, efficiency and accountability have developed across the United Kingdom. For example, the NHS in Scotland (Scottish Office, 1998) provided a list of indicators to determine whether clinical governance is working well in a trust. In the next Activity, we ask you to apply these indicators (slightly amended to make them equally relevant for health and social care) to your own area of work.

ACTIVITY 15.2

Work through the list of indicators and make a brief note for each of any evidence of good practice in your area of work.

1 Services will be provided, organised and managed in a manner that supports the delivery of high-quality care.
2 The wider environment in which care is provided will support the delivery of high-quality care. (This could include the clinical environment, the physical environment and the culture of the organisation.)

3 Effective quality assurance and improvement processes will cover all aspects of service delivery.

4 Those providing care will be appropriately trained and have the skills and competences required.

5 Continuing professional development and lifelong learning will be taking place and there will be mechanisms for further training, retraining and reassessment.

6 Poor performance that affects the quality of care will be recognised and appropriate action taken.

7 There will be mechanisms through which staff can raise concerns over any aspect of service delivery that they feel may be having a detrimental effect on the care of service users, including the performance of colleagues or the management of services, without prejudicing the principles of service user and staff confidentiality.

8 Representatives of service users and the public will be involved in quality-related activities.

9 Evidence-based practice will be in day-to-day use and (in health care) there will be an infrastructure and support for activities relating to clinical effectiveness, including appropriate information systems.

10 Techniques such as risk management will be utilised to anticipate and minimise potential problems.

11 Techniques such as clinical audit and critical incident reporting will be in use to monitor and improve existing practice.

12 Programmes of research and development will be pursued and the lessons applied.

13 Complaints will be handled in accordance with national guidance and lessons will be learned from their investigation and resolution.

14 The codes of practice on openness and on confidentiality of personal information and related statutory provisions will be applied and monitored.

Some of these indicators of good governance may involve matters over which you have little, if any, direct influence. Others, however, may have given you ideas of ways in which you could improve your area of work. For example, in relation to item 3, you might have ideas about effective mechanisms to ensure that quality is maintained and developed or about plans for improving processes. In relation to item 5, you may have some thoughts about staff development, both to ensure that your staff have the appropriate skills and competences and to support professional development and lifelong learning. These guidelines suggest taking positive approaches to recognising poor performance and taking steps to improve it, rather than creating a culture in which it is more important to find someone to blame than to remedy a problem. You will also have noted an emphasis on openness in seeking opinions and on using information to improve practice.

These important themes are frequently encountered in discussions about modernising services. They were emphasised in March 2000 with the Government's decision to increase funding to the health service but to require specific performance improvements from the allocation of additional resources. The areas identified as priorities were:

■ partnerships (to improve the integration of services)
■ performance (to improve the quality of services and to ensure that the same quality is available to service users wherever they live)
■ reducing the impact of professional boundaries
■ improving the care of service users
■ focusing on prevention.

These are all important issues in delivering and developing services. They imply that there will be an increasing expectation that managers will contribute to improvements in managing services, so we now turn to how the concepts of accountability and responsibility apply to you.

Managerial accountability

Most managers are accountable for the performance of their staff and for the use of other resources in contributing to service delivery. In many organisations in the health and social care sector, managers are accountable through a traditional hierarchical structure. Increasingly, however, managers' responsibilities for co-ordinating and controlling the work of others are exercised in more complex structural relationships. Consider the following example.

Figure 15.1 illustrates the structure of a large housing association's building and maintenance department, which includes a number of specialist support services. The department has to handle a variety of projects, each of which requires different skills at different times. Each project is therefore staffed according to its needs – as the needs change, so the teams must change.

In Figure 15.1, staff member 2, Dympna Scherelsky, is a specialist in building services (for example, electrical and plumbing work). She is temporarily assigned full-time to project manager A, although he is no more senior in the organisation – he just happens to have the skills needed to lead this project. Scherelsky reports to project manager A on matters concerning the project and he, in turn, reports to the senior architect. However, Scherelsky remains responsible to her specialist manager, the senior building officer, in respect of conditions of employment, discipline and the professional quality of her work.

Dympna Scherelsky's continuing reporting relationship to her technical chief is represented by the dotted line from the staff member 2 box to the box of the senior building officer. Similarly, all the other staff members and leaders in the project teams will be linked by dotted lines to their permanent bosses (but the diagram would become rather untidy if we showed them all).

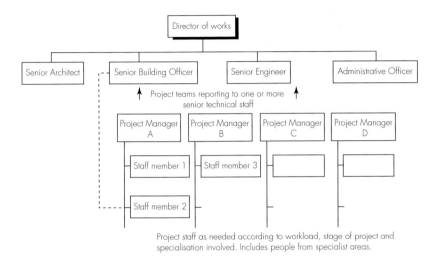

Figure 15.1 Lines of accountability in a housing association's building and maintenance department

---

ACTIVITY 15.3

To whom are you accountable?

How do you report to him or her?

Who is accountable to you?

Draw a chart showing the lines of accountability you have identified. Show the direct accountability to your line manager with a solid line. If you are accountable to other people for parts of your work (for example, to a human resources department or a finance department), show these accountabilities with dotted lines.

You may find your accountabilities listed in your job description. If your job description is not clear about your accountability, you could discuss this with your manager. You may be in a position where you are answerable to someone other than your line manager, perhaps for a particular project or for a particular area of work. If you are in this position, are your levels of authority clear to you?

It is important that you understand what you are accountable for – and to whom – so that you can keep the relevant manager informed of your achievements and your problems. You need appropriate authority to carry out your duties, but the extent of your authority is limited. If you find that your authority is not sufficient to deal with a particular situation, you would refer the matter up the line of accountability.

Organisations establish structures and frameworks to define, monitor and enforce accountability. Organisational charts, job descriptions, and some of the control processes (such as procedures) seek to define who is accountable at different levels and for what. In many social care organisations, the supervision process creates a structure of accountability throughout the organisation, from the director or chief executive to the care assistant. This is managed through regular supervision meetings between line managers and their staff to ensure that responsibilities, authority and reporting mechanisms are clear.

Personal and professional accountability

The concept of *personal responsibility* is crucial in the provision of health and social care services. Many staff at all levels work alone with patients and service users. Some are responsible for toxic substances and difficult and sometimes dangerous procedures, and some have powers to deprive vulnerable citizens of their liberty. All staff carry personal responsibilities for ensuring that they do their work to the best of their abilities, without casual mistakes or deliberate abuse. They are all expected to know what they are doing, to keep themselves up to date with best practice and to maintain service quality. They need a level of confidence in their abilities to be able to operate effectively, but also an awareness of their limitations so that they seek support when necessary. It is part of a manager's role to help staff to recognise their responsibilities.

Patients and their families place their trust in health professionals. They need to be assured that their treatment is up to date and effective, and that it is provided by those whose skills have kept pace with new thinking and new techniques.

(Department of Health, 1998)

Health and social care organisations require their staff to be able to act appropriately – and sometimes creatively and imaginatively – when working alone or under pressure. The requirements of accountability to patients, service users and the public at large tend to generate structures, frameworks, committees and inspections that can sometimes feel time-consuming and repressive. This needs to be balanced by having confidence in staff and giving them some freedom to experiment, in order to enable best practice to emerge and to develop. This is a dilemma for most organisations and is an issue you need to address in managing within your own service.

Professional bodies expect their members to be accountable for their professional conduct. This includes responsibility for continuous professional development and lifelong learning. Professional bodies provide advice and support to their members on good practice. Most of them are also involved in setting standards and some have the power to remove from the register members who consistently fail to meet the required standards.

ACTIVITY 15.4

Are the staff that you manage accountable to one or more professional bodies? If so, list the main standards to which they adhere.

Are any of your colleagues, either in your own organisation or in partner organisations, members of professional bodies? If so, list the main standards to which they adhere.

If you work alongside people who have to adhere to standards set by professional bodies, it is helpful if you understand what is required of them. Difficulties in working across professional boundaries are often caused by misunderstandings about what each profession sees as particularly important.

Where individual health professionals fail to meet the standards set by their profession, when things go wrong, people expect matters to be openly investigated, explanations provided and, where appropriate, action taken to prevent similar problems. Staff [should be] supported in their duty to report on concerns about colleagues' professional conduct and performance . . . [There should be] clear procedures for reporting concerns so that early action can be taken to support the individual to remedy the situation.

(Department of Health, 1998)

ASSESSING AND MANAGING RISK

All staff have responsibilities for health and safety. They need to know what to do if a dangerous or harmful situation occurs. They should be aware of how to protect themselves, service users and visitors, and to be confident that they can take appropriate actions. This confidence is usually developed by rehearsing situations, for example, by holding fire drills and evacuations to ensure that buildings can be cleared quickly. They are also, as we have said, responsible for keeping up to date with best practice in their area of work.

Managers, however, have a broader responsibility to ensure that neither staff nor service users are subjected to danger and harm while they are, in any way, the responsibility of the organisation. They need to be aware of potential risks that exist because of the kind of work staff are doing, or the circumstances in which they do it, as well as of risks arising from the physical or emotional state of patients, service users and carers. They are responsible for taking appropriate action to protect staff and service users from harm.

The terms 'risk', 'risk assessment' and 'risk management' are frequently heard in health and social care circles. The *New Oxford English Dictionary* defines risk as:

to hazard, to endanger; to expose to the chance of injury or loss.

Aleszewski and Manthorpe (1991) define risk rather differently, as:

> *The possibility that a given course of action will not achieve its desired outcome but instead some undesirable situation will develop.*

Both definitions are useful in the context of health and social care. Parsloe (1999) goes further:

> *Risk is closely linked to dangerousness, resulting in harm. The issue here is not about defining dangerousness, which it seems to be agreed means harm to self or others, but with the extent of harm which should constitute a risk in various situations and with different kinds of people.*

All health and social care services face risks. *Risk assessment* is about recognising and predicting the potential for a dangerous situation to occur. *Risk management* is about taking reasonable steps to avoid risk, to reduce the likelihood of risk occurring, or sometimes to accept the consequences of risk.

Different kinds of risk

Different kinds of risk require different responses. Managers need to balance the likelihood of a risk occurring with the resources that are put into preventing it. For example, if it is likely that your staff will sometimes face abuse or violence from service users, you will need to invest resources in protecting them. However, if it is extremely unlikely that your staff will face such situations, you may not need to take any action other than, perhaps, to keep the situation under review.

Your responsibilities as a manager include:

- knowing the risks involved in your area of work
- knowing the procedures that staff are expected to follow
- ensuring that all necessary safety equipment is available
- taking action on any faults or potential hazards.

Let's look briefly at two categories of risk – risks from the environment and risks arising from people's actions.

Environmental risks

The environment in which staff work, patients are treated and other members of the public visit can have a significant impact on

There are a number of potential risks in any working environment. These include the safety of the physical fabric of buildings, vehicles and equipment. Regular safety checks need to be carried out to ensure that accommodation and equipment are safe to use.

Environmental risks also include equipment and materials used in the workplace that are inherently dangerous, such as drugs, needles, high voltage electricity, radioactive sources, clinical waste and other substances that are hazardous to health, including chemicals that are volatile or may deteriorate. All health and social care organisations have procedures to protect staff, patients and service users from the dangers of such environmental risks and it is part of your job as a manager to ensure that they are followed.

ACTIVITY 15.5

1 Who takes responsibility in your organisation for preventing environmental risks?
2 What are your main responsibilities for the maintenance of a safe and healthy working environment?
3 Is there any action that you need to take to ensure that you and your staff are aware of potential risks, or any additional precautions that are necessary to avoid harm to staff, patients or service users?

---

behaviour. You should consider assessing environmental factors such as cleanliness, light, temperature, the adequacy of space, control of access and signage as well as the provision of, for example, smoking areas and private room(s). This will ensure that the physicality of a place doesn't trigger or exacerbate a stressful situation. The use of CCTV has also been well documented as a good disincentive to anti-social and/or unlawful behaviour. Local crime reduction officers are trained to offer advice on environmental factors.

(Department of Health, 1998)

If you are unsure of the policies and procedures that exist in your organisation, or suspect that they are inadequate, this is certainly something to follow up. Having explicit policies and procedures – and making sure that staff know what they are – are the first step towards safe practice and are the responsibility of every employer.

People risks

Risks associated with people tend to fit into three categories.

RISKS INHERENT IN THE WORK AND WORKING PRACTICES OF THE ORGANISATION

These include the risks to people's backs and shoulders from frequently lifting people or heavy objects, and risks incurred from working excessively long hours. The dangers here arise from not applying safe lifting techniques (not using suitable equipment such as hoists), and from accidents or mistakes caused by poor attention and fatigue. There are also potential risks in offices, for example, for those using visual display units, or from trailing leads or uneven flooring.

RISKS FROM EVENTS THAT MIGHT HAPPEN

These risks are difficult to predict. Anything might happen, but some things are more likely to happen than others. For example, stones might be thrown at ambulance drivers, staff working at night might have their cars stolen, or there might be attacks on or accidents to staff while they are carrying out their duties. It is difficult to predict occurrences like these, but precautions can be taken to reduce risks. For example, when staff are making visits away from their organisational base, information about where they are going and when they are expected to return should be left with a responsible person. It may be appropriate to keep a supply of mobile phones, torches and emergency alarms for staff to borrow. It may be possible to arrange shifts so that staff are not working alone at times of high risk.

RISKS ARISING FROM SOME IMPAIRMENT TO A PERSON'S FUNCTIONING

Much of the work of health and social care organisations involves working with people who are in pain, distressed, or under stress of one kind or another – people who may be under the influence of drugs or alcohol, people whose functioning is impaired by mental illness, or people who are unable to deal with their emotions. Sometimes risks may arise because a normally calm person is under great stress; some-times the risks may be a continuing part of the way a person is. Much of the work of social care in particular, but also of some health services, is concerned with protecting vulnerable people from abuse.

An important step that a manager can take is to ensure that there are systems to protect people from human fallibility. Memory and habit are not enough when there are risks to safety. In areas of work where safety procedures must be followed, posters on the wall can remind people. You can also set up systems to remind you to carry out safety inspections and to have equipment checked.

One of your functions as a manager is to foster attitudes in your workplace that raise awareness of safety. Once a culture of vigilance is established, everyone is at less risk because everyone is aware of potential danger to themselves and to others.

ACTIVITY 15.6

Think back over an incident in your personal, professional or manage-rial career where harm occurred. How did this situation arise? Make a note of the action you took – or could take – to minimise the likelihood of it occurring again.

We came up with the following list of contributory factors that could lead to a fairly ordinary situation becoming a hazardous one:

■ *ignorance* – not knowing that the hazard is or could be there, not knowing what type of hazard it might be
■ *incapacity* – poor judgement or loss of the ability to act, perhaps associated with tiredness, stress or error
■ *believing that nothing can be done* – hazards can occur because no attempt has been made to identify risks or take action to reduce them
■ *lack of vigilance* – staff failing to observe potential hazards
■ *lack of support* – there was no one there to help when help was needed – this can sometimes arise from a feeling of invincibility that proves to be unfounded.

We have focused on environmental risks and risks arising from people's actions. However, there are other kinds of risk.

There are also risks associated with the reputation of your organisation. As a manager, you represent your organisation to the public and you might be asked your opinion. The risk here is that, as a manager, what you offer as your personal opinion may be misunderstood to be an 'official' statement. If you are invited by a newspaper or local radio to comment about an incident in which your organisation appears to be involved, it is usually wise to seek advice from a senior manager before offering comment.

There are also financial risks in failing to anticipate essential expenditure and thus exceeding budgeted targets. In services that are responsive to demand, it is not easy to forecast expenditure accurately. However, many areas of expenditure can be anticipated by thinking ahead. For example, equipment deteriorates and needs replacing and you should be aware of approximately how long equipment will last, so that plans can be made in good time to obtain replacements. Similarly, good record keeping will enable you to plan to replace stocks of materials that are used in your area of work, avoiding the risk of running out of essential supplies.

Frameworks for the management of risk are vital to prevent unnecessary danger and harm. No matter how careful, logical and rational you are, you cannot anticipate everything that might represent a danger. However, you can take reasonable precautions and encourage vigilance. In particular, you can make sure that people are well trained and properly supervised.

Circumstances in which risk taking should be encouraged

Where would medical science be today if people had not taken risks?

There are situations in which seeking to remove all risk is counter-productive to the purposes of a service. For example, it is important for people with learning disabilities to have the opportunity to learn from experience. Learning to cross the road, for example, carries risks but is an essential part of helping people to live their lives. In the past, the consequence of removing all likelihood of risk was the development of large residential institutions which, while keeping people safe, created their own forms of hazard for residents and staff.

As a manager, you may often be asked to approve a course of action. The following list may help you to make decisions in a situation where you recognise that there may be risks.

1 Ensure that you fully understand the situation.
2 Identify the benefits of the proposed course of action and compare these with the likely benefits if no action is taken.
3 Assess the risks of the proposed course of action.
4 Generate options for alternative approaches and consider what criteria you will use to make the best choice.
5 Once the choice is made, reassess the risks associated with that course of action.
6 Decide on sensible precautions that will minimise the risks without reducing the benefits too much.
7 Review the process once the action has been taken and revise the precautions if necessary.

Assessing and managing risk are a matter of judgement, and judgement is developed through reflecting on experience. You can supplement your own judgement by seeking advice if you feel ill-equipped to make a particular decision. However, you should also feel confident about questioning an assessment of risk. It is possible that working practices have developed that are excessively defensive in avoiding risk. If you want to challenge a practice that appears to be unnecessarily risk-averse, be prepared to review a number of options and to consider evidence from past experience. Sometimes organisations become risk-averse because staff are afraid of blame if things go wrong.

There is a difference between being vigilant and safety conscious and being reluctant to do anything differently in case you are blamed if something goes wrong. Be prepared to review practices and consider other options. Be guided by your own judgement and the judgement of those with appropriate experience. Review your procedures for reporting incidents and the mechanisms for taking remedial action. Take action to reduce risks that have been identified. Develop your judgement by seeking out examples of good practice in other organisations.

■ ■ ■

We began this chapter by considering the context in which health
and social care services are planned, and looking at what is involved in
business planning. We have examined the structures that support and
reinforce public accountability for health and social care services, as
well as the concept of personal responsibility. We have also examined
the processes of risk assessment and risk management: protecting staff,
patients and service users from harm has become an increasingly
important component of the work of health and social care services.

REFERENCES

Aleszewski, A. and Manthorpe, J. (1991) 'Literature review: Measuring
    and managing risk in social welfare', *British Journal of Social Work*, 21:
    277–90.
Department of the Environment, Transport and the Regions (1998) *Modern
    Local Government: In Touch with the People*, The Stationery Office.
Department of Health (1998) *A First Class Service: Quality in the NHS*, The
    Stationery Office.
Parsloe, P. (ed.) (1999) *Risk Assessment in Social Care and Social Work*,
    Jessica Kingsley Publishers.
Scottish Office (1998) *Clinical Governance*, Scottish Office Department of
    Health.

WORKING WITH A BUDGET

You will already be aware of some of the changes that are taking place in health and social care organisations in order to make better use of finite resources in a climate of ever-increasing demand. These changes may have affected the way in which you carry out your job. For example, you may:

- have more responsibility for your decisions
- have to consider costs more carefully before making decisions
- be expected to contribute to the process of setting budgets
- be responsible for controlling the budget for your service or department
- be expected by senior managers to be more efficient
- have to account for the money you spend.

Many of these changes arise from the way in which health and social care services are now financed – in particular the separate responsibilities of those who commission services and those who provide them. But there is also a general trend in many health and social care organisations towards delegating more responsibility for budgetary matters to junior managers and team leaders.

In order to do your job more effectively in this new climate, you therefore need to develop competences that will enable you to play your part in budgetary management. We begin by examining the purposes of budgeting, and also discuss a number of different approaches to setting budgets. We then turn to some of the practicalities of budgeting: the initial stages of timetabling and preparing the ground, and the crucial stage of budget negotiation.

SETTING BUDGETS

The aims that organisations set themselves are like signposts that provide a sense of direction for both the organisation and its managers.

However, statements of aims rarely spell things out in any detail. They do not usually indicate precisely what has to be done, nor do they say what resources will be necessary to achieve the aims. The next stage has to be filling in the details. As a manager, part of your job is to work out – and to communicate – organisational expectations and available resources in detail. This is where budgets come in.

Budgets are plans that set out financial details about:

A *budget* is a detailed financial plan.

■ *income* – the resources available to an organisation and the departments within it
■ *expenditure* – the uses to which these resources will be put.

Budgets contain mainly financial data. They are usually expressed in monetary terms, but some budgets use quantities. Look at the simple budget statement in Table 16.1.

It appears from Table 16.1 that senior management have estimated an income level of £500,000 and expenditure at £450,000. They expect the organisation to make a profit of £50,000 (or to carry forward this amount into the following year as reserves).

Is there any sense of direction in these estimates? Most certainly there is. Those responsible for 'selling' the organisation's services know that they are working towards a total income of £500,000 and staff know that their salaries are expected to total £350,000. Those responsible for purchasing the organisation's supplies know that they are expected to spend £50,000 and the organisation can spend £50,000 on rent. This is a clear statement of the organisation's financial plans, which provides a sense of direction for its staff.

So budgets are a practical expression of the aims of organisations. The emphasis is on the word *practical*, because the budget determines, directs and plans the actions that follow.

One important difference between budgets and aims is the time-scale. Budgets are normally drawn up for 12 months, and are regarded as being part of an organisation's short-term or, at most, medium-term planning. By contrast, aims are designed to provide a long-term framework. The period covered could be five years or perhaps even longer.

An organisation – or a department or section within an organisation – cannot be directed in enough detail if only longer-term aims are

Table 16.1 Budget statement

Income		£500,000
Expenditure:		
Salaries	£350,000	
Purchases	£50,000	
Rent	£50,000	£450,000
Profit/reserves		£50,000

available. Direction is best thought of in much shorter planning periods. Twelve months seem to be the maximum length of time for which detailed planning can be undertaken. Indeed, the 12-month budget is usually divided into six-monthly, quarterly and monthly statements.

The purposes of budgeting

Budgeting has a number of important benefits – in other words, there are several purposes of budgeting.

Budgeting as a contribution to planning

We have already said that all managers must be fully aware of the aims of the organisation so that they can draw up detailed plans. The budgeting process involves managers in doing precisely that: planning their future activities in detail.

Budgeting as a contribution to communication

Budgeting, by its nature, involves senior management in briefing front-line managers and other staff about what is expected from them – in other words, in communicating. Since departments often work collaboratively, part of the budgeting process involves managers who are on similar levels communicating with one another across departments about their future activities.

Budgeting as a contribution to co-ordination

Communication does not, in itself, ensure that managers work together for the overall good of the organisation. Some managers may want a larger 'empire' and request more staff. Or they may want to develop a particular area of work because it is of personal interest to them. Some may be put under pressure to purchase goods and services they don't really need. In these and other ways, events may take place that do not benefit the organisation.

The budgeting process helps to influence this sort of behaviour. It forces managers to communicate with one another and co-ordinate their activities. Where departments support one another and use each other's services, the budgeting process makes sure that the right level of support is available, by identifying what resources are required and who will provide them. The intentions of managers are therefore known, and unsatisfactory behaviour can be identified and rectified. An overarching master budget, incorporating all the detailed activities, will be compiled to provide an overview for senior management, making effective co-ordination possible.

Budgeting as a contribution to motivation

All organisations – including health and social care organisations – are dependent on people and their goodwill. Staff therefore need to be encouraged to carry out their tasks to the best of their ability. Most people like 'a bit of a challenge': when budget levels are being set, a slightly optimistic view of what can be achieved may provide this. However, too challenging a budget can be demotivating if staff feel under pressure to compromise standards to achieve financial targets.

Budgeting as a contribution to control

The budget specifies future activities and directs staff towards achieving them. If the budget is staged on a monthly basis, it is possible to discover when plans are not being carried out satisfactorily and to take action to make sure that the targets are reached later on.

What we have just described is the controlling function of a budget. Actual performance is compared regularly with budgeted performance. Differences can be identified and explanations sought. Action may be taken to bring activities into line with the budget. However, this may be inappropriate in some situations. For example, if the original plans were too optimistic or inaccurate, or if circumstances have changed significantly, making the plans unachievable, it may be necessary to revise the budget.

Budgeting as a contribution to assessing performance

Managers are responsible for carrying out plans. They are expected to undertake specific tasks, make the necessary decisions and manage staff. The budget helps to assess their level of success in carrying out these responsibilities. A budget does not cover the full range of managers' responsibilities, but it is useful in assessing their performance in relation to those responsibilities that involve money.

However, too much reliance should not be placed on financial results in isolation. Managers also have responsibilities of a non-financial nature, which cannot be ignored. They need feedback on the full range of activities that they undertake, in order to build up a fuller picture of how effectively they have carried out their jobs.

APPROACHES TO BUDGETING

Budgets, then, are simply plans expressed in financial terms. They help organisations to achieve their agreed aims. Budgeting is about planning for specified levels of activity with the resources available. We now turn to the examination of some different approaches to creating

Table 16.2 Budget statement for a day-care centre

	Annual budget (£)	Planned budget to end of month 9 (£)	Actual expenditure to end of month 9 (£)	Budget variance at end of month 9 (£)
Pay costs:				
Nursing and care staff salaries	102,000	76,500	82,000	(5,500)
Technical staff salaries	30,000	22,500	18,000	4,500
Non-pay costs:				
Drugs and dressings	36,000	27,000	28,800	(1,800)
Physiotherapy and occupational therapy supplies	28,000	21,000	23,500	(2,500)
Cleaning	10,000	7,500	7,500	–
Building maintenance (including heat and light)	15,000	11,250	11,250	–
Administration costs	20,000	15,000	15,000	–
Total costs	241,000	180,750	186,050	(5,300)

budgets. We'll look at the differences between 'input' and 'output' budgeting and then at 'incremental' and 'zero-based' approaches to budgeting.

Input and output budgets

Let's look at an example of a budget.

ACTIVITY 16.1

Table 16.2 is a budget statement from a day-care centre.

You will notice that, in the final column, some figures are shown in brackets: this means that they are negative (in some budgets they are shown with a minus sign, rather than with brackets).

1 What is the total annual budget expenditure?
2 What is the single largest category of expenditure?
3 Has the actual expenditure to date exceeded the budget or been less than expected, and by how much?

4   Now make a brief note on whether you think that this statement
    provides you with a good picture of the day centre's running costs.
5   What do you think is the main weakness of this budget statement?

The annual budgeted expenditure for the day-care centre was
£241,000. The largest single category of expenditure is the salaries of
nursing staff. Up to the date of this budget statement, actual expenditure has exceeded planned expenditure by £5,300.

We think this budget probably does provide a good picture of the
running costs of the day-care centre. Its main weakness is that it does
not provide any information about the level of activity that is being
budgeted for.

That is because this is an *input* budget, with the costs grouped
by department and function. The inputs used by each function or
department – people, materials and other costs – are simply listed and
cosseted to form the budget. It is not possible, from this budget, to
calculate the cost of providing services to any particular user of the
day-care centre, so it is difficult to obtain the financial data needed to
cost the day-care centre's objectives.

The key point is that it is not the running costs of each department
or function that we need to know in order to plan effectively. We are
more interested in the *outputs* – the costs of running particular services,
which may involve many functions and departments.

As a first step in determining the overall costs of operating any
service, input budgeting can make a useful contribution to budget
construction, but the next step takes us much deeper. We have to find
out how many *workload outputs* each department or function produces
and for which customers.

Information about workload outputs and customers can be used in
a variety of ways:

■   to work out the average cost for each unit of service delivered
■   to compare the services provided with other similar services, and
    thus find out how efficient (or inefficient) they are
■   as a basis for pricing services or recharging costs to external or
    internal customers
■   to build up financial forecasts for the future.

Output budgeting analyses the activities undertaken in workload terms
to arrive at average unit costs. It is, however, necessary to exercise
caution when using average unit costs to construct a budget. The signal
for caution is the word 'average'. If the service you work in has a highly
variable mixture of work or provides services for people with very
different needs, the calculations involved in output budgeting can be
rather complex.

So how should you approach budgeting? Perhaps the best advice is:

Workload outputs are ways
of expressing in monetary
terms what a department or
service produces or deals
with.

1 Analyse your costs into those that are *fixed* – those that do not depend, to a significant extent, on the number of service users – and those that are *variable* – those that vary roughly in proportion to the number of people you provide services for.
2 Use an input-based budgeting approach for those costs that are more or less fixed.
3 Base your budget calculations on estimated unit costs and projected outputs for the costs that are variable.

If you follow this guidance, the approach to budgeting for a service might look something like that shown in Table 16.3.

ACTIVITY 16.2

Can you distinguish the input-based calculations from the output-based ones in Table 16.3? Tick the appropriate boxes.

	Inputs	*Outputs*
1 Salaries	❐	❐
2 Materials costs	❐	❐
3 Cleaning, meals served	❐	❐
4 Rents and maintenance costs	❐	❐
5 Income (services provided)	❐	❐

Table 16.3 An approach to the budget plan

Items to be budgeted	Calculation
Salary costs	Either: Actual costs × Number of staff in post or: Estimated costs on mid-salary points × Funded establishment of staff
Materials or consumables used directly by the service	Average cost per unit of activity × Volume of activity
Services supplied by other departments (e.g. cleaning, meals served)	Number of units of service provided × Average unit cost
Charges for using and maintaining buildings, land and equipment	Estimated annual charges for rents, maintenance, etc.
Income	Number of units of service 'sold' to other departments or external customers × Agreed average 'prices'

We have suggested that you employ both input and output methods in assembling your budget. Salaries, rents and maintenance costs – items 1 and 4 – can most usefully be calculated by the input method. However, the costs of materials, cleaning and meals – items 2 and 3 – should be calculated, wherever possible, on the basis of outputs. Income – item 5 – should also, if possible, be calculated by the output method.

Incremental versus zero-based budgeting

Two important techniques that can be used to create budgets are incremental budgeting and zero-based budgeting. We'll describe each technique briefly, and then attempt to evaluate their usefulness.

Incremental budgeting

This approach to budgeting is heavily reliant on what has happened in the past. The costs for the previous and current year provide the starting point for the coming budget year. Incremental budgeting involves accepting fairly uncritically what happened the previous year and then updating that year's figures. Adjustments are made to cope with:

Incremental budgeting involves updating the previous year's budget.

- pay and price rises
- the 'full year' effect of plans previously put into action
- the effect of new projects that will come on stream in the forthcoming budget year
- any planned 'efficiency savings'.

Zero-based budgeting

This approach to budgeting ignores the figures and assumptions of the previous year. Instead, it examines, from first principles, what is required to carry out the tasks expected of the organisation and its various components.

Zero-based budgeting involves rebudgeting from scratch each year.

First, a list of 'core' activities is drawn up. These form the essential base of the budget. Other activities are regarded as optional, and managers have to decide whether or not they will continue.

Then, the core activities and those optional activities that have survived the first stage are costed, and the costs are updated to take account of the effects of any new plans that will be implemented during the coming year. For example, new projects may be coming on stream that will have important financial consequences.

Which approach should you use?

The zero-based approach is better in theory, because it relates the budget directly to the tasks for which the organisation exists. But, in practice, it is difficult and time-consuming. It requires managers to be fully aware of all the tasks that have to be carried out, which can sometimes be a tall order. It also means that managers have to be completely objective when deciding which activities are essential to the delivery of the service and which are not.

Incremental budgeting is comparatively straightforward. Details of the income and expenditure in the previous year are readily available. All the manager is expected to do is to think about how the costs of the activities will change in the coming year. This is far easier than undertaking a full review. Discussion about whether current staffing is adequate and whether the heating system is efficient can be expensive in terms of time. However, no one would claim that incremental budgeting is very comprehensive.

Whichever approach you adopt, your budget will have to be submitted to senior management for final approval, and they may change the figures. Perhaps insufficient funds are available, or perhaps senior management have different priorities. Departmental managers may be involved in negotiating their budgets, but this is not the case everywhere. Some organisations impose budgets from above. It is generally considered that a 'bottom-up' approach to budgeting is more likely to encourage staff to take responsibility for managing resources. However, there is a counter-argument that, because senior management are more aware of current demands and future priorities, they should direct how the funds available should be used.

The approach taken to the allocation of funds between departments and services varies from organisation to organisation, depending to a significant extent on the management style adopted by senior staff. But inevitably, in the process of setting budgets, some departments and services will lose out while others will gain. Decisions that affect the budget can have quite profound effects on the ways in which the various parts of the organisation operate.

TIMETABLING AND PREPARING THE GROUND

The production of plans and budgets is a complex set of activities, and it needs careful organisation and timetabling. If a health or social care organisation is to secure the full commitment of its managers in building up meaningful and accurate budgets, it is vital that clear guidelines be available, showing not only where everyone fits into the budget preparation process, but also when. In order to start things moving, a timetable is essential.

Envisage yourself in a budget-planning situation. What would you want to be clear about? The range of responses that managers provide to this question is quite wide. However, the following suggestions sum up much of what people feel.

I want an overview of responsibility. For example, I'd like a list showing the name of each manager responsible for budget preparation. Then we could at least talk to each other.

It's important to know exactly what will be required of me: the sort of information I need to pull together and when it is required.

The process needs to be clear. For example, to whom should I pass information and in what form?

Speaking personally, I need some kind of plan or diagram – a picture if you like. A diagram showing where I stand in the scheme of things for preparing the budget would be very useful.

I need to know the stages in the process and the key deadline dates.

All these comments point towards the need for a clear timetable. Table 16.4 is an example of a master timetable for budget preparation and Table 16.5 is an example of the timetable for an individual budget holder.

Benefits undoubtedly arise from the fact that everyone involved in the budgeting process knows exactly what he or she is responsible for

Table 16.4 A master timetable for budget preparation

Process	Organisational level	Aug	Sept	Oct	Nov	Dec	Jan	Feb
Strategic objectives set	Commissioners/senior management	✓						
Prepare departmental and service budgets; agree recharges between departments	Departmental and service managers/ accountant				✓			
Prepare master budget; revise individual budgets	Senior management/ accountant					✓		
Issue individual budgets	Accountant							✓

Table 16.5 An individual budget preparation timetable

Service	Budget manager	Data required	Format of data and basis of collection	Date required	Required by	Budget preparation deadline
Community occupational therapy	Ms I. V. Packer	Forecast occupational therapist's travel costs for next year	Total travel costs forecast from unit personal travel records	10 Sept	Mrs O. Etoe (accountant)	16 Nov
		Forecast number of domiciliary visits for next year	Total number of visits (using sample of one quarter's figures)	5 Sept	Mrs O. Etoe (accountant)	16 Nov
		Forecast number of aids to daily living required for next year	Forecast total number of aids by type of aid (using sample of two quarters' figures)	5 Sept	Mrs O. Etoe (accountant)	16 Nov

producing, in what format, for whom and by when. A sense of direction and clarity is essential to personal motivation and commitment. In addition, the budget preparation timetable can be used by accountants and senior management to pull the budget together by the agreed deadline. It becomes the means by which control is exercised over the process of budget preparation throughout the organisation. Slippages can be monitored, and senior management can take corrective action when appropriate. The ultimate pay-off is a co-ordinated approach to the budget preparation process.

NEGOTIATING THE BUDGET

Having drawn up a timetable and identified the process by which the budget will be developed, you move into budget negotiation. In the political sphere, a poor diplomat can increase the chance of hostilities. Budget negotiation can be equally sensitive, and there are acceptable and unacceptable ways of going about it. Consider how you might apply the following guidance in your situation.

Be clear-sighted
You must be clear about the objectives of your organisation and be able to identify where your service fits in. Before going to any budget meeting, be clear about how your financial position fits into the overall budget and how your activities are likely to influence it.

Be brief
You should be prepared to state your service's aims and its financial objectives without too much elaboration. Be prepared to talk through a short report, which you should circulate well in advance to all those attending the meeting. Use this report to highlight your key objectives.

Be simple
Make your report as plain and simple as possible. Avoid too much detail, particularly arrays of figures. This can alienate people very quickly. You are not trying to score points: you are trying to make them.

Be well informed
You need to make yourself familiar with the overall financial climate and the policies of your organisation. For example, do you know the policies for financial control?

Be open
Try to be open-minded in your approach to finding new resources for your service. This means reviewing the situation in your service as a whole and

thinking about opportunities that may be available. Before going to a budget meeting, you should have taken a cool and critical look at the main features of your service. There is no need to be afraid of thinking radically.

Be factual

You must go into negotiation knowing the facts. What are the facts on your current costs and activities?

Be prepared

You need to do your homework on the information you have gathered.

Be alert

If you are aware of opportunities that exist to save money, you may be able to use them as a bargaining point. When you identify such savings, do so on the basis that you expect some share of them to be passed back to you for the development of your service. Work out the savings as accurately as you can and calculate the time-scale over which you can make them. Don't let the finance staff – or anyone else – work out these things for you: on the whole, they will be less well informed than you are. If you fail to take the initiative, unreasonable demands may be made on your service to deliver savings and cost improvements.

Be straightforward

If, at the end of the negotiation meeting, you feel that the resources necessary to run your service adequately will not be available for the forthcoming year, spell out the consequences in a clear and rational way. Be explicit about the quantitative and qualitative effects on your service. If the under-resourcing is likely to be critical, you could prepare and circulate a report to senior management, after the meeting is over, to record your analysis of the situation. An honest, straightforward presentation of the facts will at least form a launching pad for a later round of budget negotiations. If there is financial leeway, your stand may gain additional financial resources for your service later on in the financial year.

We cannot anticipate how you will have reflected on each of these points. 'Clear-sighted', 'brief' and 'simple' appeal to most of us when we look at what other managers present us with, but perhaps you also thought about how what you produce might appear to other people. For example, being open might involve recognising that you have not always achieved the best use of resources.

When it comes to being factual, managers mention a range of items: amount spent to date, income due to date, the total value of orders currently placed, the number of staff in post compared with the funded staff establishment, workload to date, projected workload and a host of others.

Being prepared involves, to some extent, reading the minds of others who will be present at the budget meeting, and perhaps having some preliminary discussions with them. One manager made this point explicitly:

> *You should project forward your income and expenditure budgets for next year. In my opinion, this gives you a head start in any negotiations with accountants, because they can see that you've already constructed your own forecast based on your specialist knowledge of the service you provide.*

These suggestions are not meant to provide an exhaustive guide. However, if you do try to use them, the process of communicating your financial concerns and needs should be made easier.

ACTIVITY 16.3

Your organisation is about to enter the budget-setting season. Your departmental head has asked for your assistance in making a case for purchasing a new piece of computing equipment. The argument for doing so is that it will achieve a net saving of £5,000 per year because the department will not have to employ a part-time clerical assistant to extract the data manually from service users' records.

Jot down some key facts that you would seek to establish about this proposal. Your ideas will form the basis for a short report, which your departmental head has been asked to take to the budget meeting. Remember to think about the sorts of question that the accountant might have in mind.

Your head of department wants some facts as a basis on which to make the case. The kinds of questions that need to be answered in the report include:

- Is the £5,000 per year saving an accurate figure? How has it been established, and by whom?
- How soon could we start saving this amount? Would it be dependent on staff redundancies?
- How much will the computer equipment cost and how long will it be before it has to be replaced?
- What would be the total forecast savings on the project after allowing for notional interest on the capital cost of the equipment?
- What are the running costs of the computer equipment?
- Will the equipment improve the output and quality of the service that we currently provide?

The answers to some of these questions may be complicated. For example, how soon you might start saving the money could be dependent on a member of staff being made redundant. If so, your figures would have to include redundancy costs. If not, the savings might have to wait for natural wastage. The last question involves deciding how you are going to demonstrate improved output and/or quality of service.

The report presented by your head of department might look something like the following.

Report on the estimated costs and financial benefits arising from the proposed acquisition of a computer for the Skin Department

I propose the acquisition of a computer, the costs and benefits of which are as follows.

Costs
Estimated capital cost: £2,400
Estimated life-span of computer: 3 years
Annualised cost = £2,400 ÷ 3 = £800
Plus 6% notional interest per year on £2,400 = £2,400 × 6 ÷ 100 = £144
Running costs (computer stationery, maintenance contract and power): £200 per year
Total cost per year = £800 + £144 + £200 = £1,144

Benefits
A part-time clerical assistant's post is currently vacant, and not filling this post would save £2,800 per year, so buying the computer will produce a net saving of £1,656 per year.

In addition, the efficiency of the department would be significantly enhanced, as data on service users would be accessible to all staff at any time.

Summary
This analysis demonstrates that the financial benefits of acquiring an Acne computer are unquestionable. The proposal enables a saving of almost £5,000 to be made over its three-year life-span.

Taj Surma, Department Manager

You will not have failed to notice the virtues of this report. First, it is brief and to the point. Second, the costs and benefits (both financial and non-financial) have been set out, showing net annual savings and total savings over the life of the project. Finally, it is presented clearly. The importance of this in making any financial case successfully cannot be overestimated.

TARGET-SETTING, MOTIVATION AND COMMUNICATION

You may have noted that budget reports are used as one means of communicating information to managers within your organisation about activity levels and the financial consequences of the previous month's activity. It may be that 'keeping within budget' is a performance criterion in your department or organisation, or you may work in a department which does not use budgets as performance targets.

Not all organisations use budgets for target-setting or motivation, although most budget holders would be deemed not to be performing well if they did not remain within their budgets. In theory, tight budgets can be used to encourage people to think more creatively about how resources are used and this may happen in your organisation. However, tight budgets can also be demotivating, particularly if the budget holders have had no say in the budget-setting process. They may feel that the constraints imposed upon them are unreasonable, or that they are not being rewarded for what they have already achieved. In either case they are unlikely to take 'ownership' of the budget, and their commitment to it may be low.

If budget reports are used as part of performance evaluation, it is important to ensure that managers are not held responsible for costs which they do not have the authority to control. Too often managers have little real control over spending. For example:

- The organisation may only allow one supplier to be used, so there is no scope for saving money by 'shopping around' for a better deal.
- Salary levels and ratios of staff to patients or service users may be fixed.
- Costs that appear in a manager's budget may be allocated from other departments (administration, cleaning, etc.) and may therefore be outside of the manager's control.

Whatever role budget reports have within your organisation, it is important to recognise that they are a form of communication. Like all communication, they need to be treated with care: they are open to differing interpretations and can have unintended consequences if their purpose is not clear to all concerned.

Budgeting and providing the financial data for setting budgets are part of the responsibilities of many managers. This is, however, a shared responsibility, as there will almost always be expert guidance readily available from accountants.

You should make the best possible use of your accountant! The two roles run together:

- Your role as a manager is to collect and validate financial information, using your experience and knowledge of the work your service does, to provide a sound basis for financial planning.
- The accountant's role is to respond to your need for sound and relevant advice, providing you with good quality financial information.

The key to success lies in establishing close, collaborative working relationships. Working together, managers and accountants can put together viable plans and produce sensible budgets.

THE FLOW OF WORK AND INFORMATION

In this chapter, we focus on the *core tasks* that need to be done in order to deliver the service(s) for which you are responsible. We are going to concentrate on the management issues that arise from the way in which these core tasks fit together, and the structures that are required to co-ordinate them.

Having relevant information is an absolute requirement for effective co-ordination. You need two kinds of information. First, you need information (relevant, clear, accurate, complete, timely and appropriate) about what is actually happening. Second, you need information about what is *supposed* to be happening. Without this second type of information (a plan or a set of standards) you cannot make sense of the first type, or make judgements about the level and quality of service that are being delivered. The relationships between those whose activities you manage – and also between them and you – must be such that both types of information are trusted by those affected, so that the decisions that are made will be accepted as legitimate by those being co-ordinated.

IDENTIFYING CORE TASKS

By 'core tasks' we mean those that constitute the rationale for your section's or department's existence. These are the essential tasks that enable your service to be delivered. There are almost certainly many other tasks that are also vital and important, but which support the main purpose of your work rather than delivering it. Figure 17.1 is based on Michael Porter's (1985) concept of a 'value chain' that demonstrates how all the activities carried out by an organisation should combine to deliver value to the service user. These activities include both support processes and core processes. The support processes include financial services, human resource services, information services and general management services. Most organisations have to put services like these in place in one way or another. However, the main purpose of any organisation in the health and social care sector is to ensure that

Figure 17.1 Core and support processes
(Source: adapted with the permission of The Free Press, A Division of
Simon & Schuster, Inc, from Competitive Advantage: Creating and
Sustaining Superior Performance, by Michael E. Porter. Copyright © 1985,
1988 by Michael E. Porter)

high-quality services are delivered to patients and service users. Its core
processes include receiving referrals and admissions, carrying out
assessments and diagnoses, delivering services to patients and service
users, and developing and improving services.

We now want you to identify the core tasks that make up your area
of responsibility, so that you can focus on the essential activities that
are involved.

ACTIVITY 17.1

Describe briefly the core tasks that you are responsible for managing
so that you have a 'picture' of all the core tasks. They are the tasks that
represent the main purpose of your job. Try to identify them as clear
and separate tasks or as clear stages in some larger task. Make a note
of whether each core task is carried out by one individual, or by a group
or team.

We are now going to focus on the interactions and flows of work and
information between these various tasks. When examining any complex
work situation, it soon becomes clear that the core tasks that form part
of any manager's responsibility can relate to one another in one of the
two main ways:

■   You may manage a process where the core tasks relate to one
     another sequentially. In this situation, each task adds or contributes

to the next one. Each needs to be completed before the next one can be started, building towards delivery of the final service. Failure to complete any one of the core tasks is likely to cause a breakdown in the chain, and thus failure to deliver the service effectively.

■ Alternatively, some of the core tasks may be carried out *in parallel*. The work pattern here is that a number of activities are carried out more or less independently of each other. Failure to complete one task does not necessarily interfere with the whole process (as in the case of sequential tasks) but is likely to reduce the volume or quality of the service that is delivered.

Let's now look at some of the issues involved in managing these two different types of situation.

THE MANAGEMENT OF SEQUENTIAL TASKS

In this situation, a number of core tasks contribute to a service, which is the sum of all these tasks. Each of the tasks constitutes a package of activity that makes sense in its own right to those who are carrying it out. All the tasks have to be completed to specified standards of performance and carried out in a particular order and in a timely way in order to deliver the total service. However well a particular task is completed, getting its timing out of phase may lead to serious disruption or even complete failure of the service. Information needs to flow from task to task, also in sequence and in time to inform the subsequent task.

An example of a sequential set of tasks might be those required to prepare an operating theatre for use by the surgical team (Figure 17.2). On a daily basis, the operating theatre is cleaned to specified standards by specialist cleaning staff (task A). Until this has been done, the theatre technicians cannot get on with their job of setting up the required equipment and resources (task B). Once task B is completed, the theatre manager checks its completion against established requirements and standards (task C). The surgical team can then use the outcome of all this activity to carry out an operation (task D). At the end of each surgical procedure, sub-routines of cleaning, restocking and preparation are carried out by the theatre staff in preparation for the next operation (task E), and so on, until the theatre is taken out of use for its next major cleaning (task A again).

Figure 17.2 Sequence of core tasks in an operating theatre

Different types of co-ordination (with some overlap between them) are required to manage a service that involves a number of core tasks and essential sequences:

- making initial plans and allocating resources
- co-ordinating tasks vertically
- ensuring that tasks are completed in a timely way
- preparing for contingencies
- co-ordinating tasks laterally
- obtaining feedback about performance.

We will consider each of these approaches to co-ordination briefly in turn, referring to the information needs as we go.

Initial planning and resource allocation

An important aspect of co-ordination is ensuring that standards are set for the performance of each task and that appropriate resources are allocated to each part of the sequence. In our operating theatre example, the theatre manager probably has a weekly schedule of planned operations, but updates and amends this daily as necessary. This allows targets and objectives to be set for the various contributing tasks and provides the cleaners and theatre technicians with their goals for the period, as well as establishing what equipment, supplies and staffing will be needed.

In sequential chains, some of the staff involved in core tasks (for example, our cleaners) do not directly encounter end-users, and may tend to become focused on their own objectives. It is therefore important for the manager to plan their tasks and the resources they need so that the service delivered to the end-user is of a high quality. In many areas of health and social care, remote or apparently self-contained activities make a crucial contribution to the delivery of services to the end-user. Careful planning of their activities is vital.

Vertical co-ordination

Initial planning and resource allocation are one aspect of vertical co-ordination. The manager's role is to have an overview of the whole chain or process. In order to control and co-ordinate effectively, managers need to be clear about what has to be done at each step in the process, as well as in the process overall, and to make plans accordingly. Vertical co-ordination includes a responsibility to ensure that the necessary information is provided to every area that needs it.

Timeliness

Each task needs to be carried out in a timely way, so that sequential activities are completed and passed along the chain of activity without delay and other dependent tasks further along the chain can be carried out. There are two aspects of co-ordination here.

First, it is important that everyone is aware of their position in the chain and understands the activities that follow on from their own. To assist in this, you might encourage staff to shadow each other to learn about each other's roles. You might even be able to introduce job rotation so that staff learn more than one job and can work flexibly in several different roles.

Second, plans and schedules are important items of information that need to be available to all those involved to help them understand how the work is intended to flow and how tasks need to be co-ordinated. Ideally, it should be possible for staff to check plans and schedules themselves, so that they can 'police' their own activities. If staff are encouraged to understand how their contribution fits into the bigger picture, they may be more willing and able to ensure that they both seek and provide information that will facilitate the flow of work.

Other structural approaches to achieve timely flows of work and information are:

- *Devising a set of rules that govern the rate of output for each task in the sequence.* Such rules become shared information that helps to co-ordinate activities. They can be based on the planning information that has already been established and an appreciation of what output is appropriate from the individual or team working on each task. This approach is particularly helpful in dealing with tasks where the outputs can be standardised, and where direct supervision or active co-ordination is more difficult.
- *Setting output targets or goals for each activity.* Targets and goals are information that helps everyone to understand what is expected and required of them. This approach may allow considerable flexibility in the way tasks are done, provided that the targets or goals are met. It may involve training staff how to achieve the desired result, or depend on the professional standards of those involved.

Preparing for contingencies

Most health and social care services are vulnerable to changes in demand. The co-ordination of sequential tasks needs to make allowances for these, in order to avoid one task producing excess output where it is not needed or another leading to a reduced output so that other subsequent tasks cannot be carried out. In this kind of situation, the co-ordination strategy of 'buffering' might pay dividends. This means thinking ahead and preparing in advance to reduce the pressure that you anticipate will come if demand exceeds your ability to meet it. In the case of the operating theatre, examples of buffers would be preparing enough sterile instrument packs in advance to cover emergencies and having additional staff on call.

Lateral co-ordination

The process of achieving co-ordination so that completion of one prerequisite task or activity is done as perfectly as possible and absolutely in time to support the next activity in the chain is at the core of just-in-time (JIT) approaches to organising work. A senior manager remarked ruefully that his organisation operates its own particular brand of JIT – just-too-late!

As we have said, there is a tendency for those involved in carrying out one core task that is part of a sequence to focus too much on their own part in the process without having a view of the overall picture and appreciating the need for co-ordination with other core tasks. This is where improvements in lateral co-ordination are needed.

The boundaries between different tasks can be smoothed in a number of ways:

■ *By making sure that those who have responsibility for a particular task get accurate and helpful information both about how they are doing and about how the whole process is going.* This is not easy to achieve. Bombarding people with information they don't need – or in a form that is hard to make sense of – often seems to be a built-in feature of organisational life and can drive people into focusing on their immediate task rather than on their part in a wider service. The guidelines to keep in mind are *simplicity, timeliness* and *relevance.*

■ *By increasing the amount and quality of communication that goes on between colleagues.* When there are difficulties to be ironed out, face-to-face communication has many advantages and there is a good deal of evidence that improving communication improves morale and goodwill.

■ *By allowing the process of 'mutual adjustment' to go on between those who are faced with the everyday problems of doing the job.* Where you can see that locally established conventions and ways of working are adding to and improving a service, find ways of building them into the system. Where they don't, make sure that staff and colleagues understand and accept why this is before trying to build something better in their place.

Obtaining feedback about performance

You need to know whether the overall sequence of core tasks you have put together is effective in delivering the service with the volume of output required, at the right time, and with the right quality. So you need a flow of performance information that enables you to compare outputs against your plan, and then to make any necessary adjustments to the way in which the core tasks are organised and resourced. But having information about performance is only the first stage: effective co-ordination depends on managing that information to good effect in making necessary improvements.

ACTIVITY 17.2

Consider each of the following examples and make notes about which of the mechanisms for co-ordination discussed earlier might help to improve the situation.

1   A social care department has a number of different units and specialist teams and there is confusion about how service users should access the services available. There are different arrangements for adults and for children/families, and there are different arrangements for each of the specialist teams. Service users are frustrated by being passed around from one unit or team to another before they find the appropriate access point. They often approach professionals that they have met previously rather than following the formal procedure for access.
2   Staff are neglecting to keep records about the service that has been delivered to each individual service user. They feel that their real work is with service users and not about keeping up with the paperwork. Some say that record keeping is their own business and records are only for their own use. Computer systems are seen as only being of benefit to managers and as the responsibility of administrative staff.

The first example is typical of situations where there is a lack of lateral co-ordination. Little attention has been paid to ensuring that services are linked in ways that make sense to service users. There also seems to be a lack of clear and helpful information so that staff and service users understand how the access systems should work.

The second example suggests that staff have a very narrow understanding of the role of record keeping. They see it only as a supporting task rather than as a core task. They are failing to recognise the contribution that their work as individual professionals makes to the delivery of organisational objectives. In particular, systematic record keeping is essential to the effective planning and resourcing of services. Records may also be used as a means of sharing information to ensure that service users are treated equitably.

THE MANAGEMENT OF PARALLEL TASKS

Another pattern of managing core tasks involves co-ordinating the output of several individuals or teams whose activities are separate from – and parallel to – each other. This separation might be in terms of the kind of service they deliver or function they carry out, or different individuals or teams might be carrying out the same core task but covering, for example, a different geographical area. This is illustrated in Figure 17.3.

At first sight, this might seem to be an easier situation to co-ordinate. Many of the problems of managing sequential core tasks do not arise, since each task is independent.

Some of the approaches to co-ordination available here are:

- collecting and using information on the demand for services in order to plan the allocation of work and to obtain and allocate the resources that are needed to achieve the service level required
- setting goals or targets for the individuals or teams charged with carrying out each of the separate tasks or services
- monitoring and using information on performance in order to plan and allocate the next phase of the work.

ACTIVITY 17.3

Consider the following example of what is basically a parallel-task operation. What co-ordination and information problems can you identify in this situation?

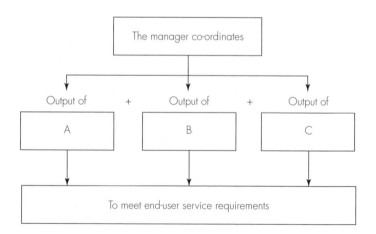

Figure 17.3 Core tasks in parallel

The community mental health team

The community mental health team is one of four serving a large northern city. It consists of five social workers (including one trainee), six community psychiatric nurses (with one vacancy), two occupational therapists (one of whom is on long-term sick leave), a number of administrative staff who support the work of the team as a whole and one team manager.

Referrals to the team come from a variety of sources, and these are channelled through the team manager. The allocation of new work is discussed at a weekly team meeting, at which the team manager works through the incoming case load and takes advice from the members of the team. Each new service user is allocated to a key worker, who carries out an initial assessment and reports back at the next team meeting. Each service user needs a different mix of skills and resources, drawn from the three professional areas within the team. It is sometimes also necessary to draw on specialist resources from outside the team. From this point onwards, the key worker is responsible for that service user, co-ordinating the input of staff and services to him or her. The key worker is supported through a process of regular supervision by the team manager and consults and liaises with colleagues both informally and at the weekly team meetings.

The team suffers from constant overloading, particularly as a result of trying to operate with only one occupational therapist. Support and help that cannot be provided from elsewhere within the team mean that the provision of some services has to be delayed or scaled down.

In addition, the limits on financial resources often mean that the treatment that a service user's key worker wishes to provide cannot be afforded, particularly if it involves bringing in support from outside the team. Key workers take requests for such resources to the team manager who, as the budget holder, makes decisions about who gets what. Thus, the professional judgement of the key worker may be overridden by the managerial judgement of the team manager because of the need to ration scarce resources.

Most team members, because of the nature of their work, spend a great deal of their time out of the office and, therefore, out of contact with their colleagues or the team manager. There is an information board on the office wall, on which team members are expected to write up their movements and locations. Although this provides some information about where team members are at any particular time and what they are doing, it rarely helps anyone to get in touch with them.

Team members are drawn from different backgrounds and operate under different professional regimes. Social workers, for instance, use a system of points to reflect the likely workload of each case they are allocated, and a particular total points score represents what is considered to be reasonable case load at any one time. Team members from a health service background are used to operating in a much more *ad hoc* way in deciding what is a reasonable workload. Because the team atmosphere is generally supportive and positive, this difference of approach is not usually a problem. On occasion, however, when everyone is under extreme pressure and there is a need for some mutual adjustment in order to get things done, the two systems do not always rub happily together.

The team is expected to deal with the demands of a fluctuating but generally increasing workload by being as flexible and co-operative as possible. Any issues that cannot be managed within the team are referred to a joint committee that co-ordinates the work of all the community mental health teams.

There are many information and co-ordination issues here, but we identified the following as being among the most significant:

- The overall workload fluctuates considerably and ways have to be found to match specialist resources with service demands. This means that the process of allocating resources has to be continuous, rather than being done once and then maintained with minor adjustments.
- The needs of each service user cannot be known accurately at the outset, so the allocation of team resources has to vary in a very flexible way and may change several times during the course of the delivery of the service.
- Key workers play an important co-ordinating role for each service user. Co-ordination is therefore not just something that happens at the top. Several key workers may require the same resources at the same time. A system is needed for co-ordination between key workers, or there is the potential for chaos.
- The co-ordination of resources seems to depend heavily on the goodwill of overworked professional staff and their willingness to help each other out. The success of the team overall depends on intangible features of the organisational structure, such as conventions, mutual adjustment and, perhaps most crucially, the climate that exists within the team and how supportive it is.
- The overload on the team's resources – especially the problem of one of the two occupational therapists being on long-term sick leave – may destroy the existing goodwill if team members begin to think they are being unreasonably and differentially exploited and if they see no signs that these problems are being dealt with.
- The team manager has both the controlling role of resource allocator (with perceived problems of fairness and equity) and also, through the supervision process, the supporting role of guide, mentor and professional coach. These controlling and supportive roles are potentially in conflict. If the manager gets the balance wrong, the structure within which the work of the team is carried out may be ineffective.

- Understanding the workload on each member of the team is made more complex by the different rules for regulating the workload of social workers and other professionals. It may be possible for the same service to be delivered by different groups of staff, but the workload rules may sometimes make sharing the burden difficult.
- There is the potential for some significant information flow problems. For example, the system used for day-to-day communication means that there is a lack of information on the location of members of the team who are out of the office. This limits the ability of key workers to co-ordinate the resources they need, and makes it difficult to share understanding, advice and good practice.

This kind of situation is one that would benefit by improving lateral co-ordination. Some mechanisms are already in place, such as weekly team meetings, but perhaps more attention might be given to helping team members to work more closely with each other, and to removing some of the barriers that restrict co-operation. Possible approaches might include:

- increasing the ease with which team members can contact each other for advice and support and to plan and agree work, for example, by providing them with mobile phones
- improving the sharing of accurate and relevant information, for example, through bulletins, team briefings and training sessions.

We have distinguished between core tasks that need to be carried out in sequence and those that can be carried out in parallel, and examined the different implications of these two ways of structuring work to ensure that the overall purposes of the service are achieved. However, even when the structures are designed to facilitate the effective flow of information, we would be very lucky if we did not occasionally encounter problems.

ANALYSING THE CAUSES OF INFORMATION PROBLEMS

In order to solve any problem, you need to identify and work on its causes, rather than just its symptoms. A useful technique for analysing the causes of a problem is to use a *cause and effect* or *fishbone* diagram. This is a way of helping you sort out and make sense of relationships between the various possible causes that may lie behind a problem. Most problems do not have a single cause, and a fishbone diagram helps you to group causes into common themes or categories, so that you can decide what needs to be done to deal effectively with each. Drawing a fishbone diagram allows you – and others – to focus on the issues involved, and to see how they might relate to each other.

Constructing a fishbone diagram

Here are the main stages involved in constructing a fishbone diagram.

1   Write the problem on the right-hand side of a large piece of paper or a whiteboard and draw a structure with a few branches that looks like the bones of a fish (Figure 17.4).
2   Brainstorm – either yourself or with your team – all the possible causes of the problem you are experiencing.
3   Write the first possible cause on one of the branches – it doesn't matter which one.
4   Then take another of the possible causes you have identified, and decide whether it is similar or related to the first one. If it is, put it alongside the first one on the same branch. If it is different or unrelated, put it on another branch.
5   Work through all the possible causes you have identified, clustering related problems on appropriate branches. You may find you need to add extra branches, or that more possible causes occur to you while you are building up the diagram. Add them in when you need to.
6   The final stage is to look at the branches, decide what categories of cause they represent, and add labels to each branch to describe the categories.

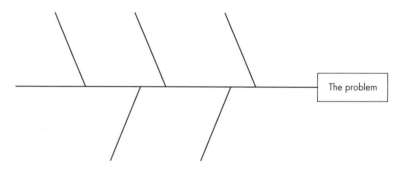

Figure 17.4 Basic fishbone diagram

An example of a fishbone diagram

Let's see how this approach might be applied to the following problem.

Initial complaint
The manager of an agency providing residential care for older people has received a letter from the son of one of the residents. The son complains that

important information about his mother's circumstances and treatment are being sent to an old address, even though he insists that he has notified the agency of his new address. On investigation, the manager finds that the son's new address was mentioned in a letter dealing with a number of other matters, and was never entered on to the agency's computer database, which still contains the old address.

Consequences
When the manager raised this complaint at the next weekly meeting of senior staff, the discussion confirmed what she already suspected – that similar errors occurred frequently. Some staff argued that this sort of problem was inevitable in the circumstances in which they were working: relatives often saw their particular problems as being the only ones that mattered. It was not uncommon for them to fail to provide information such as changes of address, no matter how often they were asked. Staff were quick to assure the manager that they always put things right as soon as a problem came to light. Indeed, they seemed to take considerable pride in their ability to fix things that had gone wrong.

After the meeting, the manager sat down to write a letter of apology. As she wrote, she began to think about the time and effort that was being wasted on 'putting things right' and wondered what she might do to get to the root causes of the problem.

To help her, the manager drew the fishbone diagram shown in Figure 17.5.

In order to keep it relatively simple, we have not included in the diagram all the possible causes that the manager thought of. There are, however, enough to demonstrate the way in which the diagram is built up. You can see that the manager grouped the possible causes under four headings – input data, input sources, processes, and people and

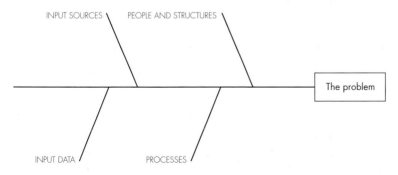

Figure 17.5 Example of a fishbone diagram

structures. Her next step was to consider what action she could take to improve the situation.

ACTIVITY 17.4

Put yourself in the manager's position, and think about the four groups of causes in turn. Which causes might she regard as 'givens' – ones that cannot realistically be changed? Which causes might she concentrate on, and what actions might she take?

Here are the manager's notes to compare with yours.

Input data

Information like this is always likely to come in a variety of forms, and will often be mixed with other information provided for other purposes. We have to accept this as a 'given'.

Input sources

Residents' relatives may sometimes make what seem like unreasonable demands. But to assume that this is the norm is to fail to empower them, and often means that we have to put a lot of effort into solving problems after the event, rather than dealing with something before it becomes a problem. We can and should work with our input sources (in this case, relatives) to build good relationships, so that the information they provide is as useful to us as possible.

Action: At the next weekly meeting, ask staff for ideas about how we might help relatives to give us the best possible information.

Processes

The database is updated twice a week by a member of the clerical staff. If changes are not notified to her in time, there will be a delay. They may even get overlooked altogether. Either way, this leads to the kind of problem we identified today. At the moment, the clerk deals only with the data that reach her. She can't be expected to go out and hunt for it. Or can she? Perhaps we can make it easier for staff to recognise information that needs to go into the database and pass it on.

Action: Devise a process for making sure that all data are sifted against a set of agreed criteria, and that relevant information then follows a simple channel into the database. We should also make the database available to all who need to use it.

I seem to have to deal with all these kinds of problems personally at the moment. If others got involved, they'd get more feedback on how well – or badly – our systems work, and they might then be encouraged to be more careful. And they've probably got some good ideas for improving things.

Action: Share and discuss difficulties regularly with staff. I've got to go about this the right way though, or they'll think I'm passing the buck.

People and structures
Our staff work hard and are often very busy. Relying on putting things right after they've gone wrong takes up the time and energy of people who should be getting on with their core jobs. If we can make changes to the system so that fewer of these problems occur, that should take some of the pressure off staff.

Action: The other action steps should have a payoff here. We could set ourselves a target for a reduction in the number of complaints about errors in our records. We need a performance indicator to tell us whether we are making progress.

But come to think of it, it's not really reducing the number of complaints that really matters: it's getting it right in the first place. What is worrying is the 'put it right afterwards' culture. We need to shift towards a culture of 'getting it right in the first place'.

Action: I need to create a climate in which information is seen as useful to everyone. This is going to take some time. Where do I start?

You may not have agreed with everything the manager said or planned to do. You may have experience that led you to suggest different actions. Also – and this is not at all unusual – the manager seems to be reasonably clear about what she wants to do in some areas, but only at the beginning of her thinking in others. Nevertheless, mapping the causes that contribute to a problem in the form of a fishbone diagram is a useful way of focusing on the major causes of an information problem and thus establishing a plan of action to improve the situation.

Categorising causes

When fishbone diagrams are used to analyse the causes of problems, the branches (or 'bones') are often not labelled at the start of the exercise. This encourages an open-ended approach and guards against making assumptions about the relationships between causes too early in the process. You often gain new insights by adding extra branches if the kinds of cause you are coming up with do not seem to relate to others you have already identified. You can always change your mind and reallocate them as your thinking develops.

However, it is often useful to label some of the branches before you start, to ensure that you focus on what you know from experience to be key areas. For instance, a typical approach when dealing with problems in service delivery would be to use branches labelled:

- people
- equipment/facilities
- materials
- methods
- environment.

You might find these categories appropriate ones to use in investigating many of the problems you encounter as a manager. In investigating information problems, however, as in our residential care example, it may be helpful to use labels for the branches that relate to the major components of an information system (Figure 17.6).

These are rather broad categories: in investigating a particular problem, you may need to subdivide them or to add extra ones. None the less, these four categories are likely to provide a useful basis for analysing causes and thus for seeking solutions. They also provide a coherent way of transferring your investigative approach – and thus also your learning – from one situation to another. They allow you to think about whether, if the causes of different information problems are similar, the solutions may also be similar.

ACTIVITY 17.5

Take each of the four categories of causes of information problems in turn, and begin to develop a checklist of the sorts of problem that might occur in a variety of different situations.

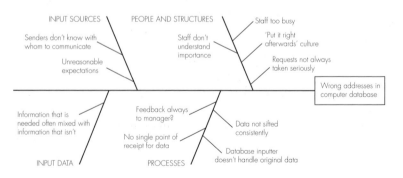

Figure 17.6 Major branches of a fishbone diagram to investigate the causes of an information problem

You will be able to add to this checklist as you build up experience in dealing with information problems and get feedback on how successful your solutions were. Here is our initial list of some of the problems that occur frequently.

Input data

■ The data you need may not exist or, if they do, they may not be being collected systematically.
■ The form in which data are collected may not be easy for you or your staff to use. For instance, the data may not be specific enough (or they may be too specific) or they might not be quantified.
■ You may have to do a lot of work to extract the data you need. This is often the case if the data have been collected for other purposes.

To generate data in a form that is as helpful as possible to all potential users, you need to understand the information needs that run throughout your organisation and the links between different people's needs for information.

Input sources

■ The people who collect or transmit data may not know what data are needed.
■ They may not understand what you intend to do with the data. If they know why you want particular information, they may be able to provide it in a more useful form.
■ Information may go astray because circulation lists are not kept up to date, or because those providing data are not made aware of changes in responsibility or function.

Keeping those who provide you with data up to date with changes in the way you are working and what the appropriate contact points and channels for information are is not easy. It is becoming increasingly complicated as those providing health and social care frequently work in partnerships across different organisations and structures. Problems may be created by major organisational changes and restructuring. It is notoriously difficult to keep track of who does what in a large organisation.

Processes

■ The procedures you have set up may not collect *all* the information you need, or may focus only on part of what you need.

■ If you trace the flow of information from input to the point at which it is used, you may find that there are:
  – *unreasonable delays* (sometimes information gets stuck in filing cabinets, on desks or in people's heads)
  – *bottlenecks* where information collects and is held up unnecessarily (you may be able to improve the speed of information flow by taking action to increase capacity at those points)
  – *dislocations* where information is passed to the wrong people.
■ The processes you have established for receiving, storing and transmitting information may be inappropriate. It may be that the system on which you are relying simply cannot deliver what you want.

Sometimes procedures for handling information are not clear or, with the best of intentions, are wrongly interpreted. By making transmission processes as clear, simple and unambiguous as possible, you reduce the risk of such misdirection. In addition, you may be relying on a process (perhaps of paper-based collection and transmission) that cannot cope effectively with the volume of information that now needs to be processed. Alternatively, you may be using a computer-based system that needs to be customised and adapted to provide you with what you need.

People and structures

■ It may not be clear who needs to know what.
■ People may not know what information they need in order to perform effectively.
■ They may not be aware of what is already available to them. What might be made available that isn't already? What would it take to achieve this?
■ They may not have the necessary skills to make effective use of the information that is available. These might include the skills to access the information (for instance, a necessary level of computer skills and confidence in their use) or the skills to handle and interpret data.
■ Attitudes towards handling and using information may not be sufficiently positive. Are staff aware of the importance of information in their jobs? Does their behaviour demonstrate this understanding? Do they actively seek out information?
■ The structures within your workplace may inhibit the transmission and use of information. People may be coping in spite of – rather than because of – the way their tasks and roles are structured. Do your structures make it harder for people to get at the information they need to do their jobs effectively?

ACTIVITY 17.6

Consider an information problem that you identify as your top priority to tackle.

1   Gather together everything you think might be useful to you in working on this problem. This might include any evidence you have about the nature of the problem (such as results, examples, opinions), as well as the analysis that led you to identify this problem as a priority.
2   Draw a fishbone diagram to help you identify the root causes of this information problem, using the four categories of input data, input sources, processes, and people and structures. You may wish to involve other people at this stage, either in suggesting possible causes or in challenging your ideas and testing your understanding of them. Involving people in thinking through a problem is a powerful way of getting them interested in solving it.
3   Work through the possible causes you have identified and select those you think are most likely to be making a major contribution to the problem. You will need to think carefully through the reasons for choosing some and not others. What evidence do you have?
4   Categorise those you have selected as:
   ■ *causes you cannot do anything about* (these are the 'givens' – whatever solutions you eventually adopt will have to take account of them)
   ■ *causes you believe you can tackle through your own actions* and through the actions of the staff you are responsible for managing
   ■ *causes where you will have to rely on other people to make changes* to bring about improvements (including senior managers, colleagues in other departments, information technology specialists, other professional colleagues, or your partners in joint working arrangements).
5   You should now be in a position to make an action plan to bring about the changes you have identified as being necessary. Decide the order in which you want to tackle issues. Some will be straightforward and the potential solutions will be fairly clear. Others will need thinking about rather more and may take longer to implement.

In moving forward from analysis into action, you have a number of factors on your side.

■ Because you can justify your identification of a priority area for action, other people are more likely to be interested in helping to bring about change.
■ You have identified the root causes in a systematic and thorough

way. This makes it easier to share understanding and agree necessary actions.

■ Where change is not possible, you will be able to explain the approach you have taken to working around the problem.

This chapter has been concerned with identifying the core tasks in your area of responsibility in order to understand the information flow and to analyse the causes of information problems. You should now be able to plan to use information more effectively in the delivery of the services for which you are responsible.

REFERENCE

Porter, M. E. (1985) *Competitive Advantage: Creating and Sustaining Superior Performance*, The Free Press.

EVIDENCE AND INVESTIGATION

This chapter introduces some of the issues involved in carrying out an investigation to collect evidence. In all areas of health and social care, there is an increasing emphasis on using evidence both to support decision making and to demonstrate the achievement of standards. We begin by considering what is meant by 'evidence' and why an understanding of the nature of evidence is important for managers. We discuss what is involved in planning an investigation, using the example of planning a consultation with service users, and we examine the advantages and disadvantages of postal surveys, face-to-face interviews and focus groups.

THE NATURE OF EVIDENCE

Evidence contributes to making something more clear or more visible. It is often used to support a statement of belief – to offer proof. However, people hold different beliefs and these are closely related to their different values and attitudes. It is often difficult to convince people of the validity of your evidence if their beliefs and values are different from yours.

If you are to base your decisions on evidence or to present evidence in support of your claims, it is important to understand the nature of evidence. It would be very reassuring to be able to say that a claim is true if there is evidence to support it. But evidence may or may not be convincing in the way it is used to support a claim. Evidence is not a truth that cannot be challenged, because it can be used in different ways for different purposes. In other words, evidence is relative. The nature of evidence and how it has been collected are important in considering how it can be used effectively.

Evidence usually takes the form of data relating to the issue under investigation. Data might include numbers, statistics, written statements, oral statements or photographs. For example, if you want to prove that you are competent in carrying out a management activity, you might present evidence including:

- memos relating to a particular occasion or event
- papers you have prepared
- witness statements from people who have seen you carry out the activity successfully
- your own statement explaining how you did it.

However, your belief that the evidence supports the claim will not necessarily be sufficient to convince others, because data do not become information until they have been interpreted in some way.

Interpretation is often personal and subjective because it relies on knowledge and experience from which beliefs and values arise. For example, you might believe that you act in an efficient and effective way in carrying out your management activities. However, your judgement is related to the knowledge and experience that you have. A more experienced person with more knowledge would be able to make a judgement that draws on a broader range of examples. He or she might corroborate your opinion or might challenge it. This is one of the reasons for the increasing interest in making comparisons in order to consider what constitutes 'good practice' or 'best value'. Interpretation is based on judgement; judgement is about comparing things and coming to a conclusion based on the comparison.

In addition, it is important to remember that data have to be collected before they are presented as evidence, and the way in which they have been collected will shape the evidence.

ACTIVITY 18.1

Imagine that it is widely known that the reception area for your service is to be moved to a new location that has yet to be agreed. Several members of your team come to you with a suggestion that it should be transferred to a site close to the new shopping centre. They are sure that this is a wonderful opportunity because it would be much more convenient for everyone. They show you evidence that service users have been consulted and agree that it is a good idea. Would you be convinced? Make notes of anything that you would want to ask them.

You would want to know how they had collected the evidence that they are presenting to support their argument. If they are so convinced by this idea, they may not have looked for any alternative ideas or even noticed if any objections were presented to them. People tend to seek out and present only data that can be interpreted to support their case. You would also want to know whom they had consulted. For example, did they seek the views of different service users, including those with mobility difficulties? Did they consult different age groups, or representatives from support services or partner or linked services? Did they consider the financial aspects? Questions such as these – and the answers – would lead you to form an opinion about the extent to which you could have confidence in the evidence presented.

Evidence is data interpreted as information and used as proof to support an argument. If you are to be convinced by the argument, you need to be convinced that the evidence is acceptable. The tests that can be applied to help you to decide whether evidence is acceptable are:

- Is it sufficient?
- Is it authentic?
- Is it valid?
- Is it current?

Sufficient evidence

Is there enough evidence to support the claim that is made? If you are told that 100 service users were asked for their views, you would want to know how many had responded. You might also want to know whether various categories of service user were represented among those that had responded – older and younger, male and female, able and disabled, and so on.

Authentic evidence

Is the evidence what it is claimed to be? In the example of relocating the reception for a service, were all those who responded users of your service? Does it matter whether they were current or past users or whether they have never used your service but would be entitled to do so if the need arose? Who collected the data? Are you seeing the raw data – in the same form as when they were collected – or have they been analysed or interpreted in any way? If so, are they still representative of the original data or have they been interpreted to present the proposal in a better light?

Valid evidence

Does the evidence demonstrate what is claimed? How was the evidence collected from the 100 respondents? Did they understand what was being asked? Were they asked whether they would like the suggested new location or were they asked which of a number of possible locations they would prefer? Their answers may depend on how the questions were asked. How closely do they represent what service users really think? How real or truthful is the evidence? Does it prove what is claimed? Could it be interpreted in any other way? Is too much being claimed on the basis of too little evidence? Have opposing views been sought?

Current evidence

Is the evidence up to date? This is important in situations where there is rapid change. What people think about an issue may depend on whether there has been a recent event that may have influenced their attitudes or opinions.

It is not easy to produce evidence that is convincing when you are investigating an issue that concerns a number of people or groups of people with potentially different interests.

PLANNING AN INVESTIGATION

Evidence is obtained by investigation. Data are collected and analysed to provide information that can be used as evidence to support decision making or to demonstrate whether standards have been met. We will introduce some approaches and techniques that can be used to carry out an investigation, using the example of planning a consultation with service users. This will help you to think through some of the issues involved in planning an investigation in which other people are involved either in giving you information and opinions or in working with you to develop ways of improving the delivery of a service. The issues are similar if you manage a support service such as finance or estate services, and are planning to consult the colleagues who are your direct service users.

In June 2000 the Government introduced a requirement for health and local authorities to develop local joint charters setting out common standards for the provision of certain services. This included a new duty to consult patients and service users – and their carers – about their experiences of receiving these services and to compare these against the standards in the local charter.

But what does it mean to *consult*? How might you go about it? What kind of evidence does consultation produce – and how useful is it?

The 'Better care, higher standards' charter

The charter for people who need long-term care – 'Better care, higher standards' – requires health, housing and social services to develop local joint standards for the provision of services. It is grounded in 'the nine principles of public service' issued by the 'Service First' unit of the Cabinet Office (Department of Health and DETR, 1999). These are that service providers should:

- set standards of service
- be open and provide full information
- consult and involve
- encourage access and promotion of choice
- treat all fairly
- put things right when they go wrong
- use resources effectively
- innovate and improve
- work with other providers.

The national charter sets out the values that should underpin the local charters:

- treating people with courtesy and honesty and respecting their dignity
- helping people to achieve and sustain as much independence as possible
- working in partnership with users and carers to provide the services they need
- involving users and carers in decisions and giving them sufficient information to make informed choices
- helping users and carers to have a voice through advocacy and other representative organisations
- treating people fairly on the basis of need and not discriminating against them on the basis of age, sex, race, religion, disability or sexual orientation
- ensuring that people feel able to complain about the standard of services they receive and that they are not victimised because they complain.

There is also a requirement to 'consult and involve users, carers and staff' and to 'build partnerships with users, carers and staff through consultation on local charters'. To find out what people think about services, you need to carry out an investigation.

ACTIVITY 18.2

What do you think are the strengths and weaknesses of each of the following approaches to planning and conducting an investigation?

Ask the questions you think should be asked and then interpret the answers that you receive.

Involve those you are consulting in deciding what questions should be asked and how the answers should be interpreted.

If you ask the questions you think should be asked, you will be focusing on the issue as you understand it. You may, however, miss some of the wider issues that concern service users. For example, you might want to ask what seems to be a simple question about whether service users can easily contact your organisation by phone. However, some service users may not have a phone and therefore prefer to visit an office; others may find it difficult to talk or to hear on the phone and prefer to meet face-to-face. Even if phones are answered promptly, some service users may have found those answering unhelpful. Some service users may prefer to access your services through a Web site or email.

If you ask a question like, 'Do you find it easy to contact this organisation by phone?', you may receive a range of different types of answer. Some people may simply say 'yes' or 'no'. That doesn't tell you what they consider 'easy' or 'difficult'. Service users are often very grateful for a service and may want to be obliging and say 'yes' rather than offer criticism. Some may say 'no' because they would prefer other means of contact rather than because there is any particular problem with using the phone.

Involving those who are being consulted in deciding what questions should be asked is often preferred because the issues may be complex and getting a range of different views and perspectives is helpful. This approach is likely to lead to a richer understanding of the range of people's feelings and opinions. From the perspective of a service provider, it is easy to make assumptions about what constitutes a 'good' service. The viewpoints of service users frequently demonstrate priorities and concerns that are different from those of providers. If you only ask people the questions that occur to you, you may only get the answers that you anticipated. If you engage people in carrying out an investigation with you, you may get some surprises and some information that is new to you.

Consultation and partnership

Consultation means asking for people's views; *partnership* implies that those views are respected and acted upon. The 'Better care, higher standards' charter says that both of these will happen:

■ the views of staff, service users and carers will be sought
■ certain actions will follow as a result.

People can be *involved* both in setting standards and in monitoring performance against standards.

Consultation implies a degree of partnership. A consultation in which the views of people are sought but then ignored would be a pointless exercise, and would not be regarded by those consulted as any kind of partnership. If service users think you have no intention of taking their views into account, they may become angry or cynical about service provision. It is important to demonstrate that their views have been heard and understood. However, this does not necessarily imply acceptance of their views. Where views are not accepted, or not acted upon immediately, you need to ensure that the reasons for the decisions you take following the consultation are explained fully and clearly.

So the first decision you need to make in planning a consultation is what you wish to consult people about. In particular, you have to think about what those consulted might expect or anticipate as a result of the consultation. Engaging in consultation has important consequences for service managers and professionals, but it also has important implications for those who are consulted, not least for their willingness to co-operate. If they are not convinced that the consultation is genuine, they are less likely to be responsive. Partnership implies a willingness to act on the information arising from a consultation which, in turn, implies that the information obtained must be in a form that can be acted on.

Planning a consultation exercise from a partnership perspective – from a perspective that regards the views of service users and carers as important – helps you to do the following:

■ think about your own and your staff's willingness and ability to listen to what service users and their carers are saying and to respond to it
■ ensure that the responses you obtain from a consultation are in a form to which you can respond
■ determine the scope of the consultation – limit it to gaining information on which you have the authority to act
■ be clear, realistic and honest about the extent to which you are prepared to share power with service users and carers
■ ensure that the consultation process is sufficiently sensitive to pick up the underlying concerns of service users and carers. For example, you might undertake a survey of satisfaction among residents in residential and nursing homes from which it is apparent that most people rate the staff and the care they receive very highly. However, you may fail to discover that most of the respondents would have preferred to be cared for in their own homes.

Attitudes to consultation

Part of the process of planning a consultation is, therefore, understanding the reasons for the consultation and making sure that all those involved understand them. This includes making sure that staff, who may be asked to adopt different working practices as a result of the consultation, understand the thinking behind it. In other words, you need to consider your own and other people's reasons for listening to service users and carers.

ACTIVITY 18.3

Jot down at least three benefits of consulting people who need long-term care about service provision.

Thinking about this puts you in a better position to judge what to ask and who should be included in a consultation. The benefits arising out of consultation might include:

- getting feedback about services
- improving services
- improving the status of patients, service users and carers
- increasing public accountability and thus contributing to clinical governance and 'best value'
- increasing the trust of service users and the general public
- getting a better understanding of the threats and opportunities facing services.

Different people may place a different emphasis on these various benefits. For example, some will recognise that there is an expectation that managers will act upon the information gained to improve services. However, others may see the requirement for consultation as just another Government initiative to which they must respond with the minimum of effort. In some organisations the responsibility for undertaking the consultation will be passed on to a policy or quality assurance unit that is somewhat removed from operational units and professionals. Either of these responses would potentially undermine the intended benefits.

Consulting service users and carers can be merely a token exercise in which the results are ignored or acknowledged with reluctance. Alternatively, it can lead to a better understanding of how services contribute positively and negatively to the quality of people's lives, and an improved understanding of the priorities of service users and carers. It can also provide valuable insights into conflicts of values and priorities that need to be better or more explicitly managed.

ACTIVITY 18.4

What value does your area of work place upon consultation with patients, service users and carers?

What are the implications of this for you and the service you manage?

WHAT KIND OF INFORMATION DO YOU NEED?

Implicit in the 'Better care, higher standards' charter are two kinds of consultation. One is concerned with obtaining feedback from patients, service users and carers about the extent to which agreed standards have been achieved. The other is a more fundamental review of whether services are meeting their needs. These require different kinds of consultations. One is asking a *closed question* – 'Did we do X?' – to which the answers are limited to 'yes' or 'no' (or perhaps 'partially'); the other is asking an *open question* – 'What do you think about X?' – to which there may be as many responses as there are respondents.

All purposeful activity relies upon feedback and evaluation to provide information about how successful it is. This is true whether the activity is striking up a friendship or delivering a service. Implicitly or explicitly, purpose is translated into action through a plan, and the information required is two types: 'Are things going according to plan?' (feedback) and 'Is the plan producing the desired results?' (evaluation). This is represented by the quality control loop in Figure 18.1.

In this model there are two sub-loops. One is relevant to managers of services who need feedback on whether their service plans are being implemented effectively. The other involves a wider range of stakeholders, including service users and carers, and is concerned with evaluating whether the plan being implemented is the right one. The first one is about the extent to which certain targets have been achieved – such as the number of patients treated or whether all service users have their own care plan. The second is about whether the treatments and care plans have delivered the desired outcomes for individuals.

Most performance management schemes involve collecting information about the achievement of targets. This is straightforward when the performance is easy to measure. For example, a standard might be that a request for assessment will be responded to within two working days: whether this standard has been achieved can be monitored by keeping a dated record of all requests and responses to them. This

Figure 18.1 The quality control loop: two kinds of involvement and consultation

record provides the evidence of achievement. Examining the record – or perhaps a statistical summary of it prepared at intervals during the year – provides feedback about achievement against the standard.

However, achievement of some standards is less easy to measure. One required by the 'Better care, higher standards' charter is:

> *Ensuring that people feel able to complain about the standard of services.*

ACTIVITY 18.5

How would you set about finding out whether patients or service users feel able to complain about your service?

1   How might you monitor performance against this standard through records kept by staff?
2   From the perspective of one of your patients or service users – or perhaps one of their carers – what would have to be in place for this standard to be met?
3   What steps might you take to monitor achievement of the standard through consultation with patients or service users?

From an internal service perspective, compliance with this standard might be based on assurances by staff that it is being complied with. This might be supported by a procedure requiring that people be informed about their right to complain, or there might be a leaflet explaining how to complain. Perhaps staff are required to keep records confirming that they have informed people about their rights. As a manager, you may be confident that members of your team are doing all they can to meet the standard.

However, from the perspective of patients or service users, your confidence may be regarded with some scepticism. In one survey of over a hundred users of social and community health services and their carers, less that 40 per cent said they knew who to contact to make a complaint. But this is not necessarily evidence that they had not been informed. A leaflet or a verbal explanation might have been given to them at some time in the past, perhaps when they were being assessed for services. This might have been at a time when they were faced with a crisis in their lives. Even in ordinary circumstances, giving information is only one half of the process of communication: information also has to be heard and understood (and perhaps also has to be readily available when it is needed) for communication to effective.

In any case, the standard refers to 'ensuring that people feel able to complain', which is a rather different matter. In the survey referred to above, less than 50 per cent of those interviewed said that they would feel confident about complaining. The reasons they gave included fear of loss of service or reprisal, and unwillingness to get their support worker (nurse, social worker, home carer, etc.) into trouble.

Using records to show that information has been provided about how to make a complaint is therefore not sufficient to demonstrate that service users feel able to complain. Records of complaints that have been made, who made them and the circumstances in which they were made are useful. But if you want to know whether your service is meeting this standard, you need to ask service users and carers for their views. Three of the principal methods for doing this are postal surveys, face-to-face interviews and focus groups. We'll consider each of these briefly in turn, and then conclude the section by considering some of the issues involved in asking questions, which apply to all of them.

Postal surveys

The problems with postal surveys are summed up in an article about the surveys of the satisfaction of users of care services, which are conducted by the Social Services Inspectorate and Audit Commission Joint Review Team:

> Professor Hasel Qureshi heads the Department of Health funded research programme into outcomes of social care at York University's Social Policy Research Unit. She points out that the joint review survey has got some important shortcomings, including an average response rate of just 42 per cent. 'As a researcher, you simply would not be able to use this data as evidence. To be seen as respectable you must have a minimum response rate of 60 per cent. It is also likely to be a biased sample – because only the views of people who are able to read and fill in a paper questionnaire are being represented.' Even leaving aside these methodological problems with the survey, Qureshi points out that previous tick-box surveys have also shown high satis-faction rates among adult users of community care services, and suggests that other approaches may elicit more useful information. 'Satisfaction is multi-dimensional. It is important to separate out people's views of the workers who help them from their views of the agency. Most people like the workers and are satisfied with them. They see them having to rush around and wouldn't want to complain or risk getting them into trouble.'
>
> (Fickford, 2000)

The critical issues raised here are the low response rate, the difficulty people may have in responding and – a point already noted – a reluctance to complain.

ACTIVITY 18.6

What are the implications of Qureshi's comments for you, as a manager, when thinking about how to obtain feedback from users and carers about your service?

First you need to be clear about what sort of information you want. Do you need to survey all the users of your service, or obtain a response rate of at least 60 per cent? If you want to know what proportion of your service users know how to complain, you do. But if you want to find out if a standard that should apply to everyone is being achieved, a smaller sample may be sufficient. Even if you survey only ten people, their feedback will provide some independent evidence to support a claim that you are meeting the standard – or to demonstrate that you are not achieving it.

It is perhaps more important to find out *why* people feel inhibited about complaining, rather than simply to discover the proportions of service users who do or do not feel inhibited. It is only by exploring the reasons that you may be able to think of ways to resolve the problem. If the type of information you require is qualitative, rather than quantitative, a low response rate to a postal survey may not necessarily be a problem. However, the type of information that postal surveys generate is an issue. They tend to ask closed questions, to which respondents have to answer 'yes' or 'no', choose between two or more alternatives or mark a point on a scale from, say, 1 to 4. Postal surveys are a good way of generating quantifiable information. If you ask 100 people if they know how to complain and 60 say 'yes', that provides a useful snap-shot about performance. But if you ask an open question in a postal survey such as 'Do you think the complaints procedure is good enough?', a hundred different replies provide you with a challenge to find a way of organising the responses other than by simply counting them.

Face-to-face interviews

A major advantage of face-to-face interviews is that they do not rely on people's ability or motivation to fill in a form. Interviews also provide opportunities to ensure that questions are understood, to cover all the questions you want to ask and to ask follow-up questions. It is possible to establish rapport and thus to gain deeper insights into people's experience as users of your service. Questions about experiences, preferences and feelings usually need to be discussed and are therefore easier to deal with by interviewing than by postal surveys.

The major disadvantage of interviews is that they are very time-consuming. It is unlikely that you will be able to obtain the views as many people by one-to-one interviews as by a postal survey – even one with a poor response rate. However, you can count responses to closed questions, as well as adding depth by asking open questions that invite people to describe their experiences and make judgements. Interviews can therefore provide both quantitative and qualitative information.

Focus groups

A focus group is a group of people who are invited to meet to discuss a particular issue.

ACTIVITY 18.7

Imagine inviting a number of users of your service to a meeting to discuss how you and your colleagues can best ensure that service users feel able to complain if they feel the need to do so. Make a note of some of the advantages and disadvantages of such an approach to consultation.

You may have thought about the difficulties of arranging for possibly severely ill or disabled people to attend a focus group. And how likely is it that people would feel able to discuss their personal experiences and feelings in such a setting? Some would, no doubt, but the meeting might be dominated by a few vocal people. So how representative would the views expressed be? You are unlikely to be able to record the number of people who agree or disagree with a certain proposition.

However, participating in a group discussion might encourage some people to have the confidence to make comments they might otherwise not make, especially if they discover that their experiences or feelings are shared by others. Focus groups can, therefore, generate useful feedback, and can help you to understand the strength of feeling about an issue that might not be apparent from one-to-one discussions.

For many service areas, advocacy groups, such as Age Concern, or support groups, such as a stroke club, can be a valuable source of information and feedback. They have a special interest in an area of work, and can be well informed about what they expect and what is good practice. However, their interest may be somewhat broader than yours as a service manager. Their role may therefore be at the second stage of the quality loop in Figure 18.1, where the emphasis is on service evaluation rather than providing feedback on current standards of practice.

How successful a meeting is in terms of getting useful feedback about your service depends on how it is structured and managed. Inviting 50 people to sit in rows in a large room is unlikely to be conducive to an open dialogue. It is easier to put people at their ease in smaller groups. A larger group can be divided into smaller discussion groups, each with a facilitator, to address a particular question or topic and then report back. As in all approaches to consultation, it is important to be clear about the purpose of the discussion, and to ask appropriate questions in appropriate ways using appropriate language.

Asking questions

A major strength of postal surveys is that they are relatively neutral and anonymous. In face-to-face discussions – whether with individuals or groups – your presence, wittingly or not, inevitably influences the consultation. Service users may not wish to give offence, and you may not want to hear negative comments. Your influence may be more limited in group settings, but it is then more difficult to control the agenda to make sure that you cover the full range of issues that you want information about. However, focus groups are more likely to generate information that you had not anticipated – what you want to know about may not be what your service users want to talk about. Face-to-face interviews can be carried out in people's homes, so that even severely disabled and ill people can be included, but in these settings it is even more difficult to avoid exerting your personal influence.

How, then, can you guard against unduly influencing people when you are consulting them? You need to consider using both open and closed questions, to be consistent in the questions you ask, to be aware that people attach different meanings to words, to ask simple direct questions and to avoid defensiveness.

Open and closed questions

It is a good idea to have a mix of open and closed questions so that you can collate the answers to closed questions, as well as obtaining more detailed views through open questions. People often feel more comfortable if you start with a closed question and follow it up with an open one.

Consistency of approach

If you are going to be able to count the answers to a specific question (such as 'Would you feel able to complain if something went wrong?'), you have to ask the same questions of everyone. This may seem obvious but, especially if there is more than one interviewer, questions may be asked with varying degrees of emphasis or slightly different wordings, and explanations about the meaning of a question might differ. All these can give rise to a lack of consistency.

The meaning of words

However you conduct a consultation, it is important to avoid professional jargon, to use everyday words as far as possible and, where difficult words are unavoidable, to explain them. For example, if you are seeking feedback about the requirement that everyone who is receiving community care services should have a care plan, it is unwise to assume that everyone knows what a care plan is.

Even more tricky is the use of everyday words that may mean different things to different people. For example, if you ask 'Did you feel involved in drawing up your care plan?', 'feel involved' is open to alternative interpretations. For some people, being informed of the nature and possible side effects of a treatment may be sufficient for them to feel involved; others may only feel involved if alternative possible courses of action are discussed with them. It may therefore be necessary to ask questions about the activities that underpin the idea of helping people to feel involved. This might include asking if service users were given a choice between different courses of action, if they think their views were taken into account when the care plan was drawn up, and so on. In this way, you can form a judgement against your professional understanding of what it is to involve people in planning their care and treatment.

Ask simple direct questions

In designing a questionnaire or drawing up a list of questions you are going to use in interviews or focus groups, you need to be clear what information you want. Consider, for example, the question 'Do you have a care plan?' There are at least three possible meanings for this apparently straightforward question depending on where the emphasis is placed and each may prompt different answers according to how it is heard by the other person:

- Do you have a *care plan*? (This might be asked as part of the process of finding out if the person knows what the term 'care plan' means.)
- Do *you* have a care plan? (This may be asking the person whether he or she has something he or she calls a care plan, which may or may not be the document that you have in mind.)
- Do you *have* a care plan? (This might mean 'Do you have a care plan in your possession?' or 'Do you know if there is one, maybe held by someone else?')

This illustrates the importance of being explicit about the purpose behind each question – of spelling out your information objectives. You need to divide the objectives into simple discrete questions and make sure that whoever is conducting the interview is clear about what information is being sought by each question. It is often helpful to try out your questions on a few colleagues and then on a few service users to ensure that they are understood in the way you intend them to be.

Avoiding defensiveness

If a question elicits a criticism, it is very easy to respond with an apology, a denial or an explanation. This may be appropriate, but it may not be. If the purpose of consultation is to obtain feedback, entering into a debate can distort the process. On the other hand, appearing indifferent to a problem or concern that has been expressed can be equally unhelpful. It is important to think through some 'What if . . . ?' scenarios so that you can be prepared – or prepare others – to handle such situations.

ACTIVITY 18.8

Select three standards (preferably from among those that are already in place for your service). Examples might be:

- all service users have a care plan
- service users are involved in planning their care
- service users feel able to complain if necessary.

Imagine that you and a colleague have set yourselves the task of interviewing 20 users of your service over the next few weeks to see if, in their experience, these standards are being met.

Design two questions – one closed and one open – that you are going to ask about each of the three standards to get this feedback.

Planning and carrying out an investigation that will be robust enough to produce reliable information are not trivial activities. They take considerable time. An investigation also demands time from other people and you have a responsibility to avoid wasting their time or raising expectations that you may be unable to fulfil. As in so many areas of management, to carry out an effective investigation you need to plan carefully, ensure that many different viewpoints have been taken into account and take time to reflect on your actions as you progress your plans.

■   ■   ■

In this chapter, we have considered the nature of evidence and the tests you can apply to decide whether evidence is acceptable – whether it is sufficient, authentic, valid and current. We have explored some of the issues involved in planning an investigation, using as an example the requirement to consult users of long-term care services and their carers. In conducting an investigation of this kind, you have three main options for collecting information – postal surveys, face-to-face interviews and focus groups – each of which has both advantages and disadvantages. All of these involve asking questions, and we concluded by examining some of the pitfalls to be avoided in designing questions.

REFERENCES

Department of Health and Department of the Environment, Transport and the Regions (1999) 'Better care, higher standards', Joint Circular, December, Service First Unit, Cabinet Office, London.

Fickford, F. (2000) 'Are customers always right?', Community Care, May, pp. 25–31.

CONTRIBUTORS

We are indebted to the many individuals who have contributed to the development of the MESOL programme 'Managing in Health and Social Care' from which the material for this book is drawn.

Alison Baker, Royal College of General Practitioners, London
Bob Baker, Salomons
Sue Balderson, De Montford University
Lawrence Benson, Bradford University
Ceridwyn Bessant, University of Northumbria
Stanley Bonthron, formerly Community Care Implementation Unit, The Scottish Office
Diane Bowler, Warwickshire Health Authority
Margaret Brand, Social Services, London Borough of Enfield
Alex Bush, Doncaster and South Humber Healthcare NHS Trust (on behalf of the MESOL National Office)
Chris Butler, Southern Derbyshire Health Authority
Peter Byrne, Salomons
Sheila Cameron, The Open University Business School
Miriam Catterall, University of Ulster
John Charles, formerly Gwynedd Community Health Trust
Andrew Clapperton, The Open University Business School
Steve Cooke, Sheffield Hallam University
David Cottam, David Cottam Consultancy
Sue Cox, Southern Derbyshire Health Authority
Sally Cray, Salomons
Nigel Crisp, NHS Executive, London
Mark Cutler, Queen Victoria Hospital, East Grinstead
Mel Daniels, Rotherham Social Services
Kathy Darby, London Borough of Enfield
Salle Dare, Cheshire Health Authority
Anne Davey, Practice Manager
Rachel Dickinson, Derby City Social Services Department
Rob Dixon, University of Northumbria

Charlotte Douglass, Development Adviser, MESOL National Office
Mervyn Eastwood, London Borough of Enfield
John Frith, Sheffield Hallam University
Alan Garland, Yorkhill NHS Trust
Neil Garret-Harris, Sheffield City Council
Lynda Gatecliffe, Bradford University
Ken Giles, The Open University Business School
Bruce Gillam, University of Northumbria
Val Glenny, Sheffield Hallam University
Jim Green, University of Northumbria
Nigel Grinstead, Partnerships for Change
Lis Haggard, King's Fund
Charles Handy
Ann Harrison, Sheffield Social Services (on behalf of the MESOL
     National Office)
Steve Harrison, University of Leeds
Joyce Healy, Training Consultant
Pat Heath, formerly Southern Derbyshire Health Authority
Nicki Hedge, The Open University Business School
Euan Henderson, The Open University Business School
Pat Honeyset, Three Boroughs NHS Trust
John Houlston, Warwickshire Health Authority
Phil Ingamells, The Open University Business School
Mark Isaac, Warwickshire Health Authority
Ken Jarrold, County Durham Health Authority
Alan Johnston, Aberdeen Royal Infirmary
Judith Johnston, Warwickshire Health Authority
Peter Key, Dearden Management Associates
Judith Knight, Warwickshire Health Authority
Jacky Korer, Barnsley Health Authority
Christa Laird, Oxfordshire Social Services Department
Hilary Lance, The Learning Agency
Carole Lawrence-Parr, Swanage Medical Practice
Penny Lawson, Three Boroughs NHS Trust
Paul Lewis, Chairman of Maidstone & Malling Primary Care Group
Penny Lewis, Sheffield Hallam University
Beryl Little, London Borough of Enfield
Brian Lund, formerly The Open University Business School
Stuart Maguire, University of Northumbria
Mike Marchmont, Warwickshire Health Authority
Gill Marsden, The Open University Business School
Philip Marsh, The Open University
Kathy Martin, University of Northumbria
Vivien Martin, The Open University Business School
Gill McDougall, formerly Southern Derbyshire Health Authority
Ian Moore, Community Health Service (North Derbyshire) NHS Trust
Elaine Mottram, Aberdeen Royal Infirmary
Peter Munro, Social Services Inspectorate

Geraldine Murrison, Central Sheffield University Hospitals NHS Trust
Steve Oliver, Southern Birmingham NHS Trust
Alice Olliver, NHS Executive, Trent
Helen Orme, Nottingham Community Health NHS Trust
Heather Paisley, Buckinghamshire Health Authority.
Andrew Paterson, Enfield Community Care NHS Trust
Marion Pearce, formerly Southern Derbyshire Health Authority
Sue Pearce, formerly The Open University Business School
Clare Perry, Bromley Health Authority
Kay Phillips, Sheffield Hallam University
Christopher Pollitt, Brunel University
Lynne Quinney, Sheffield Hallam University
Sally Ravenhall, Practice Manager
Cathy Reilly, Consultant
Colin Robinson, KPMG, Peat Marwick
John Robinson, University of Northumbria
Julia Ross, Queen Victoria Hospital, East Grinstead
Derek Rowntree, The Open University
Jill Sandford, Development Adviser, MESOL National Office
Brenda Sawyer, University of Exeter
Paul Shanahan, Gregory Harland Ltd
Jill Sharp, University of Northumbria
Gillian Smith, OLM Consulting
Joan Smith, The Open University Business School
Tony Stapleton, The Open University Business School
Geoff Stevenson, Southern Derbyshire Health Authority
Anne Tofts, Partnerships for Change
Jill Turner, Avon Health Authority
Trevor Walker, The Open University Business School
Vanessa Walker, Maidstone & Tunbridge Wells NHS Trust
Joe Walsh, The Learning Agency
Teresa Waring, University of Northumbria
Harry Watkins, De Montfort University.
Alan Watson, formerly The Development Group for the NHS in
    Scotland
Maxwell Wide, Development & Training Consultant
Jo Williams, Social Services, Cheshire County Council
Norman Woods, formerly The Open University
Heather Worsley, Queen's Court Day Centre, Buxton
Jennifer Yates, Southern Derbyshire Health Authority

ACKNOWLEDGEMENTS

Page 67, extracts from COSHE/Unison (1994) 'Code of practice for care people with mental illness', pp 47–8

Page 99, extracts from Gorman, P. (1998) *Managing Multi-Disciplinary Teams in the NHS*, Open University Press

Page 116, Figure 7.1 reprinted from Hackman, J.(1983) *Perspectives of Behaviour*, McGraw-Hill. By permission of the McGraw-Hill Companies

Page 125, Figure 7.3 adapted from Turrill, T. (1986) *Change and Innovation: A Challenge for the NHS*, Institute of Health Services Management

Page 146, 'Pain Score' Figure © BMJ Publishing Group (1997) Advanced Life Support Group; Advanced Paediatric Life Support: The Practical Approach (2nd ed)

Page 150 extracts from Wright, C. 'Are you being served' *Health Service Journal*, 02 September 1999, pp 12–13

Page 155, material from Essex, S. and Wilde, M. (1996) *A Matter for Investigation*, EBS Trust, ISBN 1 898152 15 2. EBS Trust, 36–8 Mortimer Street, London W1 7RG, tel 020 7765 4635/5087, e-mail mail@ebstrust.u-net.com

Page 162, Table 9.1 reprinted from Berry, L., Zeithaml, V. and Parasuranam, A. (1985) *A Practical Approach to Quality*, Joiner Associates Inc, materials are copyrighted by Oriel Incorporated, formerly Joiner Associates Inc and are used here with permission. Further reproductions are prohibited without written consent of Oriel Incorporated, call 1 800 669 8326

Page 173, extracts from Hands, D 'Integrated Care', in M. Lugon and J. Secker-Walker (eds) *Clinical Governance*, The Royal Society of Medicine Press, http://clinical-governance.com

Page 188, Table 10.3 reprinted from Maxwell, R. (1984) 'Quality assessment in heath' *British Medical Journal*, 13: 31–4, with permission from the BMJ Publishing Group

Pages 193 and 207, Figures 11.1 and 11.2 reprinted from Koch, H. (1991) *Total Quality Management*, Churchill Livingstone. By permission of the publisher Churchill Livingstone

Page 200, extracts from Smyth, C., Simmons, I. and Cunningham, G. (1999) *Quality Assurance in Social Work - A Standard Audit Approach for Agencies and Practitioners*, National Institute for Social Work

Pages 202–3, extracts from Department of Health (1998) 'A First Class Service: Quality in the New NHS'. Crown copyright material is reproduced with the permission of the Controller of Her Majesty's Stationery Office

Page 206, Table 11.3 reprinted from Kitson, A. 'Rest Assured', *Nursing Times*, 27 August 1986, pp 28–31

Page 236, extracts from 'Next Patient Please – the Operating Theatres Problem at Leicester General Hospital NHS Trust' Buchanan, D. and Wilson, R. in Storey, J. (ed.) *Blackwell Cases in Human Resources and Change Management*. © 1996, Blackwell

Pages 274–5, extracts from Department of Health (1988) 'Clinical Governance Extracts' Crown Copyright. Reproduced with the permission of the Queen's Printer for Scotland.

Page 304, Figure 17.1 adapted with the permission of The Free Press, A Division of Simon & Schuster, Inc, from Competitive Advantage: Creating and Sustaining Superior Performance, by Michael E. Porter. Copyright© 1985, 1988 by Michael E Porter

While the authors and the publishers have made every effort to contact copyright holders of the material used in this volume, they would be happy to hear from anyone they were unable to contact.

INDEX

Note: References to figures and tables are indicated by italics (58*f*, 78*t*).